# LEARNING AND BEHAVIOR PROBLEMS
# IN ASPERGER SYNDROME

# LEARNING AND BEHAVIOR PROBLEMS IN
# ASPERGER SYNDROME

*Edited by* Margot Prior

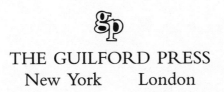

THE GUILFORD PRESS
New York    London

© 2003 The Guilford Press
A Division of Guilford Publications, Inc.
72 Spring Street, New York, NY 10012

Printed in the United States of America

This book is printed on acid-free paper.

Last digit is print number: 9 8 7 6 5 4 3 2

**Library of Congress Cataloging-in-Publication Data**
Learning and behavior problems in Asperger syndrome / edited by Margot
Prior.
    p. cm.
Includes bibliographical references and index.
  ISBN 1-57230-917-2 (alk. paper)
  1. Asperger's syndrome.   I. Prior, Margot
RJ506.A9L427 2003
371.94—dc21

                                                                    2003007549

# About the Editor

**Margot Prior, PhD, FAPS,** is Professor of Psychology at the University of Melbourne and a Fellow of the Academy of Social Sciences in Australia. She has been a lecturer, clinical psychologist, and researcher in the field of family and child development for more than 30 years at several Australian universities, as well as holding visiting appointments at the University of Padua (Italy), the University of London (England), and the University of Otago (New Zealand). Until 2002, Dr. Prior was Professor/Director of Psychology at the Royal Children's Hospital in Melbourne. She has written five books and many scientific papers on psychological disorders in childhood, and is a frequent speaker at national and international scientific meetings. Dr. Prior has specialized in research into behavioral and cognitive aspects of autism and Asperger syndrome, and has recently produced a film to help parents and teachers understand Asperger syndrome.

# Contributors

**Tony Attwood, PhD,** MacGregor Centre, Queensland, Australia

**Susan L. Calhoun, MS,** Department of Psychiatry, Pennsylvania State University College of Medicine, Hershey, Pennsylvania

**Val Gill, BEd, GDSE,** Western Autistic School, Footscray, Australia

**Patricia Howlin, PhD,** Department of Psychology, St. Georges Hospital Medical School, London, England

**Rita Jordan, PhD,** School of Education, University of Birmingham, Birmingham, United Kingdom

**Linda Kunce, PhD,** Department of Psychology, Illinois Wesleyan University, Bloomington, Illinois

**Wendy Lawson, BSS, BSW, Gdip,** private practice, Warrnambool, Victoria, Australia

**Janine Manjiviona, PhD,** Child and Adolescent Mental Health Services, Royal Children's Hospital, Parkville, Australia

**Susan Dickerson Mayes, PhD,** Department of Psychiatry, Pennsylvania State University College of Medicine, Hershey, Pennsylvania

**Margot Prior, PhD, FAPS,** Department of Psychology, University of Melbourne, Melbourne, Victoria, Australia

**Jo-Ann Reitzel, PhD,** Center for Studies of Children at Risk, Chedoke–McMaster Hospitals, Hamilton, Ontario, Canada

**Michal Shaked, MD,** Department of Psychology and School of Education, The Hebrew University of Jerusalem, Jerusalem, Israel

**Peter Szatmari, PhD,** Center for Studies of Children at Risk, Chedoke–McMaster Hospitals, Hamilton, Ontario, Canada

**Helen Tager-Flusberg, MD,** Department of Anatomy and Neurobiology, Boston University School of Medicine, Boston, Massachusetts

**Digby Tantam, MD,** Centre for the Study of Conflict and Reconciliation and Department of Psychotherapy, University of Sheffield, Sheffield, United Kingdom

**Nurit Yirmiya, PhD,** Department of Psychology and School of Education, The Hebrew University of Jerusalem, Jerusalem, Israel

# Contents

## II. Asperger Syndrome in the Schools

# Introduction

## MARGOT PRIOR

The study of autism and related disorders over the last two decades has been characterized by a marked surge of interest in a particular variant of autism known as Asperger syndrome (AS). This childhood disorder was originally described in a series of case studies by Austrian psychiatrist Hans Asperger in 1944 (Asperger, 1944/1991), but a year after Leo Kanner (1943) had outlined the features of "his" syndrome, "infantile autism." AS attracted relatively little attention at the time, and its import was overwhelmed by the rapid growth of interest during the 1940s and 1950s in classic autism, which Kanner and colleagues in the United States described with such detail, lucidity, and authority.

At the outset, Asperger conceptualized these patients, with their syndromic-like picture of symptoms and behaviors, as suffering from a "personality disorder," which was genetically determined. He used the term "autistic psychopathy" in his paper, in which he presented four detailed case studies (see translation of this paper in Frith, 1991). Key features in the original AS presentations were onset before the age of 2 years; persistence of symptoms throughout life; characteristic peculiarities of eye gaze; lack of gestural and facial expression; a variety of abnormalities in expressive language; creativity and originality in intelligence and in language; narrow, isolated, and circumscribed interests; problems in attention and learning; lack of clear-sightedness; self-absorption, especially with regard to their own bodies and bodily functions; impaired social relationships; and overall abnormality in their interactions with all aspects of the environment. Asperger also noted stereotypic behaviors, the existence of pronounced likes and dislikes, abnormal relationships with objects, poor self-care skills, egocentric behavior, impaired ability to understand other people, along with aggression, conduct problems, and "delinquent acts."

Despite the categorization of these problems at this time as a personality disorder, and the evident wide range of problems inherent in the presentation, the core connections with autism were very clear. Indeed Asperger published a number of articles comparing infantile autism with his syndrome, noting both the commonalities of symptoms in social and communicative domains and the differences in cognitive and personality domains.

In interpreting Asperger's writings of almost 60 years ago, we need to take into account the social meaning of childhood and its behavioral mores at this time in history, in conjunction with the different approach to child psychiatry than the context in which we currently assess, diagnose, and treat troubled children. Although AS may have been an appropriate categorization in the 1940s in Europe, the question of whether it could be considered a personality disorder has never been developed or thoroughly explored. However, Wolff (1996) presented a translation of a paper published in Germany by Ssuchewa in 1926 (i.e., almost 20 years before Asperger's time) that described cases of schizoid personality disorder in six boys ages 10–13 years. Included in these fascinating case descriptions we find a number of Asperger-like symptoms and behaviors. Although we might not go so far as to rediagnose these boys with AS, the parallels in the two sets of cases are notable. Wolff (1995) and her colleagues have examined the overlap between AS and schizoid personality disorder, as well as the persistence of the latter over time and the possible relationship to the emergence of schizophrenia in later life, without, however, coming to any definitive conclusions about their connections. In light of the viewpoints about mental disorders in the 1920s, the diagnosis of schizoid personality disorder was probably apposite at that time, but it is interesting to wonder how those same boys would be categorized by mental health clinicians today. Nagy and Szatmari (1986) also made comparisons between children with AS and people with a diagnosis of schizotypal personality disorder, demonstrating some common characteristics between these two disorders, such as social isolation, lack of empathy, difficulties in understanding social rules, and impairments in emotional expression. They did not, however, suggest that it was difficult to discriminate between these disorders.

Such papers illustrate the degree to which perceptions and interpretations of symptoms and pathology are influenced by psychiatric thinking of the time and thereby contribute to the inexactitude of clinical science. Miller and Ozonoff (1997) have argued that the kinds of children attracting a diagnosis of AS in contemporary clinical practice are different from those presented by Asperger in his early writings.

In our contemporary context, the framework of autism has dominated the study of AS, with a great deal of current research focused on the questions relating to the diagnostic relationship between AS and autism. AS, as a distinct disorder, received cursory international attention in the literature, until researchers such as Wing (1981), Schopler (1985), Tantam (1988), and Gillberg (1989) published papers that effectively reengaged interest in identifying and understanding individuals with the disorder. Since the seminal writings by Wing, researchers have become sensitized to the existence of children who have the core features of autism but who are different in subtle ways. A growing number of researchers has sought to understand and categorize children with these symptoms and behaviors, and to differentiate them from other kinds of odd, eccentric, and socially inept children. Clinical and research interest then moved toward attempts to distinguish between children with AS and those diagnosed with autism who were intelligent, competent in language, and able to talk about their problems in a way that was rare in the majority of the population diagnosed with autism.

Despite substantial research and a number of comparisons differentiating children diagnosed with autism and those diagnosed with AS, the field is still somewhat uncertain about how to conceptualize the nature of this disorder. The latest versions of the major diagnostic manuals, the *Diagnostic and Statistical Manual of Mental Disorders—Fourth Edition* (DSM-IV; American Psychiatric Association, 1994) and the *International Classification of Diseases and Disorders—Tenth Edition* (ICD-10; World Health Organization, 1993), include specified criteria for autism and AS separately; the major differentiating criterion is a presumed history of normal language development in AS. This recommended differentiating criterion has not proved satisfactory, as will be seen in the arguments presented in this book. In current clinical practice as well as a substantial proportion of research studies, the diagnosis of AS is being used for children who display a milder form of autism, normal or near-normal intelligence, and well-developed language. The diagnostic system recommendation regarding normal development of language appears to be ineffective as a characteristic that can discriminate reliably between two distinct disorders (Eisenmajer et al., 1998).

Empirical and clinical evidence reported thus far supplies no reliable, consensual ways of clearly distinguishing between children with a diagnosis of autism who are high functioning, and those with a diagnosis of AS. It is an underlying premise of this volume that the notion of a continuum or spectrum of autistic conditions is the most logical position to take, given the evidence. This spectrum includes a range of characteristics, from extremely withdrawn and low-functioning cases at one end, to socially aware, articulate, and intelligent children who nevertheless share the core social and communicative impairments that are the hallmark of autism, at the other. Attempts to identify empirical and clinical subgroups within the autism spectrum have been reported over several decades (Prior et al., 1998; Schopler, 1985; Waterhouse et al., 1996) but have had very limited utility. Frith (1991, p. 2) has discussed the "developmental diversity of autism" in this context and suggests that AS is the first plausible variant on the spectrum. A further variant, "pervasive developmental disorder, not otherwise specified" (PDD-NOS), still eludes definition but seems to refer to sub-threshold or mild autism. There is evident confusion in the diagnostic assignment of PDD-NOS versus AS that has not yet been addressed.

A growing number of research studies has focused on the search for identifiable differences between autism and AS in core domains of cognition and behavior, with limited success (e.g., Ozonoff, South, & Miller, 2000; Szatmari, Archer, Fisman, Streiner, & Wilson, 1995; for reviews, see Mayes & Calhoun, Chapter 1, and Tager-Flusberg, Chapter 4, this volume). Contributors to this book vary somewhat in their views regarding the place of AS in the autism spectrum, but all agree that the current diagnostic guidelines need clarification and reconsideration.

## PREVALENCE

Given the ongoing debates regarding the status of AS within or outside the autism diagnostic category, it is not surprising that prevalence estimates are varied and changing. Many researchers believe that the prevalence of AS is much higher than for classic autism, with estimates currently varying between 10–26 per 10,000 (see Wing & Potter, 2002). In fact, answers to the questions of incidence and prevalence of autism spectrum disorders (ASD) are a moving feast. Many more children are being diagnosed, it is true, but whether this increase represents a real rise in the rates of these disorders remains to be established (Charman, 2002). A number of authors have reviewed the reasons for the apparent increase in prevalence of ASD, most recently, Wing and Potter (2002). Greater public awareness of autism may be leading to concerns about unusual developmental features earlier in life and foster an increased willingness of parents to present a puzzling child for assessment. Broadening of the diagnostic criteria, including AS within the autism spectrum, and greater professional knowledge of the conditions also may underpin the increase in numbers of children diagnosed with AS. Perhaps many of these children were formerly dismissed as odd, eccentric, socially awkward, difficult, loners, etc., within their schools. Now teachers are more likely to be aware that children who have distinctive social and communicative impairments that separate them from their classmates could be children with AS. Ascertainment rates also may be affected by the willingness of medical and educational systems to recognize and (sometimes) provide educational support for these children. The relative domination of psychodynamic approaches to assessment and therapy with troubled children appears to have diminished, opening the way for a more empiricist approach to assessing, categorizing, and comparing collections of symptoms and behaviors that may have gone unlabeled in former times.

It is now widely accepted that autism and AS are sometimes associated with a range of other neurodevelopmental conditions. In previous decades, before this association was recognized, children who were not "pure" (nonorganic) cases might have been excluded from research studies. Moreover, it is now accepted that autistic traits can be associated with other psychiatric conditions, including obsessive–compulsive disorder, Tourette syndrome, anxiety and depression, and attention-deficit/hyperactivity disorder (Tantam, 1988). This further widens the gates for an ASD or AS diagnosis. Prevalence estimates rarely consider primary and secondary diagnoses, especially if service issues are in question, producing additional effects on prevalence rates that have not been assessed. In previous decades, too, numbers of undiagnosed children could be found in institutions or special facilities for intellectually disabled children; or, in adulthood, among the population diagnosed with mental illnesses such as schizophrenia and personality disorder. As long as debate regarding the status of AS vis-à-vis ASD remains, and there is some level of uncertainty about its defining characteristics, we will continue to question its prevalence as a subgroup or separate disorder.

## BACKGROUND

The terms "AS" and "HFA" (high-functioning autism) are both used in this book, reflecting the starting premise that these terms are an adaptive way to write about children with high-functioning autism as well as those diagnosed with AS, with their special problems—problems that are common and need understanding and treatment, no matter what label the children have been given. The needs of these children and the concomitant educational resource implications have become ever more pressing, as we have grown more aware and skilled in recognizing, understanding, and treating the condition.

This volume focuses on the behavioral and educational issues pertinent to understanding the common features of the disorder and to providing effective intervention for children with AS. Although there is a reasonably well-integrated literature that describes and analyzes the characteristics of the syndrome and details methods of assessment and diagnosis (e.g., Klin, Volkmar, & Sparrow, 2001), there is a need for an up-to-date compendium that identifies and documents the key behavioral and learning difficulties children have at school and work and provides adaptive ways of helping them to overcome the challenges they face. Providing educators with a resource that would offer them increased understanding of these children was also a motivating factor in preparing this volume.

The many questions and dilemmas in all these domains served as the foundation for the selection of topics:

> Do children with AS have particular problems with learning in the regular classroom, and if so, can they be usefully characterized?
>
> Are they vulnerable to the development of "specific learning difficulties"?
>
> What are the effects of the idiosyncratic and eccentric behaviors on the children's capacities to integrate themselves into school settings and to profit from education?
>
> How should unusual and sometimes very challenging behaviors be managed?
>
> What are the major problems faced by teachers and caregivers in providing the best ways to teach such children so that their undoubted abilities can be optimized?
>
> How can schools work with parents to foster the best possible outcome?
>
> Is it best to label such a child; to inform the teachers, the classroom peers, and the child him- or herself about the nature of the disorder; or to allow the child and family to manage the differences as best they can, without reference to a "medical" condition?
>
> Is inclusion in the regular school system in the best interests of children with AS, and what problems does inclusion engender?
>
> What happens to these children when they reach the end of formal education; what careers and employment prospects do they have, and how might their opportunities be enhanced?

The contents of this volume reflect the wealth of knowledge and skills that has developed over 50 years of searching for the best ways to help children with ASD. The wisdom gained in this journey of search, trial, and evaluation offers valuable insights into the most strategic, benign, and acceptable interventions that are available. It must be acknowledged that research on treatment evaluation has been small in quantity and inconclusive in outcomes, but more is appearing each year, and a clearer picture is emerging of the principles involved in providing successful interventions for these children from the earliest years through adulthood.

The international selection of contributors from the United States, Canada, the United Kingdom, Israel, and Australia provides expertise from their subspecialty areas as researchers, clinicians, and teachers. Wendy Lawson, an extraordinarily articulate adult who has lived with the disorder, provides an enlightening picture of her experiences as she grew up and had to cope with the mysteries of the school environment.

## ORGANIZATION OF THIS VOLUME

Part I of the book addresses some of the basic issues pertinent to working effectively with children who have AS. These include diagnostic challenges, cognitive assessment, analysis, interpretation, and relationship to intervention, as well as the implications of specific learning difficulties for the education of these children. The latter half of this section focuses on the emotional and behavioral problems that are characteristic of the syndrome, with some emphasis on how these should be treated, in order to maximize the potential of these children and adolescents in their educational and social worlds. Part II examines the challenges posed by school systems that currently have little scope with which to fully understand and accommodate the individual differences of the kind presented by children with AS. The viewpoints of teachers, students, and educational theorists are represented here. The longer-term outlook for students with AS is also reviewed in the final section. The book concludes with an overview of the ongoing challenges facing researchers, clinicians, educators, and parents who wish to understand children with AS and to help them flourish in a complex and demanding social world.

The difficulties of differentiating diagnostically between AS and high-functioning autism are addressed in the first chapter by Mayes and Calhoun, who provide a clear and thoroughly researched evaluation of the current situation, with conclusions and suggestions for future diagnostic system development that might reduce puzzlement and dissatisfaction among clinicians and teachers.

Asperger himself asserted that most of these children have learning difficulties, and he noted the difficulties of attending to their needs in school (Asperger, 1944/1991, as translated by Frith, 1991). Two chapters present the cognitive and learning characteristics of children with AS, using case studies and long-term follow-up data on children in school.

Reitzal and Szatmari address the methodology involved in the assessment of learning difficulties and emphasize the need for a comprehensive approach covering all domains of functioning. They review the relatively few studies that delineate cognitive profiles in AS and HFA and evaluate the extent to which these have any specificity to either group. In addition, they report the most recent follow-up results regarding academic achievement in a sample of children (ages 4–13 years) studied longitudinally by Szatmari's group. They propose a new and interesting interpretation of their findings, which addresses the current debate on the relations between AS and HFA.

Manjiviona draws on a wealth of experience in clinical assessment, diagnosis, and educational liaison to illustrate some of the learning difficulties experienced by children with AS. Her work illustrates the value of expert analyses and interpretation of assessment results, the range of tests that can be brought to bear on the analyses of learning problems, and the need to assess in a comprehensive manner. Through three case studies, she conveys the varying presentations encountered in clinical practice and exemplifies the process of conducting a detailed assessment, including cognitive and neuropsychological analyses and their implications. These assessment findings can be used to better inform the family members and teachers, as they struggle to find ways to help these children participate in satisfying academic learning experiences. Manjiviona notes the therapeutic value of a comprehensive assessment for the family.

In Chapter 4, language development and its idiosyncrasies are reviewed and analyzed by Tager-Flusberg. She builds a compelling case for the invalidity of differentiating between AS and HFA on the basis of language development features. She offers insights into how children with AS can make use of their cognitive and language abilities to overcome some of their social, adaptive, and educational difficulties, through developing compensatory strategies to process information that is important in learning about the world.

Shaked and Yirmiya review the social problems of individuals with AS and how these deficits affect their efforts to gain acceptance by their peers and cope with the contingencies of the various school contexts. They describe teaching and training techniques that provide learnable strategies for reducing the mystification of a complex and unpredictable social world, and which can help children with AS navigate that world, especially in the context of their educational experiences. A somewhat less commonly investigated feature of children with AS is their intense preoccupation with specific idiosyncratic interests. Attwood documents and analyzes a range of individual expressions of this highly significant aspect of their lives. He provides vivid examples of the preoccupations these children develop and suggests ways of managing—and, indeed, benefiting from—these special interests.

Tantam reminds us that the diagnosis of AS is not the whole story. These young people often have to cope with associated problems connected to, but not necessarily explained by, their autistic features. In his overview of the frequent connections between AS and problems such as attention deficits, hyperactivity, and anxiety, illustrated by case examples, Tantam analyzes what underlies the often extreme reactions of people with AS, and suggests helpful interventions, including the judicious use of medication in some instances.

Part II focuses more intensely on educational experiences—a complicated enough pathway for children with unexceptional developmental histories but a hugely demanding experience for children with AS. Lawson and Gill, as former student and teacher, respectively, set the scene for the focus on educational matters by giving compelling first-hand accounts of their experiences.

Wendy Lawson underwent all the trials of schooling without anyone knowing that she was suffering from AS; indeed, as is often the case with this disorder, no one understood her condition and the challenges she faced. She vividly recalls her experiences and extracts from these a range of mature understandings of the nature of the syndrome and the specific difficulties involved in trying to understand and deal with the world. She writes eloquently of her fear and confusion in this "other world," where she must struggle to translate the meanings of people's behavior into a form she can understand. Her insights can help us develop empathy for the often silent struggles taking place in children with AS. We also learn ways in which we might better "read" their behaviors. Her insights and suggestions are highly instructive for those parents, clinicians, and teachers who are engaged in efforts to understand the autistic world and to make connections with the children and adolescents for whom they care. These insights and suggestions are in accordance with the recommendations made by authors in the following chapters, which discuss flexible adaptations for school environments and teaching styles to better accommodate the needs of children with AS.

Gill is the principal of a large school for children with autism and AS. Children attend this school's specialist programs for varying periods of time. The purpose of these programs is to prepare them for successful integration into either mainstream regular school programs or special schools, depending on their needs and levels of functioning, as well as on parental choice, of course. The wisdom and expertise that Gill has acquired in her career in special education shines through her often moving account of the problems she encounters in assisting children and adolescents with AS to acquire rich experiences in both academic and social domains.

Jordan gives us a vivid picture of the learning difficulties encountered by children with AS in regular school settings and takes us through all the major subject areas of the secondary school curriculum, providing comprehensive, detailed, and insightful analyses of their particular challenges. She shows how solutions tailored to individual needs can be crafted with creative ideas and strategies.

Kunce accepted the challenge of providing a chapter addressing the topic of what would constitute the "ideal classroom" for children with AS. Based on the most recent research, she gives us a comprehensive construction of such a classroom, including all the essential elements: key persons needed, adaptive and facilitative structures and strategies, individualization of curricula, and a focus on both short- and long-term goals for students with AS. Acceptance and support for the implementation of her model would, no doubt, enormously improve the current situation for these students and their teachers and parents, and would contribute to a less stressful school career and more satisfying outcomes for these young people.

In recent years, Howlin has made a unique and invaluable contribution to the study of adult outcomes in ASD; in her chapter she focuses on longer-term outcomes for young people with AS. She notes the paucity of research studying children/adolescents in secondary school settings in contrast to the more numerous published studies of pre- and primary school teaching and training. She reviews the common challenges encountered by young people with AS as they move through school, university, or work training into adult life and employment, and she includes a summary of international follow-up studies that report on adult outcomes. Making supported employment and independent living work for these individuals is a key task for families and professionals working in this field.

## REFERENCES

American Psychiatric Association. (1994). *Diagnostic and statistical manual of mental disorders* (4th ed.). Washington, DC: Author.

Asperger, H. (1991). Autistic psychopathology in childhood. In U. Frith (Ed.), *Autism and Asperger syndrome* (pp. 37–92). Cambridge, UK: Cambridge University Press. (Original work published in German 1944)

Charman, T. (2002). The prevalence of autism spectrum disorders: Recent evidence and future challenges. *European Child and Adolescent Psychiatry, 11*(6), 249–256.

Eisenmajer, R., Prior, M., Leekam, S., Wing, L., Ong, B., Gould, J., & Welham, M. (1998). Delayed language onset as a predictor of clinical symptoms in pervasive developmental disorders. *Journal of Autism and Developmental Disorders, 28,* 527–533.

Frith, U. (Ed.). (1991). *Autism and Asperger syndrome.* Cambridge, UK: Cambridge University Press.

Gillberg, C. (1989). Asperger syndrome in 23 Swedish children. *Developmental Medicine and Child Neurology, 31,* 520–531.

Kanner, L. (1943). Autistic disturbances of affective contact. *Nervous Child, 2,* 217–250.

Klin, A., Volkmar, F. R., & Sparrow, S. S. (Eds.). (2001). *Asperger syndrome.* New York: Guilford Press.

Mayes, S. D., & Calhoun, S. L. (2001). Non-significance of early speech delay in children with autism and normal intelligence and implications for DSM-IV Asperger's disorder. *Autism, 5,* 81–94.

Miller, J., & Ozonoff, S. (1997). Did Asperger's cases have Asperger's disorder? A research note. *Journal of Child Psychology and Psychiatry, 38*(2), 247–251.

Nagy, J., & Szatmari, P. (1986). A chart review of schizotypal personality disorders in childhood. *Journal of Autism and Developmental Disorders, 16*, 351–367.

Ozonoff, S., South, M., & Miller, J. N. (2000). DSM-IV-defined Asperger Syndrome: Cognitive, behavioral, and early history differentiation from high-functioning autism. *Autism, 4*, 29–46.

Prior, M., Eisenmajer, R., Leekam, S., Wing, L., Gould, J., Ong, B., & Dowe, D. (1998). Are there subgroups within the autistic spectrum? A cluster analysis of a group of children with autistic spectrum disorders. *Journal of Child Psychology and Psychiatry, 39*(6), 893–902.

Schopler, E. (1985). Convergence of learning disability, higher-level autism, and Asperger's syndrome. *Journal of Autism and Developmental Disorders, 15*, 359.

Szatmari, P., Archer, L., Fisman, S., Streiner, D. L., & Wilson, F. (1995). Asperger's syndrome and autism: Differences in behavior, cognition, and adaptive functioning. *Journal of the American Academy of Child and Adolescent Psychiatry, 34*, 1662–1671.

Tantam, D. (1988). Lifelong eccentricity and social isolation: II. Asperger's syndrome or schizoid personality disorder? *British Journal of Psychiatry, 153*, 783–791.

Waterhouse, L., Morris, R., Allen, D., Dunn, M., Fein, D., Feinsten, C., Rapin, I., & Wing, L. (1996). Diagnosis and classification in autism. *Journal of Autism and Developmental Disorders, 26*, 59–86.

Wing, L. (1981). Asperger's syndrome: A clinical account. *Psychological Medicine, 11*, 115–129.

Wing, L., & Potter, D. (2002). The epidemiology of autism spectrum disorders: Is the prevalence rising? *Mental Retardation and Developmental Disabilities Research Reviews, 8*, 151–161.

Wolff, S. (1995). *Loners: The life path of unusual children.* London: Routledge.

Wolff, S. (1996). The first account of the syndrome Asperger described? *European Child and Adolescent Psychiatry, 5*, 119-132.

World Health Organization. (1993). *International classification of diseases and disorders* (10th ed.). Geneva: Author.

# I

Assessment
and Management
of Behavioral
and Learning Difficulties

# 1

# Relationship between
# Asperger Syndrome
# and High-Functioning Autism

SUSAN DICKERSON MAYES
SUSAN L. CALHOUN

Many experts now agree that autism is a spectrum disorder and that Asperger syndrome (AS) is high-functioning or mild autism (Attwood, 1998; Eisenmajer et al., 1996; Manjiviona & Prior, 1995; Miller & Ozonoff, 2000; Myhr, 1998; Ozonoff, South, & Miller, 2000; Prior et al., 1998; Schopler, 1996, 1998; Wing, 1998). However, controversy persists, and "Asperger syndrome" remains a popular term used by clinicians and parents alike. This chapter (1) provides an historical overview of Asperger syndrome relative to autism, (2) assesses the validity of the DSM-IV diagnostic criteria for Asperger's disorder, (3) reviews studies attempting to determine if AS is separate and distinct from high-functioning autism, (4) summarizes the impact of IQ and age on autistic symptoms, and (5) discusses the reliability of the DSM-IV pervasive developmental disorder subtypes.

## HISTORICAL OVERVIEW

The first published descriptions of autism appeared in the 1940s. Leo Kanner (1943) in the United States and Hans Asperger (1944/1991) in Germany independently wrote about a group of individuals that each described as having "autism." Specifically, Kanner used the term "early infantile autism" and Asperger used "autistic psychopathy." Asperger's original description of symptoms is consistent with what the DSM-IV defines as "autistic disorder." The DSM-IV divides its diagnostic criteria for autism into three categories: social impairment, restricted and repetitive behavior and interests, and communication impairment. Asperger stated that "autistic individuals" have profound social problems, are socially isolated, and make poor eye contact. According to Asperger, these individuals have abnormal fixations, special interests, ritualized behaviors, and stereotyped play and movements. They also have language abnormalities, including unusual use of speech, atypical voice quality, and problems with conversational speech. Asperger noted other symptoms that match the associated features of autism summarized in the DSM-IV. These include special abilities, difficulty with attention, behavior problems, and unusual sensory responses (e.g., dislike of certain sounds, tactile sensations, and foods). According to both Asperger and the DSM-IV, individuals with autism can have below- to above-normal intelligence. Asperger stated that his patients encompassed "all levels of ability from the highly original genius . . . to the . . . mentally retarded individual" (1944/1991, p. 74).

Wing first used the term "Asperger syndrome" in 1976 and defined it in a 1981 publication. Her criteria for AS differed somewhat from Asperger's original descriptions. Wing proposed that the label "Asperger syndrome" be applied to "children and adults who have autistic features, but who talk grammatically and who are not socially aloof" (1981, p. 124). In other words, the original definition of Asperger syndrome was autism with better social and language functioning.

Before Asperger's disorder appeared in the DSM-IV, early proponents (Ghaziuddin, Tsai, & Ghaziuddin, 1992b; Gillberg, 1985, 1989, 1991a; Gillberg & Gillberg, 1989; Klin, 1994; Szatmari, 1991; Szatmari, Tuff, Finlayson, & Bartolucci, 1990; Tantam, 1988; Wing, 1981) contended that individuals with AS displayed the core features of autism, including impaired social interaction, restricted and repetitive behavior and interests, and communication impairments. In contrast to individuals with autism, individuals with AS demonstrated better language and social skills (Frith, 1991; Gillberg, 1985; Klin, 1994; Szatmari, 1991; Tantam, 1988; Wing, 1991), higher (but not necessarily normal) IQs (Gillberg, 1985; Gillberg & Gillberg, 1989; Klin, 1994; Tantam, 1988; Wing, 1991), fewer symptoms such as stereotypies or sensory abnormalities (Klin, 1994; Szatmari, 1991; Wing, 1981, 1991), and more unusual or intense interests and preoccupations (Klin, 1994; Wing, 1981). Some researchers and clinicians proposed that gross motor incoordination was a symptom of AS (Gillberg, 1991a; Gillberg & Gillberg, 1989; Tantam, 1988; Wing, 1981, 1991), whereas others felt this was not always true (Ghaziuddin, Tsai, & Ghaziuddin, 1992a; Ghaziuddin et al., 1992b; Klin, 1994; Szatmari, 1991).

In 1985, Schopler cautioned against the premature use of the label "Asperger syndrome" and maintained that what people were describing as AS was really high-functioning autism. In 1991, Wing stated that there may not be a difference between AS and high-functioning autism, and she proposed that autism be considered a spectrum disorder, from mild to severe, with AS or high-functioning autism at the mild end.

## DSM-IV ASPERGER'S DISORDER

The 1994 publication of the DSM-IV listed "Asperger's disorder" as one of the five pervasive developmental disorder (PDD) subtypes. The DSM-IV criteria for Asperger's disorder versus autism differed from previous conceptualizations of AS in the literature. Social impairment and restricted and repetitive behavior and interests were included as core features, but the DSM-IV (1) did not specify that social skills were less impaired in AS than in autism and (2) did not include communication impairment as a symptom of Asperger's disorder. Furthermore, the DSM-IV required the absence of significant cognitive and speech delays for a diagnosis of Asperger's disorder. Although the DSM-IV provided an official definition for Asperger's disorder, it has not been universally accepted. Proponents of AS disagree with the DSM-IV, contending that individuals with AS have abnormalities of language (Ghaziuddin, Weidmer-Mikhail, & Ghaziuddin, 1998; Gillberg & Ehlers, 1998; Klin & Volkmar, 1995; Siegel, 1996), may have an early history of speech delay (Eisenmajer et al., 1996; Manjiviona & Prior, 1995; Siegel, 1996; Twachtman-Cullen, 1998), have better language and social skills than individuals with autism (Eisenmajer et al., 1996; Myhr, 1998; Siegel, 1996; Szatmari, Archer, Fisman, Streiner, & Wilson, 1995), and may have below-normal IQs (Klin & Volkmar, 1995; Siegel, 1996).

Since the publication of the DSM-IV, researchers and clinicians have continued to disagree about the criteria for AS or even the existence of AS as separate and distinct from autism (Eisenmajer et al., 1996; Ghaziuddin, Leininger, & Tsai, 1995; Gillberg & Ehlers, 1998; Hooper & Bundy, 1998; Kunce & Mesibov, 1998; Manjiviona & Prior, 1995; Myhr, 1998; Prior et al., 1998; Schopler, 1998; Szatmari, 1998, 2000; Szatmari et al., 1995; Volkmar & Klin, 1998; Young & Brewer, 2002). As stated by Schopler (1998), "It becomes increasingly difficult to arrive at a useable classification system as increasing numbers of authors introduce their own variations in criteria" (p. 389). This variability is very evident in research studies that attempt to compare individuals with "Asperger syndrome" to individuals with "high-functioning autism." For example, Szatmari, Bartolucci, and Bremner (1989) used criteria for AS that were "adapted from Wing" (p. 710). In another study (Szatmari et al., 1995), diagnostic criteria for AS were "not identical with" those proposed by the DSM-IV (p. 1663). In the same year, Klin, Volkmar, Sparrow, Cicchetti, and Rourke (1995) published a study using "modified" (p. 1131) ICD-10 criteria for AS. Ozonoff, Rogers, and Pennington (1991) also used a "modified version" (p. 1109) of ICD-10 AS criteria. In later studies (Miller & Ozonoff, 2000; Ozonoff et al., 2000), DSM-IV criteria were applied. All of the children with a diagnosis of Asperger's disorder had autistic symptoms but fewer than the six required for a DSM-IV diagnosis of autism. Previously these children would have been diagnosed with pervasive developmental disorder not otherwise specified (PDD-NOS). Finally, Gilchrist and colleagues (2001) used the presence versus absence of early speech delay to distinguish high-functioning autism from AS. Children who spoke in phrases by age 3 were included in the AS group, even if they met criteria for autism. In short, all of these studies used different criteria, making it impossible to compare and interpret findings.

## VALIDITY OF DSM-IV ASPERGER'S DISORDER

Research studies have now shown that most children with clinical diagnoses of Asperger syndrome or disorder actually fulfill DSM-IV diagnostic criteria for autism and not Asperger's disorder. Miller and Ozonoff (1997) analyzed Asperger's (1944/1991) original case presentations and found that all fulfilled the DSM-IV criteria for autism and not Asperger's disorder. In another study, DSM-IV criteria were applied to children who had received clinical diagnoses of AS (Eisenmajer et al., 1996). All 69 children met DSM-IV criteria for autism. Similarly, a study of 12 children previously diagnosed with AS (Manjiviona & Prior, 1995) indicated that all children had social impairments, restricted and repetitive behavior and interests, and a language impairment, consistent with the DSM-IV symptoms for autism. Szatmari and colleagues (1995) studied preschool children with pervasive developmental disorder, including 21 who were diagnosed by the authors as having AS. Only one of the 68 children met the DSM-IV criteria for Asperger's disorder.

Most recently, Mayes, Calhoun, and Crites (2001) studied a sample of 157 children with clinical diagnoses of autism or AS to determine if any of these children fulfilled DSM-IV diagnostic criteria for Asperger's disorder. As shown in Table 1.1, if a child with no significant cognitive or speech delay (the latter defined by the DSM-IV as "single words used by age 2 years, communicative phrases used by age 3 years"; American Psychiatric Associ-

**TABLE 1.1. DSM-IV Diagnostic Criteria**

| Autistic disorder | Asperger's disorder |
|---|---|
| **Development** | |
| 1. "Delays or abnormal functioning in ... social interaction, ... social communication, ... or ... imaginative play" and "onset prior to age 3" (may or may not have normal IQ or speech delay) | 1. "No clinically significant ... delay in language ... [or] cognitive development" |
| **Symptoms (minimum required)** | |
| 1. "Impairment in social interaction" (2) | 1. "Impairment in ... social interaction" (2) |
| 2. "Restricted repetitive ... behavior, interests" (1) | 2. "Restricted repetitive ... behavior, interests" (1) |
| 3. "Impairments in communication" such as "impairment in the ability to initiate or sustain a conversation" or "stereotyped and repetitive use of language or idiosyncratic language" (1) | 3. Does not meet criteria for autistic disorder |
| **Minimum total number of symptoms required** | |
| 6 | 3 |

ation, 1994, p. 77) has the required number of symptoms (six or more) in the three DSM-IV core areas (i.e., "impairment in social interaction," "restricted repetitive ... behavior, interests," and "impairments in communication"), with onset before age 3, the child's DSM-IV diagnosis is autistic disorder. If a child has no significant cognitive and speech delay, two or more social impairment symptoms, one or more restricted behavior and interests symptoms, and either no communication impairment or fewer than six symptoms in all areas, the child's diagnosis is AS. A licensed psychologist and a board-certified child psychiatrist independently determined that all children in the study met DSM-IV criteria for autistic disorder and none met criteria for Asperger's disorder. All children had the required number of symptoms for autism, and all children (including those with normal IQs and no history of speech delay) had "impairment in social interaction" and "restricted repetitive ... behavior, interests" (required by the DSM-IV for both autism and Asperger's disorder) *and* "impairments in communication" (i.e., "impairment in the ability to initiate or sustain a conversation" or "stereotyped and repetitive use of language or idiosyncratic language"; American Psychiatric Association, 1994, p. 70).

This finding is not surprising; a child who has a social impairment and restricted and repetitive interests is also likely to have difficulty sustaining a conversation and to use repetitive language, thus fulfilling DSM-IV criteria for autism, not Asperger's disorder. Furthermore, all previous definitions of AS included abnormalities of language as a symptom (Ghaziuddin et al., 1992a; Gillberg, 1985, 1989, 1991a; Gillberg & Ehlers, 1998; Gillberg & Gillberg, 1989; Klin, 1994; Klin & Volkmar, 1995; Manjiviona & Prior, 1995; Siegel, 1996; Szatmari, 1991; Szatmari et al., 1990; Tantam, 1988; Twachtman-Cullen, 1998; Wing, 1981). In summary, research suggests that Asperger's disorder, as defined by the DSM-IV, may not exist and that Asperger syndrome is really another name for high-functioning autism. Children previously considered by clinicians to have AS actually meet DSM-IV criteria for autism (Eisenmajer et al., 1996; Mayes et al., 2001; Miller & Ozonoff, 1997). Is the DSM always correct? No. If it were, we would not have a DSM-I, -II, -III, -III-R, -IV, and -IV-TR. The DSM is a diagnostic system that is being revised continuously. The DSM proposes diagnostic categories, which then must be validated or modified according to the results of empirical research.

## NONSIGNIFICANCE OF EARLY SPEECH DELAY

One of the DSM-IV distinctions between Asperger's and autistic disorder is the absence of significant speech delays in children with Asperger's disorder, whereas children with autism may or may not have these delays. However, the significance of early speech delay in autism is questionable. In a study by Eisenmajer and colleagues (1998), the presence versus absence of early language delay was not significantly related, overall, to later autistic symptoms in children with autism spectrum disorder (ASD). Similarly, a study of empirically derived autism spectrum subtypes (Prior et al., 1998) failed to show differences in early language development between subgroups. In a recent study of 47 children with normal intelligence and clinical diagnoses of autism or AS (Mayes & Calhoun, 2001), those with early speech delay did not differ significantly on any of the 71 variables assessed, including autistic symptoms, from those without this delay. Autistic symptoms were measured by the Checklist for Autism in Young Children (Mayes & Calhoun, 1999; see appendix at the end of this chapter), which lists 30 symptoms that include all of the DSM-IV criteria for autism as well as symptoms mentioned in the DSM-IV as associated features of autism. Children with, versus without, a significant speech delay did not even differ on language variables. At the time of the study (mean age 6 years, 1 month), all children with normal intelligence had acquired speech. Children with an early speech delay had a mean Verbal IQ of 95.4, which was consistent with that for children who did not have a speech delay (94.5). Most of the children in both groups had difficulty initiating and sustaining a conversation, and they had similar atypical vocal or speech patterns, which included abnormal voice quality or modulation; screeching or making other odd noises; repetitive vocalizations; idiosyncratic jargon; echolalia; rote phrases uttered out of context; improper use of pronouns; or idiosyncratic, perseverative, sporadic, and infrequent or nonsensical speech. Therefore, early speech milestones may not be predictive of later speech development in children with high-functioning autism or AS.

Nonsignificant differences between children with and without a speech delay were found for all of the remaining variables as well, including complications during pregnancy, labor, delivery, or the neonatal period; gestational age; birth weight; age at acquisition of motor milestones (both groups walked at a mean age of 12–13 months); Full Scale IQ (both groups had a mean IQ in the average range); Verbal–Performance IQ discrepancy; type or frequency of splinter skills; and parent and teacher rating scale scores for anxiety, depression, oppositional and aggressive behavior, and motor incoordination. These results suggest that early speech delay may be irrelevant to later childhood outcome in children who have ASD and normal intelligence, and that the absence of a speech delay as a DSM-IV criterion for Asperger's disorder (vs. autism) may not be justified.

## DIFFERENCES IN AUTISTIC SYMPTOMS AS A FUNCTION OF IQ AND AGE

Another DSM-IV distinction between Asperger's disorder and autism is the absence of a clinically significant delay in cognitive development in Asperger's disorder, which may or may not be the case in autism. Research suggests that autistic symptoms are influenced by IQ and age. Autistic symptoms decrease with increasing IQ (Bartak & Rutter, 1976; Eaves, Ho, & Eaves, 1994; Miller & Ozonoff, 2000; Myhr, 1998; Prior et al., 1998; Sevin et al., 1995; Szatmari, 2000; Tantam, 1988; Tsai, 1992; Volkmar, Cicchetti, Cohen, & Bregman, 1992; Waterhouse et al., 1996; Wing, 1981) and increasing age (Bartak & Rutter, 1976; Church & Coplan, 1995; Mayes & Calhoun, 1999; Wing, 1976). Furthermore, children with higher IQs are likely to be identified as having autism at a later age, because of their milder symptoms, than children with lower IQs (Gillberg, Nordin, & Ehlers, 1996; Mayes & Calhoun, 2003a). In a study of 157 children with ASD (Mayes & Calhoun, 2003a), the 110 children with below-normal IQs (< 80) had a significantly greater total frequency of autistic symptoms (i.e., a higher composite score on the Checklist for Autism in Young Children) and more problems with social interaction than did children who had an IQ of 80 or above ($n$ = 47). However, these differences were no longer significant when the effects of IQ and age were statistically removed. Therefore, differences between the two groups could be explained simply by differences in IQ and age and not some intrinsic difference related to autism.

A study that attempted to empirically identify autism spectrum or pervasive developmental disorder subtypes (Prior et al., 1998) also found that symptom differences could be explained by differences in intelligence and/ or age. These results fail to support the DSM-IV's use of normal cognition as one criterion for Asperger's disorder versus autism. It does not seem logical for the DSM-IV to subdivide a psychological disorder on the basis of intelligence. The DSM-IV does not do this for any other disorder that occurs in childhood (e.g., attention-deficit/hyperactivity disorder, major depression, or the anxiety disorders). Furthermore, the purpose of the Axis II designation is to denote normal intelligence versus mental retardation. To incorporate the presence or absence of mental retardation into an Axis I diagnosis violates one rationale for creating separate Axis I and II diagnoses—which is that any psychiatric disorder can occur with or without mental retardation. There is growing support among clinical researchers for the view that AS is high-functioning autism. If this is true, "Asperger's disorder" should be deleted from the next version of the DSM. High-functioning autism would continue to be indicated by an Axis I diagnosis of autism, without an Axis II diagnosis of mental retardation.

## DIAGNOSTIC RELIABILITY

According to Rutter and Schopler (1987), "of all the psychiatric syndromes arising in childhood, autism is much the best validated by empirical research" (p. 180). Diagnostic agreement for the presence versus absence of ASD or pervasive developmental disorder (PDD) is far higher than agreement for the DSM-IV PDD subtypes (Mahoney et al., 1998; Stone et al., 1999; Volkmar et al., 1994). To compromise diagnostic validity by introducing empirically unsubstantiated and unreliable subtypes is unfortunate. In our clinical experience, children with autism who have mild symptoms and relatively high IQs may receive different diagnoses from different clinicians, including Asperger's disorder or syndrome, high-functioning autism, mild autism, or PDD-NOS. This disparity causes much confusion for professionals and parents alike, and it implies that these diagnoses represent separate and distinct disorders that differ in clinically meaningful ways—

which has not been proven empirically. For example, Szatmari (1998) notes, "there is very little information on empirical distinctions that can be made between Asperger syndrome, autism, and other disorders within the PDD spectrum" (p. 62). Similarly, Volkmar and Klin (1998) state, "There is little disagreement that Asperger syndrome is on a continuum with autism. . . . What is less clear is whether the condition is qualitatively different from high-functioning autism" (p. 113).

## AUTISM SPECTRUM

In 1998, Wing concluded that AS and high-functioning autism were one and the same, stating, "Asperger syndrome and high-functioning autism are not distinct conditions" (p. 23). Research attempting to differentiate autism, AS, and PDD-NOS suggests that these subgroups differ only in symptom severity or IQ (Miller & Ozonoff, 2000; Myhr, 1998; Ozonoff et al., 2000). Therefore, these groups fall along a single spectrum representing the same disorder. In contrast, Rett's disorder and childhood disintegrative disorder are unique and rare disorders that should not be considered among the autism spectrum subtypes (Myhr, 1998). Furthermore, many experts oppose the use of the term "pervasive developmental disorder" instead of "autism spectrum," including Baird, Wing, Mesibov, and 13 others (Baird et al., 1991), Gillberg (1991b), Happé and Frith (1991), Myhr (1998), and Szatmari (2000). Baird and colleagues (1991) contend that the introduction of the PDD label was "a serious mistake" (p. 363), and Happé and Frith (1991) describe it as an "inappropriate and uninformative term" and "an unhelpful label since it does not take advantage of the hard-won public awareness of autism" (p. 1167).

Unfortunately, use of euphemisms such as PDD may delay the provision of intensive intervention for young children with autism. Even today, parents say they have been mislead by the term PDD and would have pursued intensive early intervention for their children if clinicians had diagnosed *autism* instead of PDD. Ultimately, these parents are angered and distressed by missed opportunities that might have improved their child's long-term prognosis. Carefully controlled research studies demonstrate that intensive behavioral intervention during the preschool years can significantly improve the long-term outcome for young children with autism (Birnbrauer & Leach, 1993; Lovaas, 1987; McEachin, Smith, & Lovaas, 1993; Ozonoff & Cathcart, 1998; Sheinkopf & Siegel, 1998; Smith, Groen, & Wynn, 2000). Outcome is considerably better when intensive intervention is initiated before age 4 or 5 (Fenske, Zalenski, Krantz, & McClannahan, 1985; Harris & Handleman, 2000).

Instead of multiple subtypes, it seems logical to conceptualize autism as a single spectrum disorder, from mild to severe. Research indicates that as IQ increases, children with autism have fewer and milder symptoms. Children at the severe end of the autism continuum may be socially avoidant and resist contact with others. In contrast, children at the mild end of the spectrum may be socially awkward, able to interact with others but lacking the social skills to do so appropriately. These are the children long ago referred to by Wing and Gould (1979) as socially "active but odd." The speech of children at the mild end of the continuum may be well developed in terms of sentence length, syntax, and vocabulary; however, these children have difficulty with reciprocal conversational speech, and their speech may be repetitive and idiosyncratic. In contrast, children at the lower end of the spectrum may lack speech altogether or communicate only when they need something.

Children at the high and low ends of the continuum both have restricted interests and obsessive preoccupations, but these may differ according to the child's level of intelligence. Children with high-functioning autism, for example, may talk incessantly about dinosaurs or spend hours drawing detailed pictures of the solar system. In contrast, lower functioning children with autism may spend hours spinning the wheels on cars or lining up toys. Splinter skills are also found in both low- and high-functioning children with autism but, as with other symptoms, these differ according to level of intelligence. One child with autism and a low IQ could not comprehend any spoken language, but he could memorize it. He could not follow simple verbal requests, such as "sit down" or "come here," but if his parents changed the words in books when reading to him, he became very upset. Spoken words were stored but not processed or understood. High-functioning children with autism also tend to have exceptional memories but with a more sophisticated focus. These children may amass scientific, historical, or other factual information. Some of these children are aware of their differences. One boy stated, "I have a photographic memory, but it has overnight developing." When asked to explain what he meant, he said, "My brain is like a computer. Everything I put in it is stored, but it takes a while to get processed." This is similar to the child with a low IQ who could memorize but not comprehend language, but at a much higher level.

Developmental and ability profiles also differ in children with autism as a function of IQ and age. The majority of children with autism have normal motor and delayed speech milestones. This pattern is true for both children with low and high IQs (Mayes & Calhoun, 2003a). In a cross-sectional study of 164 children with autism, ages 3–15 years, verbal IQ continued to lag behind nonverbal IQ during the preschool years, but by school age, the gap had closed (Mayes & Calhoun, 2003a). Group nonverbal and verbal IQs steadily increased during the preschool years, verbal more so than nonverbal. The nonverbal–verbal discrepancy thereby decreased with time and was no longer significant by ages 6–7 for children in the high IQ ( 80) group and by ages 9–10 for children in the low IQ (≥ 80) group.

Analyses of scores on tests measuring IQ (Stanford–Binet: IV and WISC-III), visual reasoning (Leiter and Test of Nonverbal Intelligence), graphomotor skills (Developmental Test of Visual–Motor Integration), and academic achievement (Woodcock–Johnson Tests of Achievement and Wechsler Individual Achievement Test) also showed that profiles varied somewhat as a function of IQ and age (Mayes & Calhoun, 2003a, 2003b). Preschool children with low IQs had strengths in visual reasoning, visual–motor skills (e.g., completing formboards) and rote memory (e.g., counting and identifying letters) and weaknesses in language and attention. School-age children with low IQs also had strengths in visual reasoning, visual–motor skills (e.g., assembling puzzles), and rote memory (e.g., high scores on reading decoding and spelling tests). Attention was again a weakness, but these children no longer had a global verbal weakness. Instead, they performed relatively well on WISC-III subtests measuring lexical knowledge, including Information (recall of facts), Vocabulary (word definitions), and Similarities (categorical terms). In contrast, they performed poorly on the WISC-III Comprehension subtest, which measures both language comprehension and social reasoning. At the other end of the spectrum, preschool children with high IQs had strong visual and rote memory skills and weak verbal, attention, and graphomotor skills. The group of high IQ school-age students showed relative weaknesses in attention, graphomotor, and compositional writing skills. Verbal abilities were split; students demonstrated relatively high lexical knowledge and low comprehension and social reasoning.

Academic achievement test scores also were analyzed. In the low IQ school-age group, mean academic achievement tests scores in reading, math, and spelling were higher than the group's mean IQ of 67. These children performed especially well in reading decoding (standard score 81) and spelling (78), reflecting their relative strengths in rote memory. Mean academic achievement test scores for school-age children with high IQs were all in the average range and consistent with their mean IQ of 103, with the exception of a significant weakness on the Wechsler Individual Achievement Test (WIAT) Written Expression subtest, which measures compositional writing skills. In the subgroup of school-age children with autism and normal IQs, 63% showed a specific learning disability in written expression (i.e., the WIAT Written Expression subtest score was significantly lower than predicted, based on IQ). Learning disabilities in math were relatively uncommon (22%), and a learning disability in either reading decoding or reading comprehension was rare (7%).

## SUMMARY

Autism is best described as occurring on a continuum, from mild to severe. IQ and age have an impact on the frequency and severity of autistic symptoms and the cognitive profiles of children with autism. Many clinicians and researchers are now in agreement that autism is a spectrum disorder and that AS is not a separate and distinct condition but is high-functioning or mild autism (Attwood, 1998; Eisenmajer et al., 1996; Manjiviona & Prior, 1995; Miller & Ozonoff, 2000; Myhr, 1998; Ozonoff et al., 2000; Prior et al., 1998; Schopler, 1996, 1998; Wing, 1998). Even Wing (1998), who first introduced and defined the term "Asperger syndrome," now maintains that AS and high-functioning autism are the same. Research has failed to support the validity of the DSM-IV's diagnostic criteria for Asperger's disorder (Eisenmajer et al., 1996; Mayes et al., 2001; Miller & Ozonoff, 1997). The children in these studies who had received previous clinical diagnoses of AS all met DSM-IV criteria for autism. A study by Szatmari and colleagues (1995) yielded similar results, and the authors concluded that a DSM-IV diagnosis of Asperger's disorder was "virtually impossible" (p. 1669). Experts still do not agree on the diagnostic criteria for AS (Eisenmajer et al., 1996; Hooper & Bundy, 1998; Manjiviona & Prior, 1995; Myhr, 1998; Schopler, 1998; Szatmari et al., 1995; Volkmar & Klin, 1998). Indeed researchers studying differences between individuals with "Asperger syndrome" and "high-functioning autism" have used different diagnostic criteria for AS (Gilchrist et al., 2001; Klin et al., 1995; Miller & Ozonoff, 2000; Ozonoff et al., 1991; Szatmari et al., 1989, 1995). When differences between the two groups are reported, these differences are explained simply by differences in IQ or symptom severity; such explanations do not support the external validity of AS (Miller & Ozonoff, 2000; Myhr, 1998; Ozonoff et al., 2000). Furthermore, diagnostic reliability for autism spectrum (or PDD) is excellent, whereas agreement is considerably lower for the PDD subtypes (Mahoney et al., 1998; Stone et al., 1999; Volkmar et al., 1994). Different labels are often used for the same children, creating much confusion for parents and professionals. For example, high-functioning children with autism are variously referred to by different clinicians as having AS or disorder, high-functioning autism, mild autism, autistic features, or PDD-NOS. If high-functioning autism and AS are one and the same, Asperger's disorder should be deleted from the next edition of the DSM. High-functioning autism would continue to be denoted by an Axis I diagnosis of autism, without an Axis II diagnosis of mental retardation. Children who have some autistic symptoms but not enough for a diagnosis of autism would receive, as before, a diagnosis of PDD-NOS.

## APPENDIX
## Checklist for Autism in Young Children, by Susan Mayes, PhD

**Problems with social interaction**

___ Social isolation, withdrawal

___ Limited eye contact, reciprocal interaction, social smile, sharing, showing

___ Self-absorption, oblivious to others, in own world

___ Socially indiscriminate behavior (e.g., going with strangers or invading personal space such as touching or climbing on people), lack of stranger and separation anxiety

___ Social skills deficit

**Perseveration**

___ Narrow or unusual range of interests and play behaviors, obsessive preoccupations (e.g., videos, toys with wheels such as trains, or symbols such as letters or shapes), attachment to and holding particular objects

___ Stereotyped and repetitive play (e.g., spinning, flicking, throwing, lining up, sorting, opening and closing)

___ Upset with change, difficulty with transitions, idiosyncratic or ritualized patterns or routines, desire to maintain sameness and order, things must be a certain way or done a particular way

___ Stereotypies (e.g., repetitive or self-stimulating movements or vocalizations such as rocking, head shaking, body tensing, toe walking, teeth grinding or clenching, hand or finger movements, facial grimacing, repetitive running, twirling, hand flapping or jumping when excited, pacing, playing with saliva, picking at skin, hyperventilating)

**Somatosensory disturbance**

___ Love of movement, frolic play, tickling, climbing, rocking, swinging

___ Unresponsive at times to verbal input (e.g., not reacting when name called, hearing may be questioned even though normal)

___ Hypersensitivity to some sounds (e.g., distress or covering ears in response to loud noise, sounds made by appliances or motors, or certain songs, commercials, or voices)

___ Distress with commotion, crowds

___ Fascination with specific visual stimuli such as spinning or rhythmic movements, details, fingers, lights, shiny surfaces, linear patterns (e.g., credits on TV, fans, "Wheel of Fortune")

___ Abnormal sensory inspection (e.g., mouthing, smelling, scratching, rubbing, visually scrutinizing objects or fingers close to eyes, placing ears against things that vibrate or hum, pressing objects against face)

___ Tactile defensiveness (e.g., dislike being touched, touching certain things, wearing clothes, having face washed, teeth brushed, hair combed)

___ High tolerance for pain (e.g., not crying when hurt)

___ Sleep disturbance (e.g., difficulty falling asleep, awaking early or during the night)

___ Feeding disorder (e.g., limited food preferences, hypersensitivity to textures, retaining food in mouth, inconsistency in eating over time, pica)

## Atypical developmental pattern

___ Possible developmental regression or slowing at approximately 1–2 years of age (e.g., loss of words)

___ Nonverbal skills higher than language, especially during the preschool years

___ Expressive language disorder: (1) no speech or absence of communicative speech with nonverbal communication at a higher level than verbal (e.g., pulling others by the hand and leading to what wants) or (2) limited reciprocal conversational speech (vs. communication in stress- and need-related situations, self-directed verbalizations, or speaking on topics of interest to self)

___ Atypical vocalizations such as unusual voice quality or modulation, screeching, odd noises, repetitive vocalizations, echolalia, idiosyncratic jargon or speech, perseverative speech, sporadic speech (e.g., uttering a word or phrase once and rarely or never saying it again), rote phrases out of context (from the past or videos), nonsensical speech, pronoun substitutions

___ Splinter skills: specific abilities significantly above the child's mental age that often involve (1) rote memory (e.g., identification of numbers, letters, shapes, logos, and colors; singing or humming tunes; memorizing car routes; counting; saying the alphabet; reading; spelling; reciting segments from videos or books), (2) visual, manipulative, or mechanical skills (e.g., completing puzzles, matching shapes, using a computer or VCR), or (3) gross motor skills

## Mood disturbance

___ Overreactivity, irritability, agitation, tantrums, aggression, self-injurious behavior (e.g., distressed by input or occurrences most children can tolerate, such as intrusions, activity interruptions, proximity, confinement, performance demands)

___ Emotional lability, with mood changes sometimes internally triggered (e.g., laughing or becoming upset for no apparent reason)

___ Flat affect, unresponsive in some situations

___ Unusual fears (e.g., elevators, steps, toilets)

## Problems with attention and safety

___ Selective attention, situational overactivity (e.g., hyperfocused on activities, objects, or topics of interest to self and inattentive at other times)

___ Recklessness, limited safety awareness, oblivious to danger (e.g., climbing on things that are unstable or unsafe, wandering about house at night, running off by self, going into traffic or water, pulling objects over on self such as lamp, TV, or kettle)

## ACKNOWLEDGMENTS

We wish to thank the Wells Foundation; Oxford Foundation; Children, Youth, and Family Consortium; and Children's Miracle Network for their generous support of this research.

## REFERENCES

Asperger, H. (1991). Autistic psychopathology in childhood. In U. Frith (Ed.), *Autism and Asperger syndrome* (pp. 37–92). Cambridge, UK: Cambridge University Press. (Original work published in German 1944)

Attwood, T. (1998). *Asperger's syndrome: A guide for parents and professionals.* Philadelphia: Kingsley.

Baird, G., Baron-Cohen, S., Bohman, M., Coleman, M., Frith, U., Gillberg, C., Gillberg, C., Howlin, P., Mesibov, G., Peeters, T., Ritvo, E., Steffenburg, S., Taylor, D., Waterhouse, L., Wing, L., & Zapella, M. (1991). Autism is not necessarily a pervasive developmental disorder. *Developmental Medicine and Child Neurology, 33,* 362–364.

Bartak, L., & Rutter, M. (1976). Differences between mentally retarded and normally intelligent autistic children. *Journal of Autism and Childhood Schizophrenia, 6,* 109–120.

Birnbrauer, J. S., & Leach, D. J. (1993). The Murdoch Early Intervention Program after two years. *Behavior Change, 10,* 63–74.

Church, C. C., & Coplan, J. (1995). The high-functioning autistic experience: Birth to preteen years. *Journal of Pediatric Health Care, 9,* 22–29.

Eaves, L. C., Ho, H. H., & Eaves, D. M. (1994). Subtypes of autism by cluster analysis. *Journal of Autism and Developmental Disorders, 24,* 3–22.

Eisenmajer, R., Prior, M., Leekam, S., Wing, L., Gould, J., Welham, M., & Ong, B. (1996). Comparison of clinical symptoms in autism and Asperger's disorder. *Journal of the American Academy of Child and Adolescent Psychiatry, 35,* 1523–1531.

Eisenmajer, R., Prior, M., Leekam, S., Wing, L., Ong, B., Gould, J., & Welham, M. (1998). Delayed language onset as a predictor of clinical symptoms in pervasive developmental disorders. *Journal of Autism and Developmental Disorders, 28,* 527–533.

Fenske, E. C., Zalenski, S., Krantz, P. J., & McClannahan, L. E. (1985). Age at intervention and treatment outcome for autistic children in a comprehensive intervention program. *Analysis and Intervention in Developmental Disabilities, 5,* 49–58.

Frith, U. (1991). Asperger and his syndrome. In U. Frith (Ed.), *Autism and Asperger syndrome* (pp. 1–36). Cambridge, UK: Cambridge University Press.

Ghaziuddin, M., Leininger, L., & Tsai, L. (1995). Brief report: Thought disorder in Asperger syndrome: Comparison with high-functioning autism. *Journal of Autism and Developmental Disorders, 25,* 311–317.

Ghaziuddin, M., Tsai, L. Y., & Ghaziuddin, N. (1992a). Brief report: A comparison of the diagnostic criteria for Asperger syndrome. *Journal of Autism and Developmental Disorders, 22,* 643–649.

Ghaziuddin, M., Tsai, L. Y., & Ghaziuddin, N. (1992b). Brief report: A reappraisal of clumsiness as a diagnostic feature of Asperger syndrome. *Journal of Autism and Developmental Disorders, 22,* 651–656.

Ghaziuddin, M., Weidmer-Mikhail, E., & Ghaziuddin, N. (1998). Comorbidity of Asperger syndrome: A preliminary report. *Journal of Intellectual Disability Research, 42,* 279–283.

Gilchrist, A., Green, J., Cox, A., Burton, D., Rutter, M., & Le Couteur, A. (2001). Development and current functioning in adolescents with Asperger syndrome: A comparative study. *Journal of Child Psychology and Psychiatry, 42,* 227–240.

Gillberg, C. (1985). Asperger's syndrome and recurrent psychosis: A case study. *Journal of Autism and Developmental Disorders, 15,* 389–397.

Gillberg, C. (1989). Asperger syndrome in 23 Swedish children. *Developmental Medicine and Child Neurology, 31,* 520–531.

Gillberg, C. (1991a). Clinical and neurobiological aspects of Asperger syndrome in six family studies. In U. Frith (Ed.), *Autism and Asperger syndrome* (pp. 122–146). Cambridge, UK: Cambridge University Press.

Gillberg, C. (1991b). Debate and argument: Is autism a pervasive developmental disorder? *Journal of Child Psychology and Psychiatry, 32,* 1169–1170.

Gillberg, C., & Ehlers, S. (1998). High-functioning people with autism and Asperger syndrome: A literature review. In E. Schopler, G. B. Mesibov, & L. J. Kunce (Eds.), *Asperger syndrome or high-functioning autism?* (pp. 79–100). New York: Plenum Press.

Gillberg, C., & Gillberg C. (1989). Asperger syndrome—some epidemiological considerations: A research note. *Journal of Child Psychology and Psychiatry, 30,* 631–638.

Gillberg, C., Nordin, V., & Ehlers, S. (1996). Early detection of autism: Diagnostic instruments for clinicians. *European Child and Adolescent Psychiatry, 5,* 67–74.

Happé, E., & Frith, U. (1991). Is autism a pervasive developmental disorder? Debate and argument: How useful is the "PDD" label? *Journal of Child Psychology and Psychiatry, 32,* 1167–1168.

Harris, S. L., & Handleman, J. S. (2000). Age and IQ at intake as predictors of placement for young children with autism: A four- to six-year follow-up. *Journal of Autism and Developmental Disorders, 30,* 137–142.

Hooper, S. R., & Bundy, M. B. (1998). Learning characteristics of individuals with

Asperger syndrome. In E. Schopler, G. B. Mesibov, & L. J. Kunce (Eds.), *Asperger syndrome or high-functioning autism?* (pp. 317–342). New York: Plenum Press.

Kanner, L. (1943). Autistic disturbances of affective contact. *Nervous Child, 2,* 217–250.

Klin, A. (1994). Asperger syndrome. *Child and Adolescent Psychiatric Clinics of North America, 3,* 131–148.

Klin, A., & Volkmar, F. R. (1995). Autism and the pervasive developmental disorders. *Child and Adolescent Psychiatric Clinics of North America, 4,* 617–630.

Klin, A., Volkmar, F. R., Sparrow, S. S., Cicchetti, D. V., & Rourke, B. D. (1995). Validity and neuropsychological characterization of Asperger's syndrome: Convergence with nonverbal learning disabilities syndrome. *Journal of Child Psychology and Psychiatry, 36,* 1127–1140.

Kunce, L., & Mesibov, G. B. (1998). Educational approaches to high-functioning autism and Asperger syndrome. In E. Schopler, G. B. Mesibov, & L. J. Kunce (Eds.), *Asperger syndrome or high-functioning autism?* (pp. 227–261). New York: Plenum Press.

Lovaas, O. I. (1987). Behavioral treatment and normal educational and intellectual functioning in young autistic children. *Journal of Consulting and Clinical Psychology, 55,* 3–9.

Mahoney, W. J., Szatmari, P., MacLean, J. E., Bryson, S. E., Bartolucci, G., Walter, S. D., Jones, M. B., & Zwaigenbaum, L. (1998). Reliability and accuracy of differentiating pervasive developmental disorder subtypes. *Journal of the American Academy of Child and Adolescent Psychiatry, 37,* 278–285.

Manjiviona, J., & Prior, M. (1995). Comparison of Asperger syndrome and high-functioning autistic children on a test of motor impairment. *Journal of Autism and Developmental Disorders, 25,* 23–39.

Mayes, S. D., & Calhoun, S. L. (1999). Symptoms of autism in young children and correspondence with the DSM. *Infants and Young Children, 12,* 90–97.

Mayes, S. D., & Calhoun, S. L. (2001). Non-significance of early speech delay in children with autism and normal intelligence and implications for DSM-IV Asperger's disorder. *Autism, 5,* 81–94.

Mayes, S. D., & Calhoun, S. L. (2003a). Ability profiles in children with autism: Influence of age and IQ. *Autism, 6,* 65–80.

Mayes, S. D., & Calhoun, S. L. (2003b). Analysis of WISC-III, Stanford–Binet: IV, and academic achievement test scores in children with autism. *Journal of Autism and Developmental Disorders, 33,* 329–341.

Mayes, S. D., & Calhoun, S. L. (in press). Influence of IQ and age in childhood autism: Lack of support for Asperger's disorder. *Journal of Developmental and Physical Disabilities.*

Mayes, S. D., Calhoun, S. L., & Crites, D. L. (2001). Does DSM-IV Asperger's disorder exist? *Journal of Abnormal Child Psychology, 29,* 263–271.

McEachin, J. J., Smith, T., & Lovaas, O. I. (1993). Long-term outcome for children with autism who received early intensive behavioral treatment. *American Journal on Mental Retardation, 97,* 359–372.

Miller, J. N., & Ozonoff, S. (1997). Did Asperger's cases have Asperger disorder? A research note. *Journal of Child Psychology and Psychiatry, 38,* 247–251.

Miller, J. N., & Ozonoff, S. (2000). The external validity of Asperger disorder: Lack of evidence from the domain of neuropsychology. *Journal of Abnormal Psychology, 109,* 227–238.

Myhr, G. (1998). Autism and other pervasive developmental disorders: Exploring the dimensional view. *Canadian Journal of Psychiatry, 43,* 589–595.

Ozonoff, S., & Cathcart, K. (1998). Effectiveness of a home program intervention for young children with autism. *Journal of Autism and Developmental Disorders, 28,* 25–32.

Ozonoff, S., Rogers, S. J., & Pennington, B. F. (1991). Asperger's syndrome: Evidence of an empirical distinction from high-functioning autism. *Journal of Child Psychology and Psychiatry, 32,* 1107–1122.

Ozonoff, S., South, M., & Miller, J. N. (2000). DSM-IV-defined Asperger syndrome: Cognitive, behavioral and early history differentiation from high-functioning autism. *Autism, 4,* 29–46.

Prior, M., Eisenmajer, R., Leekam, S., Wing, L., Gould, J., Ong, B., & Dowe, D. (1998). Are there subgroups within the autistic spectrum?: A cluster analysis of a group of children with autistic spectrum disorders. *Journal of Child Psychology and Psychiatry, 39,* 893–902.

Rutter, M., & Schopler, E. (1987). Autism and pervasive developmental disorders: Concepts and diagnostic issues. *Journal of Autism and Developmental Disorders, 17,* 159–186.

Schopler, E. (1985). Convergence of learning disability, higher-level autism, and Asperger's syndrome. *Journal of Autism and Developmental Disorders, 15,* 359–360.

Schopler, E. (1996). Are autism and Asperger syndrome (AS) different labels or different disabilities? *Journal of Autism and Developmental Disorders, 26,* 109–110.

Schopler, E. (1998). Premature popularization of Asperger syndrome. In E. Schopler, G. B. Mesibov, & L. J. Kunce (Eds.), *Asperger syndrome or high-functioning autism?* (pp. 385–399). New York: Plenum Press.

Sevin, J. A., Matson, J. L., Coe, D., Love, S. R., Matese, M. J., & Benavidez, D. A. (1995). Empirically derived subtypes of pervasive developmental disorders: A cluster analytic study. *Journal of Autism and Developmental Disorders, 25,* 561–578.

Sheinkopf, S. J., & Siegel, B. (1998). Home-based behavioral treatment of young children with autism. *Journal of Autism and Developmental Disorders, 28,* 15–23.

Siegel, B. (1996). *The world of the autistic child: Understanding and treating autistic spectrum disorders.* New York: Oxford University Press.

Smith, T., Groen, A. D., & Wynn, J. S. (2000). Randomized trial of intensive early intervention for children with pervasive developmental disorders. *American Journal on Mental Retardation, 105,* 269–285.

Stone, W. L., Lee, E. B., Ashford, L., Brissie, J., Hepburn, S. L., Coonrod, E. E., & Weiss, B. H. (1999). Can autism be diagnosed accurately in children under 3 years? *Journal of Child Psychology and Psychiatry, 40,* 219–226.

Szatmari, P. (1991). Asperger's syndrome: Diagnosis, treatment, and outcome. *Psychiatric Clinics of North America, 14,* 81–93.

Szatmari, P. (1998). Differential diagnosis of Asperger disorder. In E. Schopler, G. B. Mesibov, & L. J. Kunce (Eds.), *Asperger syndrome or high-functioning autism?* (pp. 61–76). New York: Plenum Press.

Szatmari, P. (2000). The classification of autism, Asperger's syndrome, and pervasive developmental disorder. *Canadian Journal of Psychiatry, 45,* 731–738.

Szatmari, P., Archer, L., Fisman, S., Streiner, D. L., & Wilson, F. (1995). Asperger's syndrome and autism: Differences in behavior, cognition, and adaptive functioning. *Journal of the American Academy of Child and Adolescent Psychiatry, 34,* 1662–1671.

Szatmari, P., Bartolucci, G., & Bremner, R. (1989). Asperger's syndrome and autism: Comparison of early history and outcome. *Developmental Medicine and Child Neurology, 31,* 709–720.

Szatmari, P., Tuff, L., Finlayson, M. A. J., & Bartolucci, G. (1990). Asperger's syndrome and autism: Neurocognitive aspects. *Journal of the American Academy of Child and Adolescent Psychiatry, 29,* 130–136.

Tantam, D. (1988). Asperger's syndrome. *Journal of Child Psychology and Psychiatry, 29,* 245–255.

Tsai, L. Y. (1992). Diagnostic issues in high-functioning autism. In E. Schopler, G. B. Mesibov, & L. J. Kunce (Eds.), *Asperger syndrome or high-functioning autism?* (pp. 11–40). New York: Plenum Press.

Twachtman-Cullen, D. (1998). Language and communication in high-functioning autism and Asperger syndrome. In E. Schopler, G. B. Mesibov, & L. J. Kunce (Eds.), *Asperger syndrome or high-functioning autism?* (pp. 199–225). New York: Plenum Press.

Volkmar, F. R., Cicchetti, D. V., Cohen, D. J., & Bregman, J. (1992). Brief report: Developmental aspects of DSM-III-R criteria for autism. *Journal of Autism and Developmental Disorders, 22,* 657–662.

Volkmar, F. R., & Klin, A. (1998). Asperger syndrome and nonverbal learning disabilities. In E. Schopler, G. B. Mesibov, & L. J. Kunce (Eds.), *Asperger's syndrome or high-functioning autism?* (pp. 107–121). New York: Plenum Press.

Volkmar, F. R., Klin, A., Siegel, B., Szatmari, P., Lord, C., Campbell, M., Freeman, B. J., Cicchetti, D. V., Rutter, M., Kline, W., Buitelaar, J., Hattab, Y., Fombonne, E., Fuentes, J., Werry, J., Stone, W., Kerbeshian, J., Hoshino, Y., Bregman, J., Loveland, K., Szymanski, L., & Towbin, K. (1994). Field trial for autistic disorder in DSM-IV. *American Journal of Psychiatry, 151,* 1361–1367.

Waterhouse, L., Morris, R., Allen, D., Dunn, M., Fein, D., Feinstein, C., Rapin, I., & Wing, L. (1996). Diagnosis and classification in autism. *Journal of Autism and Developmental Disorders, 26,* 59–86.

Wing, L. (1976). Diagnosis, clinical description and prognosis. In L. Wing (Ed.), *Early childhood autism: Clinical, educational and social aspects* (2nd ed., pp. 15–64). Oxford, UK: Pergamon.

Wing, L. (1981). Asperger's syndrome: A clinical account. *Psychological Medicine, 11,* 115–129.

Wing, L. (1991). The relationship between Asperger's syndrome and Kanner's autism. In U. Frith (Ed.), *Autism and Asperger syndrome* (pp. 93–121). Cambridge, UK: Cambridge University Press.

Wing, L. (1998). The history of Asperger syndrome. In E. Schopler, G. B. Mesibov,

& L. J. Kunce (Eds.), *Asperger syndrome or high-functioning autism?* (pp. 11–28). New York: Plenum Press.

Wing, L., & Gould, J. (1979). Severe impairments of social interaction and associated abnormalities in children: Epidemiology and classification. *Journal of Autism and Developmental Disorders, 9,* 11–29.

Young, R., & Brewer, N. (2002). Diagnosis of autistic disorder: Problems and new directions. *International Review of Research in Mental Retardation, 25,* 107–134.

# 2

# Cognitive and Academic Problems

JO-ANN REITZEL
PETER SZATMARI

Learning is an incredibly complex task and can be particularly challenging for children with special needs. In the classroom, the demands of the curriculum, the limitations of the physical setting and the materials, and the expectations of dedicated teachers can all have an influence on how children with special needs learn. Classroom learning is also nested within an educational system and society at large. Both convey enormous expectations for academic achievement. As a result, children with Asperger syndrome (AS) often experience considerable stress in the classroom. Although all children bring their own individual strengths and weaknesses to learning opportunities, those with AS may bring unique challenges as well. What do we know about the learning characteristics of children with AS? Are there specific learning patterns among children with AS? Are there peaks and valleys in their learning profiles? Does the learning profile change with age? Do children with AS also have specific learning disabilities? These questions are crucial in understanding how children with this type of autism spectrum disorder (ASD) cope with the demands of the classroom, a place where they spend so much of their time.

Although there has been much interest in investigating if and how AS differs from autism on a variety of cognitive, linguistic, social–cognitive, and neuropsychological measures, only a few studies have been conducted on the learning characteristics of this type of ASD. In this chapter, we examine three sources of what is known. The assessment process used in clinical practice provides a methodology that assists us in identifying cognitive and academic strengths and weaknesses. First we synthesize data from other fields to suggest a battery of useful tests to assess learning in children with AS. Next a systematic review of the literature summarizes the empirical findings, to date, on the learning characteristics of children with AS. Finally, we present data from an ongoing follow-up study we have been conducting for several years, on the learning characteristics of persons with AS at different ages.

## THE METHODOLOGY FOR ASSESSMENT OF LEARNING CHARACTERISTICS IN CHILDREN

### Psychological Assessment and Testing

Many of the learning problems seen in AS are not unique. Children with other disabilities or disorders (such as attention-deficit/hyperactivity disorder, nonverbal learning disabilities, etc.) can exhibit similar learning difficulties. Academic achievement and maintaining passing grades in certain subjects may be problematic for any child with special needs. For instance, math may be harder than reading for some children, or vice versa. Social learning situations with other adults and peers also may be difficult. But the underlying reasons for difficulties in learning may be varied and the assessment of learning progress requires a comprehensive perspective. Visual and movement distractions as well as noise can make attending and focusing difficult. A quiet and somewhat isolated work space may be helpful for some children in getting tasks completed, but this isolation may occur at the expense of opportunities to learn in the integrated class setting with typical peers. Organization and self-monitoring skills may be weak; however, some independence is required in the organization of space, materials, and belongings during the early primary grades. Less structured times, such as free play, recess, and group activities, may not provide optimal consistency and predictability. When a child with AS and weak learning skills is placed in a demanding learning situation, problem-solving and coping skills may be lacking, and anxiety or frustration may become heightened; in turn, the stress may negatively affect the student's learning.

Children who are experiencing learning problems are assessed with psychological tests for clinical and diagnostic purposes (for a comprehensive review of child assessment, see Sattler, 2002a, 2002b). Assessment leads to recommendations for treatment and education. There is an important distinction between psychological testing and psychological assessment. *Testing* refers to the administration of tests, and the resulting findings are limited in interpretation to the scope of the test. Testing is one component of a comprehensive psychological assessment that also takes contextual factors into account. The assessment also includes gathering history and information from interviews with relevant persons involved in the child's life, observing the child in a variety of learning situations, and administering questionnaires relevant to the child's age, stage of development, and context. Ideally, assessment results are interpreted in a manner that is meaningful to the child's predicament.

After relevant background information is gathered, a battery of tests is administered to assist in answering a referral question. Although the battery of tests may vary and the results may be analyzed differently, depending on the purpose of the assessment, the procedures for administration of the test remain standard. The test battery typically includes measures of cognitive functioning, academic skills, and behavioral functioning, whose purpose is to identify the nature and severity of the learning problem and to assist in developing an educational program (Sattler, 2002a, 2002b). Since these tests often do not reveal *why* children with AS do poorly in school, other tests of more basic skills, such as those that measure complex problem solving and executive functioning (see below), may need to be administered.

Intellectual functioning is assessed by a comprehensive measure of both verbal and nonverbal abilities. Tests commonly used are the Wechsler Intelligence Scale for Children—Third Edition (WISC-III; Wechsler, 1991) or the Stanford–Binet Intelligence Scale—Fourth Edition (Thorndike, Hagen, & Sattler, 1986). Test results are analyzed using standardized procedures and statistical comparisons. Cognitive tests are analyzed to determine the overall level of intellectual functioning from the Full Scale score, as well as any significant discrepancies between Verbal and Performance (nonverbal) scale scores. These scores are compared to norms for defined age ranges. The Wechsler scales of intelligence are also analyzed in terms of factor scores for Verbal Comprehension and Freedom from Distractibility on the Verbal scale as well as Perceptual Organization and Processing Speed on the Performance scale (Kaufman, 1994). Significant strengths and weaknesses within each of the verbal and performance domains are also determined. At another level, individual subtest scores from the Verbal or Performance domains can be compared to an average of the subscale scores in each domain, to determine if there is variability in the skills within that domain.

Intellectual assessments may be supplemented by the administration of tests specially designed to assess visual and nonverbal problem solving (Sattler, 2002b). These tests provide particularly useful information when there is reason to believe that the child's Full Scale score on a comprehensive test may not be the best estimate of cognitive functioning. Additional tests are often administered to measure more specific skills that may be important in the cognitive profile, such as fine and gross motor skills, paper-and-pencil copying tests of visual–motor integration, verbal learning, receptive vocabulary, expressive vocabulary, executive functioning, and memory abilities. These additional analyses allow for a more comprehensive description of cognitive strengths and weaknesses, which then assist in providing a more accurate overview of the child's learning style, information-processing skills, long-term retention capacity, and short-term memory and working memory capacities.

Academic tests of reading comprehension and word recognition, spelling and story writing, as well as arithmetic calculations and problem solving are typically administered in a comprehensive assessment. Common tests include the Wechsler Individual Achievement Test (Psychological Corporation, 1992), Wide Range Achievement Test—Revision 3 (Wilkinson, 1993), and Woodcock Reading Mastery Tests—Revised (Woodcock, 1987). The scores of academic tests are compared to norms for specified age levels. To determine if there are areas of significant academic strengths or weaknesses, the scores of each academic test are compared to the best estimate of the child's cognitive functioning, as determined by the intellectual assessment results. The most reliable estimate of cognitive functioning may be the Full Scale score or, if there is a significant discrepancy between the Verbal and Performance scores, the higher score may be the best estimate of cognitive functioning (Kaufman, 1994), however, the interpretation of the significant Verbal–Performance discrepancy needs to take many other factors into consideration.

Assessment of adaptive and maladaptive behavioral characteristics is obtained by gathering information from self-reports and from informed persons such as teachers and parents. This information comprises an important part of the learning profile needed to describe the associated social, emotional, and behavioral characteristics of the child being assessed. Measures of day-to-day communication, socialization, self-care and motor skills, as well as maladaptive behaviors are typically obtained. Common scales include the Vineland Adaptive Behavior Scales (Sparrow, Balla, & Cicchetti, 1984), the Child Behavior Checklist (Achenbach & Edelbrock, 1986a), and the Teacher Report Form (Achenbach & Edelbrock, 1986b). Scores are compared to norms; for the Vineland Adaptive Behavior Scales—Survey Edition, supplementary norms for special populations have been gathered, allowing the opportunity to compare scores to others with the same disorder (Volkmar et al., 1987). Areas of statistically significant strengths and weaknesses are determined by comparisons of scores with these norms.

## The Diagnosis of Learning Disabilities

Another step in the assessment process may be to identify whether a child meets criteria for other diagnoses, such as those for a learning disability. The definition of learning disabilities has developed since the 1960s (Wong, 1996). A definition, written in 1988 by a National Joint Committee on Learning Disabilities, has been fairly well accepted, and there is agreement on the four main features of the definition:

1. The person shows "significant difficulties in the acquisition and use of listening, speaking, reading, writing, reasoning or mathematical abilities" (Hammill, 1993, p. 4).
2. The primary characteristics of the learning disability are considered to be CNS (central nervous system) processing problems; however, the psychological processes have not been identified, due to a paucity of definitive psychological processing tests.
3. Sensory, environmental, emotional, developmental, or cultural conditions are ruled out as the primary cause of the learning disability.
4. Secondary characteristics, such as motor impairments, are associated features, but these are not the reason(s) for the significant learning weaknesses.

Learning disabilities (LD) are also included in the DSM-IV (American Psychiatric Association, 1994). They are diagnosed as disorders of reading, written expression, and mathematics. Key features of these diagnoses are related to the definition. A "substantial" discrepancy is required between the child's assessed level of intellectual functioning on a standardized measure of intelligence and his or her academic functioning on standardized tests of reading, written language, and arithmetic. Sensory problems cannot account for the learning difficulties, and the discrepancy between the person's potential to learn and his or her achievement must interfere significantly with academic achievement or activities of daily living. However, the actual criteria for determining a discrepancy are not clear (Stanovich, 1991), and several definitions are currently being used in different settings by different professions.

Research into subtypes of learning disabilities can be used to define more homogeneous groups of children with shared problems. This research also helps to better understand the nature of the relationship between academic and nonacademic features of the learning disability. One subtype is based on language-processing difficulties. There is convergent validity from over 20 years of studies indicating that children with limited phonological processing skills have difficulty learning to read (Stanovich, 1991; Wong, 1996). A lack of sensitivity to phonology (i.e., the sounds comprising words) makes it difficult for the child to learn the sound–symbol correspondences needed to decode reading. The phonological core-deficit model asserts that the phonological processing difficulties are associated with significant academic deficits in reading, spelling, writing, and arithmetic. This model does not suggest that all reading-disabled children would have this problem, only that phonological problems are one plausible explanation. A second learning disability subtype (Rourke & Tsatsanis, 2000) is based on nonverbal or visual–spatial processing difficulties. Rourke (1989) described a nonverbal learning disability (NLD) that was associated with difficulties in visual organization, tactile-perceptual, psychomotor, nonverbal problem solving, and concept formation abilities. These weaknesses, Rourke noted, contrasted with the cognitive strengths in language-based skills such as verbal rote learning, sound–symbol matching, and amount of verbal output. In addition, Rourke reported variability in academic achievement profiles, wherein reading/word recognition and spelling skills were strong, whereas arithmetic skills were significantly deficient. Finally, social judgment and interpersonal skills also were described as impaired.

## COGNITIVE PROFILES IN ASPERGER SYNDROME

A systematic search of the relevant literature was conducted, using the PubMed and PsycINFO databases. "Asperger syndrome" was a keyword used in each of the searches. The term was joined to each of the following keywords: "neuropsychological profiles," "cognitive profiles," and "learning profiles." The result of the search revealed eight studies that reported cognitive as well as academic, neuropsychological, or behavioral tests.

A few factors complicate the interpretation of these studies. First, some of these studies were conducted prior to the establishment of the diagnostic criteria in the DSM-IV for AS in 1994. This fact makes comparisons between studies difficult. Second, it is important to note that although these studies collected cognitive, language, academic, or behavioral data for children with AS, their purpose, most often, was to determine whether AS could be distinguished from high-functioning autism (HFA), based on data that were independent of the diagnostic criteria. The research was not aimed at studying the specific learning characteristics of children with AS, using a broad range of academic measures. The studies included in this review are summarized in Table 2.1, and the main findings are discussed below.

The study by Szatmari, Tuff, Finlayson, and Bartolucci (1990) was designed to answer two questions: (1) whether the neuropsychological profiles of children with AS were similar to those of children with HFA, and

(2) whether the primary cognitive deficit in AS was language-related or in abstract problem solving. Wechsler intelligence tests, the Wide Range Achievement Test (WRAT), and motor speed tests were administered to participants with AS, HFA, and matched controls with other psychiatric conditions (OPC). The cognitive profiles analysis revealed that the Verbal IQ and Performance IQ scores of both the AS and HFA groups were in the low-average range and were significantly lower than OPC group scores. When subtests were analyzed, it was found that the AS group scored significantly higher than the HFA group on the Similarities subtest of the Wechsler scales, and the HFA group scored significantly higher than the AS group on a test of motor speed. Academic achievement was also assessed: (1) There were no differences between the three groups on the WRAT reading and arithmetic tests; (2) there was no evidence of a learning difficulty in terms of significantly weak scores in reading, spelling, or arithmetic on the WRAT subtests in comparison to the Full Scale IQ scores. In fact, the AS and HFA groups scored approximately 10 points higher on the reading and arithmetic tests in comparison to their Full Scale IQ.

The study by Ozonoff, Rogers, and Pennington (1991) was designed to investigate possible differences in neuropsychological profiles of persons with AS and HFA. Wechsler intelligence tests revealed that although the Full Scale IQs were comparable for both groups, the AS group's Verbal IQ was in the average range of functioning and significantly higher than the HFA group's. The Verbal, Performance, and Full Scale IQs were all in the average range for the AS group, and there was no significant difference between Verbal and Performance IQs.

Klin, Volkmar, Sparrow, Cicchetti, and Rourke (1995) compared the neuropsychological profiles of AS and HFA participants. Clinical records of standardized tests were reviewed for Verbal–Performance IQ differences and evidence of nonverbal learning disability (NLD). They found no significant differences between the HFA and AS Full Scale IQs, which were in the average range. However, Klin, Volkmar, Sparrow, Cicchetti, and Rourke (1995) found a significant difference between the average range Verbal IQs and the low-average range Performance IQs for the AS group. Furthermore, the NLD profile of assets and deficits was found in the AS, but not the HFA, group. The NLD profile of cognitive assets and deficits correctly identified 18 of 21 of the AS participants. The profile of assets and deficits included gross and fine motor skills, visual–motor integration, visual–spatial perception, visual memory, and weaknesses in nonverbal concept formation. Klin and colleagues concluded that, from a "clinical" viewpoint, the AS and NLD groups were similar.

Szatmari, Archer, Fisman, Streiner, and Wilson (1995) completed a study designed to examine pervasive developmental disorder (PDD) subtype vari-

**TABLE 2.1. Review of Studies**

| Authors | AS diagnoses | AS sample size | AS age (yr) | Group cognitive results | | |
| --- | --- | --- | --- | --- | --- | --- |
| | | | | Overall test scores | Factor scores | Subtest scores |
| Szatmari et al. (1990) | Modified DSM-III-R | n = 25 | Mean CA = 14 Range 8–18 | FSIQ = VIQ = PIQ = low-average range | None reported | AS > HFA on Similarities |
| Ozonoff et al. (1991) | Modified ICD-10 language criteria | n = 10 | Mean CA = 12.38 Range 8–20 | FSIQ = VIQ = PIQ = average range | N/A | N/A |
| Klin et al. (1995) | ICD-10 and DSM-IV field trial criteria and motor clumsiness | n = 21 | CA = 16.11 SD = 8.27 | FSIQ = average Average range VIQ > low-average range PIQ (from record review) | N/A | N/A |
| Szatmari et al. (1995) | ICD-10 and DSM-IV | n = 21 | CA (mo) = 68.6 SD (mo) = 9.1 | Nonverbal IQ (Leiter) = average | N/A | N/A |
| Ehlers et al. (1997) | Gillberg et al. (1989) criteria and motor clumsiness | n = 40 | CA = 9.9 SD = 2.9 | FSIQ = VIQ = average range PIQ = low-average range | Verbal Comprehension and Perceptual Organization = average range | Information, Similarities, Vocabulary, Comprehension = average range |

| Study | Criteria | n | Age | IQ profile | Freedom from Distractibility | Subtest pattern |
|---|---|---|---|---|---|---|
| Manjiviona & Prior (1999) | DSM-IV | n = 26 | CA = 10.4 Range 6–17 | FSIQ = VIQ = PIQ = average range (but considerable variability at the within-individual level) | Freedom from Distractibility = low-average range | Object Assembly, Arithmetic, Coding = low-average range; Block Design strength = high-average to average range; Digit Span and Coding weakness = low-average range |
| Gilchrist et al. (2001) | ICD-10 | n = 20 | CA = 13.75 Range 11–19 | FSIQ = VIQ = PIQ = average range; VIQ > PIQ for 50% of AS group and none had VIQ lower than PIQ | N/A | Block Design strength compared to Performance score; Comprehension weakness compared to Verbal score |
| Miller & Ozonoff (2000) | DSM-IV | n = 14 | CA = 10.14 SD = 1.93 | FSIQ = VIQ = high-average to superior range; PIQ = average range VIQ > PIQ for 57% but disappeared when IQ was controlled | N/A | None reported |

*Note.* AS, Asperger syndrome; HFA, high-functioning autism; CA, chronological age; FSIQ, Full Scale IQ; VIQ, Verbal IQ; PIQ, Performance IQ.

ables that were considered to be relatively independent of diagnostic criteria. (*Note*: this sample was different from the one used in the Szatmari et al., 1990, study.) Two groups of children were identified (HFA and AS), using inclusion criteria that were consistent with, but not identical to, the DSM-IV diagnostic criteria. Essentially, the two groups differed on whether there was a history of "delayed and deviant language development" in the group with HFA (Szatmari et al., 1995, p. 1662). Exclusionary criteria were established to select children with PDD who were above the IQ cutoff for mental retardation. Still, the AS group's score on the Leiter International Performance Scale (Levine, 1986) test (a nonverbal measure of cognitive functioning) was 99.3, which was somewhat higher than the HFA group's score of 86.6. Szatmari and colleagues found the two groups to be similar on some measures but different on others. The AS group scored significantly better than the HFA group on a composite of expressive and receptive language and communication tests, but there were no differences on motor skills and various nonverbal cognitive measures. It appeared that the AS group lacked the language impairment so commonly seen in autism.

The study by Ehlers and colleagues (1997) examined WISC subtest profiles for children with AS, HFA, and/or attention deficit. They hypothesized that AS shared executive functional deficits with the other disorders. Intragroup differences for the AS group revealed WISC scores in the average range for the children with AS. Verbal scale strengths were evident on tests of Information, Similarities, Comprehension, and Vocabulary. Performance scale weaknesses were found on tests of Object Assembly and Coding. Arithmetic was weaker than other Verbal subtests. In addition, the AS group scored higher than the autism group on verbal abilities, as measured by the Verbal IQ, on the Verbal Comprehension factor, and specifically on the Comprehension and Vocabulary subtests. The Performance IQ scores, as well as the Perceptual Organization and Freedom from Distractibility factor scores of both groups were comparable. From the grouped data, the researchers concluded that "only a minority (albeit a large one) of each diagnostic group showed the highly characteristic profile" (Ehlers et al., 1997, p. 215). AS was associated with better verbal abilities (with the exception of Arithmetic) and weak performance abilities, primarily due to weak Object Assembly skills.

Gilchrist and colleagues (2001) studied the cognitive and social functioning in adolescents with AS, HFA, and conduct disorder (CD), to determine whether the socialization impairments of AS were different from the social problems of children in these other groups. The Full Scale IQ was in the average range for the AS group, and the Performance IQ was > 70 for the HFA group. Fifty percent of the AS group had a significantly higher Verbal IQ than Performance IQ, and none had a significantly lower Verbal IQ than Performance IQ. A subtest analysis was done to determine the contribution of each subtest score to the scale scores. Both the AS and HFA groups were stronger than the CD group on Block Design, relative to their overall Performance scores. In the verbal domain, the AS and HFA groups were weaker than the CD group on the Comprehension test relative to the Verbal scale score.

Miller and Ozonoff (2000) also tried to distinguish DSM-IV-diagnosed AS from HFA using cognitive and neuropsychological data. The AS group showed significantly higher Full Scale IQ and Verbal IQ as well as significantly greater discrepancy in verbal performance scores in the cognitive profiles compared to the HFA group. However, when IQ was controlled, the group differences disappeared. There were no differences between the two groups on the measures of executive functioning and motor skills. The authors concluded that AS may be better characterized as a "high IQ" autism rather than a separate diagnosis.

The final study, by Manjiviona and Prior (1999), attempted to determine if neuropsychological information would be helpful in differentiating children with AS from those with HFA. They examined neuropsychological profiles of children clinically diagnosed with HFA and AS, according to DSM-IV and ICD-10 criteria—that is, with and without language delay. On average, the children were age 10 years, 8 months old. There were two main findings. First, the AS group had a significantly higher Full Scale IQ scores than the HFA group. Second, when comparing the neuropsychological profiles of the two groups for similarities and differences on the WISC-R, the authors found no significant difference between the groups on the Verbal IQ and Performance IQ scores; however, the standard deviations were large, which indicates a great deal of scatter in the Verbal and Performance domains for both groups. They also found no significant difference between the WISC-R Verbal Comprehension and Perceptual Organization factor scores; however, both groups were weakest on the Freedom from Distractibility factor, which measures attention, working memory, short-term recall, and mental arithmetic skills. Due to the high standard deviations in the between-group analysis, individual cognitive profiles were examined for the presence of a Verbal–Performance discrepancy, defined as a difference of 12 or more points. In the AS group three children had Verbal IQs > Performance IQs and five children had Performance IQs > Verbal IQs. In the HFA group three children had Verbal IQs > Performance IQs and four had Performance IQs > Verbal IQs. This comparison showed that there was no difference between the proportion of children from each group who had a significant Verbal–Performance discrepancy, and the authors suggested that this proportion may not be different from the incidence of this same discrepancy in the normal population. A subtest analysis revealed consistent patterns of cognitive skills in both groups, with relative strength in Block Design and weaknesses in Digit Span and Coding. They concluded that there was no evidence for differentiating between the two groups, based on the Verbal and Performance scores of the WISC-R—at least, for this clinically diagnosed sample.

## Summary of Literature Review

There are few studies on neurocognitive profiles in children with HFA and AS, and a specific focus on academic achievement is even more sparse. Two conclusions, however, can be made. First, neurocognitive profiles in both groups (i.e., AS and HFA) are very uneven. That is, these children have a number of specific deficits in information processing but also a number of age-appropriate skills. It is perhaps the unevenness of the cognitive profile that places academic achievement at risk. Although deficits are apparent, it is not clear whether there is a specific neurocognitive profile associated with AS that is different from that seen in HFA. Children with HFA have specific difficulties in verbal comprehension, or general understanding of both verbal and nonverbal concepts, and relative strengths in visual–motor and visual–spatial processing. Most studies agree that language skills in the AS group are in the average range (albeit low-average range, in some circumstances) and better than in the HFA group. Whether there are specific deficits in visual–spatial and visual–motor functioning is less clear. If anything, a pattern of higher Performance IQ than Verbal IQ is seen in children with autism, not AS, but the pattern is certainly not seen universally in the former group, by any means. We now turn to a more specific examination of academic achievement in these two ASD subtypes.

## ACADEMIC ACHIEVEMENT IN ASPERGER SYNDROME AND HIGH-FUNCTIONING AUTISM

In this section we present results from our own ongoing follow-up study of children with HFA and AS. The objective of this study was to conduct longitudinal assessments on measures of cognitive functioning, autistic symptoms, and adaptive behavior. Because there are no outcome data available on children with AS, this study was conducted to ascertain whether children with AS have a different outcome than those with autism. An "inception cohort" was assembled when the ASD children were 4–6 years of age; this term means that the sample was selected very close to the time of initial diagnoses. This temporal factor is an important prerequisite for follow-up studies, whereby those at very different stages of the disorder are not combined under a false assumption that they represent a homogeneous group. We also sampled the group in this manner to ensure that those with a very good outcome, or those with a very poor outcome, were not lost. The group was assembled from six different centers in Southern Ontario to ensure that those from both university and non-university-based settings were included. The facilities were all regional diagnostic centers involved in the assessment and treatment of very young children with an ASD. The children were then followed up when they were between 6 and 8 years of age (Szatmari et al., 2000), and a second time when they were between 9 and 13 years of age (Szatmari, Bryson, Boyle, Streiner, & Duku, 2003).

Full details of the sampling and diagnostic procedures are available in previous publications (Szatmari et al., 1995). In brief, all children were defined as high functioning if they had an IQ score above 70 on either the Leiter International Performance Scale (Levine, 1986) or the Stanford–Binet Intelligence Scale—Fourth Edition (Thorndike et al., 1986). The Autism Diagnostic Interview (ADI; Le Couteur et al., 1989; Lord, Rutter, & Le Couteur, 1994) was used to provide information on the differentiation of autism from AS. We did not rigidly follow the ADI algorithm rules, because these were not designed to distinguish autism from AS. To qualify as children with autism, examples of impairments in reciprocal social interaction, in verbal and nonverbal communication, and of repetitive stereotyped activities, behaviors, or interests were necessary. To qualify as children with AS, the same impairments were necessary, but these were differentiated from the autism criteria on the basis of two key absences: (1) no indications of a clinically significant language delay (operationally defined as the onset of spontaneous free speech with a verb prior to 36 months of age), and (2) an absence of persistent deviant language development (operationally defined as persistent delayed echolalia, pronoun reversal, and neologisms). These criteria follow those outlined in DSM-IV very closely, except that DSM-IV does not mention "deviant language development," and it also includes a hierarchy rule; that is, children who meet criteria for *both* autism and AS are given a diagnosis of autism. If we had simply applied the ADI algorithm to diagnose autism according to DSM-IV, most of the children with AS would have met the criteria. In order to secure a large enough sample of children with AS, and to reflect current clinical practice, we reversed the hierarchy rule so that if children met criteria for both disorders, they were preferentially given a diagnosis of AS. We, and now others, have found it very difficult to identify children as having AS when they also do not meet ADI criteria for autism (Leekam, Libby, Wing, Gould, & Gillberg, 2000; Miller & Ozonoff, 1997).

In order to focus on learning disabilities and academic achievement, we have restricted the analysis in this chapter to those who had Leiter IQ scores greater than 70 at both follow-up assessments. Some children with autism had IQs greater than 70 at inception, but their scores dip below 70 at the follow-up points, primarily because the demands of the test change over time and require more complex problem-solving abilities than developmentally earlier items of the test. There were 30 children with autism, 27 boys and three girls; their mean age at the first follow-up was 7 years, 6 months, and at the second follow-up, 12 years. There were 21 children with AS in the original cohort, but we added more (*n* = 6) at the second follow-up to increase sample size. There were 4 girls in the AS sample. This supplemental sample was identified using the same criteria as in the original sample. The mean age of the AS group was only 2 months older than the autism group. We selected measures of IQ, language abilities, reading and arithmetic abilities, and visual–motor and motor performance. Data are presented from both the 6- to 8-year assessments and the 9- to 13-year assessments.

## Results

Table 2.2 provides the results at the first follow-up assessment, when the children were between the ages of 6 and 8. There is no difference between the groups on nonverbal IQ (the Leiter scale) or on their Visual–Motor Integration (VMI; Beery, 1987); scores was virtually identical. Children with

**TABLE 2.2. Psychometric Profile at Time 1: Autism versus Asperger Syndrome**

| Measure | Autism | | Asperger | | |
| --- | --- | --- | --- | --- | --- |
| | Mean | SD | Mean | SD | p |
| Leiter IQ | 91.97 | 12.89 | 95.00 | 11.86 | .42 |
| TOLD Picture Vocabulary | 6.63 | 3.69 | 8.72 | 3.59 | .06 |
| TOLD Grammatical Understanding | 5.70 | 3.68 | 8.11 | 3.99 | .04* |
| TOLD Grammatical Comprehension | 4.47 | 2.18 | 6.61 | 3.66 | .02* |
| TOLD Word Articulation | 7.40 | 3.33 | 8.39 | 2.50 | .28 |
| McCarthy Oral Vocabulary Test | 4.68 | 4.87 | 11.44 | 5.34 | .00* |
| Visual–Motor Integration | 6.80 | 2.51 | 6.50 | 2.85 | .71 |
| Peabody Picture Vocabulary Test | 65.10 | 22.72 | 84.94 | 30.77 | .01* |
| WRAT-R2 Arithmetic | 77.66 | 21.12 | 79.89 | 24.15 | .73 |
| Test of Auditory Comprehension | 73.33 | 10.90 | 85.50 | 16.53 | .00* |
| Verbal Articulation | 83.14 | 31.63 | 92.72 | 27.30 | .29 |
| Woodcock–Letter Identification | 89.77 | 34.04 | 85.17 | 21.43 | .61 |
| Woodcock–Word Identification | 96.87 | 27.81 | 96.56 | 31.07 | .97 |
| Woodcock–Word Attack | 86.93 | 26.87 | 86.89 | 24.61 | .99 |
| Woodcock–Word Comprehension | 79.71 | 25.66 | 84.28 | 26.57 | .56 |
| Woodcock–Passage Comprehension | 73.75 | 29.94 | 80.17 | 30.66 | .48 |
| Woodcock–Readiness | 88.86 | 31.20 | 87.89 | 24.42 | .91 |
| Teacher Vineland–Communication | 77.28 | 14.64 | 87.39 | 15.12 | .03* |

*Note.* TOLD, Test of Language Development; WRAT, Wide Range Achievement Test.
*p < .05.

autism, however, had substantially lower scores on measures of language, including the McCarthy Oral Vocabulary Test (McCarthy, 1972), the Peabody Picture Vocabulary Test (PPVT; Dunn & Dunn, 1981), two subtests from the Test of Oral Language Development (TOLD; Newcomer & Hammill, 1988), and the Test of Auditory Comprehension (Carrow-Woolfolk, 1985). In contrast, there was no difference between the groups on measures of either academic achievement in Arithmetic (from the WRAT) or in reading achievement tests from the Woodcock. It is worth noting that the standard deviations on these reading tests are quite large, indicating that a large difference between the groups or a much larger sample size would be needed to find significant differences. Nevertheless, the mean scores indicate that, for many of the tests, there was little difference in academic achievement for the children in these two groups at this point in their development.

A somewhat different picture emerges when comparing the groups at the second follow-up assessment (Table 2.3) when the children were 9–13 years of age. There remain no differences between the groups on nonverbal IQ or VMI scores. Differences on their language skills remain such that those with AS have better language skills then those with autism. What has changed, however, are their differences on academic achievement. At this follow-up assessment, children with AS have significantly *better* scores on Arithmetic and on Passage Comprehension from the Woodcock. Sizable differences exist on Word Comprehension and Passage Comprehension. It is also interesting to note that the standard deviations have lessened consid-

**TABLE 2.3. Psychometric Profile at Time 2: Autism versus Asperger Syndrome**

| Measure | Autism | | Asperger | | |
|---|---|---|---|---|---|
| | Mean | SD | Mean | SD | p |
| Leiter IQ | 86.89 | 14.04 | 96.81 | 19.51 | .06 |
| TOLD Grammatical Understanding | 20.39 | 4:87 | 23.29 | 2:37 | .03* |
| TOLD Grammatical Comprehension | 18.00 | 9:44 | 25.29 | 6:56 | .01* |
| McCarthy Oral Vocabulary | 13.73 | 5:07 | 17.06 | 2:77 | .02* |
| Visual–Motor Integration | 7:39 | 3:70 | 8:56 | 3:44 | .31 |
| Peabody Picture Vocabulary Test | 71.79 | 24.04 | 94.41 | 24.81 | .00* |
| WRAT-R2 Arithmetic | 73.96 | 18.57 | 87.18 | 23.18 | .04* |
| Woodcock–Word Identification | 90.75 | 16.91 | 95.63 | 18.34 | .39 |
| Woodcock–Word Attack | 93.83 | 18.48 | 97.81 | 15.55 | .48 |
| Woodcock–Word Comprehension | 83.63 | 15.58 | 92.44 | 22.37 | .15 |
| Woodcock–Passage Comprehension | 79.91 | 15.26 | 92.94 | 21.18 | .03* |
| Teacher Vineland–Communication | 76.12 | 17.60 | 82.27 | 15.19 | .32 |

erably, suggesting that there is now more homogeneity in the scores as a group over time.

In order to understand how these differences have appeared over time, paired *t*-tests were conducted to compare scores obtained at the second follow-up to those obtained at the first follow-up in each of the groups. The children with autism showed a significant *decrease* in scores of nonverbal IQ (Leiter IQ; $t = 3.43$, $p = .001$), an *increase* in PPVT scores ($t = -2.65$, $p = .012$), but no substantial change on arithmetic and reading scores, except that the Word Identification scores went down (from 96.87 to 90.75; $t = 4.04$; $p < .001$). In the AS group, on the other hand, there were no changes in IQ or VMI scores, no changes in arithmetic, but significant *increases* on most reading tests (Word Attack, $t = -3.84$, $p = .001$; Word Comprehension, $t = -2.42$, $p = .03$; Passage Comprehension, $t = -.2.26$, $p = .04$). In other words, on their academic achievement, the groups have diverged over time, leading to clinically and statistically significant differences at the second follow-up assessment.

Finally, we calculated rates of "general" and "specific" learning disabilities at the 9- to 13-year follow-up in the two groups. A general LD was defined as a standard score below 80 on either the WRAT Arithmetic score or the reading composite score from the Woodcock. A specific LD was defined as a Leiter score above 80 and a 15-point discrepancy between IQ and academic achievement on the WRAT Arithmetic or Woodcock reading composite (roughly, a standard deviation difference). *General* LDs appeared to be more common in the HFA group: 73% of this group showed a general math LD, and 45%, a general reading LD, compared to 35% and 18% respectively in the AS group. On the other hand, *specific* LDs were more common in the AS group: 46% for math and 21% for reading, compared to 12% and 3%, respectively, in the HFA group.

## DISCUSSION

What can we conclude from these results and from the literature review carried out earlier? First, it is useful to point out that the mean academic achievement scores of the children with AS were all in the average range (i.e., they have scores within a standard deviation of the mean, ≥85). Almost half the AS group has a specific LD in math, and a fifth in reading. Thus LDs, as defined psychometrically, are not universally present in children with AS. This finding does *not* mean that these children were not having difficulties at school. In fact, the vast majority of children with AS were having difficulties in school and their performances were below that expected of their age-matched peers. However, the kinds of difficulties they were experiencing were not reflected in standardized academic achievement

scores. Both parents and teachers reported difficulties in academic performance related to inattention and lack of focus, an inability to complete
homework, and weak areas in problem solving, abstract conceptual learning, and generating creative solutions to complex problems. These kinds of
difficulties are not reflected in the simple tests of academic achievement but
are perhaps more reflective of the kinds of executive function deficits that
have been described in children with AS and autism (see Ozonoff et al.,
1991).

The second important implication of these results is that developmental
stages influence the similarities and differences found in children with HFA
and AS. If we had only reported data at the first follow-up assessment, no
significant differences in academic achievement would have been apparent. It
was only at the second follow-up assessment that those differences began to
emerge. Any study seeking to assess similarities and differences between
autism and AS needs to factor in developmental stage as a variable.

These data support our model of the relationship between autism and
AS (Szatmari, 2000). Previously we have argued that the relationship between these clinical conditions cannot be reduced simplistically to a number of "different" pervasive developmental disorders or a "single" underlying spectrum of autism disorders. Rather the ASDs need to be viewed in a
developmental context. We have proposed that, prior to 3 years of age,
ASD children are relatively undifferentiated; at least, they cannot be divided into different subtypes. With the onset of useful phrase speech, one
subgroup emerges on a particular developmental trajectory (i.e., the AS trajectory). Those who do not display phrase speech at that age are now on a
different developmental pathway (i.e., the HFA pathway) and obtain lower
scores on a number of neurocognitive tests in language. The relatively early
onset of language in those with AS opens up a number of new opportunities for them, so that over time, they are able to learn basic academic skills
and acquire better social and communication skills. However, it is also true
that some children with autism develop phrase speech and fluent language,
but they commonly do so after 3 years of age. Those that do so are able to
"jump" to the developmental trajectory of those with AS, so that the differences between them become smaller. Those who continue with significant
language delay stay on their initial developmental trajectory and fall further
and further behind their age cohort. This summary might suggest why the
variances in the two groups diminish over time and significant differences
emerge at the second follow-up assessment and not at the first. These PDD
subtypes become more and more differentiated and "canalized" with ongoing development.

It is also worth pointing out that these data do not support the idea
that children with AS have a specific cognitive deficit characterized by a
nonverbal learning disability or specific problems in motor coordination,

visual–spatial processing, and visual–motor skills. In fact, in our data (and in most others) they were equal to those with autism on visual–motor performance. Children with autism appeared to have a specific deficit in language comprehension. This observation provides a novel retort to the often-asked question, "Isn't Asperger syndrome really a form of high-functioning autism?" In fact, based on these data, we would argue that autism is *really* AS with a specific language impairment. AS can be thought of as the primary deficit. Autism occurs when a deficit in language development is superimposed on AS. Children with autism and AS share impairments in social reciprocity, in pragmatics of communication (in the widest sense), and show a preference for repetitive, stereotyped behaviors. The difference is that, in autism, there is an *additional handicap* of mental retardation or specific language impairment. We believe that this interpretation provides a better explanation for the results reported in the literature and in our own data than either the different disorder model or the spectrum model.

These results carry several clinical implications. First, academic difficulties are to be expected in the majority of children with AS. However, a reliance on simple tests of academic achievement and IQ generally will not reveal the specific nature of these difficulties. Instead more complex tests of problem solving and executive function need to be administered, and special attention given to the types of attentional difficulties experienced by children with AS. Second, remediation strategies should focus on these attentional difficulties. Unfortunately, there are no studies that support the use of specific teaching techniques that could deal with these problems. Clearly a great deal more research needs to be conducted in this area. A more precise description of the types of learning difficulties and impairments in academic achievement encountered by individuals with AS across the lifespan certainly needs to be constructed. In addition, rather than focusing exclusively on specific neurocognitive impairments, there needs to be a greater appreciation for the types of academic difficulties these children experience on a daily basis.

## REFERENCES

Achenbach, T. M., & Edelbrock, C. S. (1986a). *Child Behavior Checklist and Youth Self-Report*. Burlington, VT: Author.

Achenbach, T. M., & Edelbrock, C. S. (1986b). *Teacher Report Form*. Burlington, VT: Author.

American Psychiatric Association. (1994). *Diagnostic and statistical manual of mental disorders* (4th ed.). Washington, DC: Author.

Beery, K. E. (1987). *Developmental Test of Visual–Motor Integration*. Chicago: Follett.

Carrow-Woolfolk, E. (1985). *Test of Auditory Comprehension of Language.* Allen, TX: DLM Teaching Resources.

Dunn, L., & Dunn, L. (1981). *Peabody Picture Vocabulary Test—Revised Manual for Forms L and M.* Circles Pines, MN: American Guidance Service.

Ehlers, S., Nyden, A., Gillberg, C., Sandberg, A. D., Dahlgren, S. O., Hjelmquist, E., & Oden, A. (1997). Asperger syndrome, autism and attention disorders: A comparative study of the cognitive profiles of 120 children. *Journal of Child Psychology and Psychiatry 38,* 207–217.

Gilchrist, A., Green, J., Cox, A., Burton, D., Rutter, M., & Le Couteur, A. (2001). Development and current functioning in adolescents with Asperger syndrome: A comparative study. *Journal of Child Psychology and Psychiatry, 42,* 227–240.

Hammill, D. D. (1993). A timely definition of learning disabilities. *Family Community Health, 16,* 1–8.

Kaufman, A. S. (1994). *Intelligent testing with the WISC–III.* New York: Wiley.

Klin, A., Volkmar, F. R., Sparrow, S. S., Cicchetti, D. V., & Rourke, B. P. (1995). Validity and neuropsychological characterization of Asperger syndrome: Convergence with nonverbal learning disabilities syndrome. *Journal of Child Psychology and Psychiatry, 30,* 1127–1140.

Le Couteur, A., Rutter, M., Lord, C., Rios, P., Robertson, S., Holdgrafer, M., & McLennan, J. (1989). Autism diagnostic interview: A standardized investigator-based instrument. *Journal of Autism and Developmental Disorders, 19,* 363–387.

Leekam, S., Libby, S., Wing, L., Gould, J., & Gillberg, C. (2000). Comparison of ICD-10 and Gillberg's criteria for Asperger syndrome. *Autism, 4,* 11–28.

Levine, M. L. (1986). *The Leiter International Performance Scale: Handbook.* Los Angeles: Western Psychological Services.

Lord, C., Rutter, M., & Le Couteur, A. (1994). Autism Diagnostic Interview—Revised: A revised version of a diagnostic interview for caregivers of individuals with possible pervasive developmental disorders. *Journal of Autism and Developmental Disorders, 24,* 659–685.

Manjiviona, J., & Prior, M. (1999). Neuropsychological profiles of children with Asperger syndrome and autism. *Autism, 3,* 327–356.

McCarthy, D. (1972). *Manual for the McCarthy Scales of Children's Ability.* New York: Psychological Corporation.

Miller, J. N., & Ozonoff, S. (1997). Did Asperger's cases have Asperger disorder? A research note. *Child Psychology and Psychiatry, 38,* 257–251.

Miller, J. N., & Ozonoff, S. (2000). The external validity of Asperger syndrome: Lack of evidence from the domain of neuropsychology. *Journal of Abnormal Psychology, 109,* 227–238.

Newcomer, P. L., & Hammill, D. D. (1988). *Test of Language Development–2.* Toronto: Psycan.

Ozonoff, S., Rogers, S. J., & Pennington, B. F. (1991). Asperger's syndrome: Evidence of an empirical distinction from high-functioning autism. *Journal of Child Psychology and Psychiatry, 32,* 1107–1122.

Psychological Corporation. (1992). *Manual for the Wechsler Individual Achievement Test.* San Antonio, TX: Author.

Rourke, B. P. (1989). *Nonverbal learning disabilities: The syndrome and the model.* New York: Guilford Press.

Rourke, B. P., & Tsatsanis, K. D. (2000). Nonverbal learning disabilities and Asperger syndrome. In A. Klin, F. R. Volkmar, & S. S. Sparrow (Eds.), *Asperger syndrome* (pp. 231–253). New York: Guilford Press.

Sattler, J. M. (2002a). *Assessment of children: Behavioral and clinical applications* (4th ed.). La Mesa, CA: Author.

Sattler, J. M. (2002b). *Assessment of children: Cognitive applications* (4th ed.). La Mesa, CA: Author.

Sparrow, S. S., Balla, D. A., & Cicchetti, D. V. (1984). *Vineland Adaptive Behavior Scales.* Circle Pines, MN: American Guidance Service.

Stanovich, K. E. (1991). Discrepancy definitions of reading disability: Has intelligence led us astray? *Reading Research Quarterly, 26,* 7–29.

Szatmari, P. (2000). The classification of autism, Asperger's syndrome, and pervasive developmental disorder. *Canadian Journal of Psychiatry, 45,* 731–738.

Szatmari, P., Archer, L., Fisman, S., Streiner, D. L., & Wilson, F. (1995). Asperger's syndrome and autism: Differences in behavior, cognition, and adaptive functioning. *Journal of the American Academy of Child and Adolescent Psychiatry, 34,* 1662–1671.

Szatmari, P., Bryson, S. E., Boyle, M. H., Streiner, D. L., & Duku, E. (2003). Predictors of outcome among high functioning children with autism and Asperger syndrome. *Journal of Child Psychology and Psychiatry, 44*(1), 1–9.

Szatmari, P., Bryson, S. E., Streiner, D. L., Wilson, F., Archer, L., & Ryerse, C. (2000). Two-year outcome of preschool children with autism or Asperger syndrome. *American Journal of Psychiatry, 157,* 1980–1987.

Szatmari, P., Tuff, L., Finlayson, M. A. J., & Bartolucci, G. B. (1990). Asperger's syndrome and autism: Neurocognitive aspects. *Journal of the American Academy of Child and Adolescent Psychiatry, 29,* 130–136.

Thorndike, R. L., Hagen, E. P., & Sattler, J. M. (1986). *Guide for administering and scoring the Stanford–Binet Intelligence Scale: Fourth Edition.* Chicago: Riverside.

Volkmar, F. R., Sparrow, S. S., Goudreau, D., Cicchetti, D., Paul, R., & Cohen, D. J. (1987). Social deficits in autism: An operational approach using the Vineland Adaptive Behavior Scales. *Journal of American Academy of Child Psychiatry, 26,* 156–161.

Wechsler, D. (1991). *Manual for the Wechsler Intelligence Scale for Children— Third Edition.* San Antonio, TX: Psychological Corporation.

Wilkinson, G. S. (1993). *Wide Range Achievement Test 3.* Lutz, FL: Psychological Assessment Resources.

Wong, B. Y. L. (1996). *The ABC's of learning disabilities.* San Diego, CA: Academic Press.

Woodcock, R. W. (1987). *Woodcock Reading Mastery Tests—Revised.* Circle Pines, MN: American Guidance Services.

# 3

# Assessment of Specific
# Learning Difficulties

## JANINE MANJIVIONA

The recognition and treatment of comorbid problems in children[1] with Asperger syndrome (AS) is now relatively common. Progress in this area has undoubtedly been slow, due in part to the complexities involved in the diagnosis of AS, such as the lack of uniformity among professionals in how the diagnosis is made. However, families and professionals are becoming increasingly aware of other problematic conditions, such as anxiety, attention deficits or attention-deficit/hyperactivity disorder, depression, and behavioral problems, and appropriate treatments (e.g., behavioral interventions and educational supports) continue to emerge that improve the quality of life of the children and families concerned.

It is well known that the environment in which children with AS are most likely to feel stressed and anxious is the school milieu, where they encounter a multitude of social, cognitive, and behavioral demands that may be exceedingly taxing for some students. Children with AS are expected to conform to social codes of behavior in areas that are fundamentally difficult for them, such as using and interpreting conventional social language (both verbal and nonverbal cues) in the classroom and playground, and appropriately interacting with teachers and peers. There is the erroneous expectation that, like most children, these children will intuitively know and

---

[1]In this chapter, the term "children" is used to avoid repeating "children and adolescents," but much of the text relates to school-age children *and* adolescents.

understand the "rules" of social interaction—which are largely unwritten, subtle, and constantly changing. In addition to their difficulties in coping with the complexity of the social demands that school entails, a significant source of these children's distress often comes from the academic curriculum, which is usually oriented toward the "typical" student.

## SPECIAL PROBLEMS RELATED TO ASPERGER SYNDROME

The presence of "specific learning difficulties" in children with AS is an area that has not received much attention, although some empirical data are now available (Klin, Sparrow, Marans, Carter, & Volkmar, 2000; Mayes & Calhoun, Chapter 1, this volume) that attest to this frequently occurring phenomenon. Despite their cognitive strengths, the presence of learning difficulties in children with AS, including information-processing difficulties and specific weaknesses in academic areas, makes success in the classroom extremely difficult. This can be a major source of distress and disruption not only for the children but also for their teachers, peers, and families. Children often "give up" in class, some becoming troublesome, not because they do not want to succeed, but because they become discouraged through repeated experiences of failure. Convincing clinical and empirical evidence (e.g., Klin et al., 2000) indicate that children with AS are at high risk for specific learning difficulties.

One of the misleading claims sometimes made by professionals working in this area is that children with AS have a distinctive cognitive profile, usually with higher verbal IQ compared to nonverbal IQ. Assuming such a distinction is a controversial issue, however. Indeed the empirical findings have been mixed (see, e.g., Klin, Volkmar, Sparrow, Cicchetti, & Rourke, 1995; Manjiviona & Prior, 1999; Szatmari, Tuff, Finlayson, & Bartolucci, 1990), even taking into account the complexities and variability in samples of children with a diagnosis of AS. The combined research data suggest that the promotion of a unique and diagnostically relevant profile in AS is not justified, at least not at the present time. The danger that lies within such a simplification is that children with AS will be perceived as having a particular pattern of strengths and deficits in common with one another, and thus a general set of interventions could be promoted. The point that needs to be strongly emphasized is that even though children with AS may share some common difficulties, they vary enormously in their profiles of skills and deficits. Only a comprehensive individualized assessment (that does more than provide IQ scores) can properly inform the choice of interventions that should be implemented in order to improve children's success at school, both academically and socially.

For the purpose of clarity, an explanation of the way in which the term "learning difficulty" is defined is provided. Children who score in the intellectually disabled range of functioning on standardized measures of intelligence are sometimes referred to as "learning disabled." Although no professional would disagree with this attribution, the pertinent issue is that the IQ deficits of the child with an estimated level of intelligence more than two standard deviations below the mean (i.e., IQ below 70) usually provide sufficient explanation of the child's slowness and difficulties with learning. The definition used here, in association with AS, relates to "specific learning difficulties." That is, the specific learning difficulties cannot be explained by the child's level of cognitive functioning, which is in the average range; nor can they be explained by inadequacies related to the child's schooling. Often, there is an element of surprise that the learning difficulties are present in this particular child, given his or her overall cognitive capacities. In this chapter, the term "specific learning difficulty" (SLD) is defined as performance on tests of academic achievement (e.g., reading, spelling, mathematics) that is substantially below what would be expected, given a child's level of cognitive functioning (i.e., IQ greater than 80); and that is associated with specific cognitive impairments (such as short-term auditory memory problems, visual-perceptual problems). In the literature, this level of impairment is usually defined as two standard deviations below the mean, or two grade levels below the child's current grade level at school (Prior, 1996).

The negative effects of undiagnosed SLDs appear in their most severe and salient form in secondary schooling, where the complexity of work increases and flexibility to alter the curriculum diminishes. In primary school, the common strengths in areas such as rote memory and visual skills mean that children with AS often excel in some subjects and may even be among the top in their class. In clinical practice, it is not uncommon to find children in grades 2 or 3 who are reading at a year 6 level (i.e., hyperlexic). However, the demands of the educational curriculum in secondary schooling rely more upon higher-level organizational skills as well as more complex verbal reasoning skills, social reasoning, text interpretation, and writing skills. In one recent study, 63% of school-age children with autism and normal IQ (presumably many with a diagnosis of AS) were found to have an SLD in written expression (Mayes & Calhoun, Chapter 1, this volume).

Given the vast array of stresses with which many children with AS cope throughout their lives, it is vital that educators, parents, and professionals are aware of the nature of SLDs so that targeted interventions can be implemented to help these children achieve optimal educational outcomes. The fact that the majority of children with AS do not qualify for specialist assistance in schools, largely because their adaptive behavior and/ or communication skills are outside the range of the eligibility criteria required by education departments for integration support (at least, this is true within the Australian context), means that parents often have to act as advocates for their children, appealing for their education within the mainstream system.

A major task parents face is that of negotiating for modifications to the academic curriculum for their children. This task can be extremely challenging, especially since many educators fail to understand how a child of average IQ, with intact verbal skills (at least superficially), who may display an encyclopedic knowledge of various subjects (e.g., the solar system), can fail to understand a teacher's subtle meanings in his or her instructions, or may be unable to perform what would seem to be relatively simple tasks (such as how to complete assignments satisfactorily and on time).

Comprehensive assessment of children's strengths and weaknesses in learning makes it possible to develop and apply targeted remediation strategies based on each child's particular profile of skills and deficits. This information can then be used to shape an individualized education program to enhance the child's learning potential. The ongoing monitoring of children's progress is critical so that goals can be set, outcomes assessed, and adjustments can be made, if necessary.

## ASSESSMENT PROCEDURE

Assessment of learning difficulties in children with AS begins with a lengthy clinical interview with parents to obtain detailed information about the child's developmental history. Areas covered include medical, pediatric, and language histories, vision and audiology, concentration/attention, medication history, family history, independent living skills (i.e., adaptive behavior), emotional and behavioral issues, and, most importantly, educational history (i.e., performance).

Comprehensive assessment for SLDs requires a multidisciplinary approach involving a psychologist or neuropsychologist and other professionals including educator and speech pathologist, all contributing their skills and expertise at various stages of the assessment process. Generally, the main areas of intellectual functioning assessed are academic achievement, attention and memory, language skills, visual–spatial ability, and motor-speed capacity. In addition, tests of social cognition and organization and planning skills (i.e., executive functioning) often provide informative data that can be incorporated into interventions within the school context.

In practice, the actual assessment for SLDs proceeds from a more general assessment of cognitive functioning, the results of which help to generate specific hypotheses to investigate in further assessment. Equally as important as test scores are the qualitative data accumulated during the administration of an IQ test. Observing how children respond to the various tasks is essential. For example: how they perform under time constraints, how they plan and organize their approach to the tasks, how they behave when faced with difficult tasks, whether they show evidence of tangentiality on verbal tasks, impulsivity and/or distractibility, or rigid, inflexible behaviors. All this information is extremely valuable and, at a later stage, may be integrated into specific avenues of intervention. These observations also provide the clinician with a rich source of information that can guide decisions about further testing. After the IQ assessment is completed, the decision for further testing is made on the basis of particular hypotheses (e.g., evidence of memory difficulties), and additional tests are selected for this defined purpose. Throughout the assessment it is important to be alert to detecting the differences between behaviors such as a lack of concentration (easily observable) and lack of motivation. Children with AS sometimes appear to be unmotivated; in fact, their motivation to avoid failure is high, but they anticipate poor performance on a particular task.

It is quite common for children with AS to demonstrate information-processing difficulties in the auditory and/or the visual domains as well as attentional problems and organizational difficulties that significantly impact their ability to learn within the classroom. Given the social communication difficulties of children with AS, tests of pragmatic language skills are often indicated. Many children are very reluctant to perform written assignments, because the actual task of writing is such a major effort for them. Motor clumsiness is not uncommon, so that assessing the child's fine motor skill development also may be helpful, especially when writing skills appear to be poorly developed.

Since there has been little documented research of the SLDs associated with AS (see Reitzal & Szatmari, Chapter 2, this volume), no particular group of tests has been promoted as essential for such an assessment. The following material provides a brief summation of tests found to be useful. However, issues of cultural appropriateness and the extrapolation from normative standards (including grade equivalents) from one country to another must be considered.

## Measures of Intellectual Functioning

The Wechsler scales are generally considered to be the best instruments available for the evaluation of cognitive profiles in children with AS: either the Wechsler Intelligence Scale for Children—Third Edition (WISC-III; Wechsler, 1991), suitable for ages 6 years–16 years, 11 months, or the Wechsler Preschool and Primary Scale of Intelligence—Revised (WPPSI-R; Wechsler, 1989) for children ages 3 years, 6 months–6 years. (The Stanford–Binet: IV is an excellent alternative when practice effects on the

Wechsler scales need to be avoided.) The main purpose of this portion of the assessment is to obtain an estimate of cognitive functioning and a profile of strengths and weaknesses across verbal and nonverbal domains. However, careful interpretation of the results is required. For example, the Full Scale IQ may not be the best way of capturing an overview of a child's functioning; there may be a significant difference between verbal and nonverbal abilities and/or a marked scatter of scaled scores. Interpretation of factor scores in relation to verbal comprehension, perceptual organization, freedom from distractibility, and processing speed (Kaufman, 1994) may better reflect the child's functioning, but even then a single inflated or depressed score may disproportionately influence the results.

Detailed analysis of the results is required. For example, differences between the child's forward and backward digit span processing capacity are important to note, because weak performance on the latter may indicate working memory impairments ("working memory" refers to the ability to mentally manipulate information). Although there is no definitive pattern of results on the subtests, the research data suggest that the relative profile of strengths and weaknesses may alter according to the IQ and age of the child. The subtest of Information (general knowledge), which depends upon memory for factual information, is often a strength, as is performance on the Similarities subtest, which measures verbal conceptualization skills (i.e., identifying how two objects are alike). Despite the children's difficulties in behaving appropriately in a variety of social situations, their results on the Comprehension subtest are often within the normal range, particularly for children who are 10 years or older (although this finding does not mean that they are free of difficulties in social understanding and behavior in everyday life). Children who have difficulty with auditory-processing tasks (including working-memory impairments) may score poorly on the Arithmetic and Digit Span subtests. As is the case with lower functioning children who have autism, children with AS often show a relative weakness on the Coding subtest, due to the combination of attentional and graphomotor demands in the context of time constraints. Weak performance on the Picture Arrangement subtest is not uncommon, but often children are able to use their verbal reasoning skills to help them score well within the normal range. Performance on Block Design is usually strong. Incorporating the qualitative information gathered throughout the administration of the test is useful when analyzing a child's learning style.

## Key Areas of Academic Assessment

Key areas of academic assessment include reading accuracy, reading comprehension, spelling, written composition, and mathematics. It is essential to check reading comprehension, considering that many children with AS are reported to be hyperlexic, with excellent word recognition skills, and yet fail to understand what they have read. The Neale Analysis of Reading Ability—Third Edition (Neale, 1999) assesses reading accuracy, comprehension, and rate, and can be used with readers of primary/elementary school age (tables of norms are provided for children ages 6–12 years). The Wide Range Achievement Test 3 (WRAT3; Wilkinson, 1993) provides a quick screen in word recognition, spelling, and mathematics and is suitable for individuals ages 5–75 years. The KeyMath–R: Diagnostic Arithmetic Test (Connolly, Nachtman, & Pritchett, 1989) covers three content areas (i.e., basic concepts, operations, and applications) and provides more comprehensive testing of mathematical ability in primary school-age children. Additional comprehensive tests include the Wechsler Individual Achievement Test—Second Edition (WIAT-II; Psychological Corporation, 2001) and the Woodcock–Johnson Psychoeducational Battery—Third Edition (WJ-III; Woodcock, McGrew, & Mather, 2001). The WIAT-II assesses the achievement of children ages 5 years to 19 years, 11 months. A wide variety of academic skills can be assessed with the eight WIAT-II subtests: Basic Reading, Reading Comprehension, Mathematics Reasoning, Numerical Operations, Listening Comprehension, Oral Expression, Spelling, and Written Expression. The Written Expression test is particularly useful because many students with AS have difficulty generating written work. The Reading Comprehension test assesses several important skills: recognizing stated cause and effect, recognizing stated detail, sequencing, and making inferences. A short form of the test is suitable as a brief screening instrument (using Basic Reading, Spelling, and Mathematics Reasoning).

In brief, the WJ-III provides a wide survey of academic achievement and cognitive abilities and an in-depth assessment of strengths and weaknesses, covering the age range 2–90+ years. One of the advantages of the WJ-III is its flexibility of usage; assessments can be comprehensive or targeted, depending on the purpose.

Given that many children with AS are reported to have difficulties with handwriting, the Handwriting Speed Test (Wallen, Bonney, & Lennox, 1996) is a useful tool that provides an objective and reliable assessment (for students in grades 3–12). The test takes only about 10 minutes to complete; the results could be utilized, for example, to provide evidence to support the need for extra time allocation in examination situations.

## Speech and Language Assessment

At the present time, the majority of speech and language tests used in clinical settings is less than ideal in providing clinically relevant information for the child with AS. The most commonly used tests include the two versions of the Clinical Evaluation of Language Fundamentals—Third Edition

(CELF; Semel, Wiig, & Secord, 1995) for individuals ages 6 years–21 years, 11 months, and the CELF—PreSchool version (Wiig, Secord, & Semel, 1992), suitable for children ages 3 years–6 years, 11 months; and the Test of Oral Language Development—Primary (TOLD-P: 3rd ed.; Newcomer & Hammill, 1997). The CELF consists of six subtests that examine different aspects of receptive and expressive language, such as (1) the ability to use and comprehend complex sentences involving words with strong grammatical meaning, (2) understanding the association between similar and dissimilar words, and (3) understanding time and spatial relationships. Because many children with AS score extremely well (or within the average range, at least) on these tests, other measures (or more informal approaches by experienced clinicians) are required to tap into the child's sometimes very subtle deficits in social communication language skills (commonly referred to as "pragmatic skills"; see Tager-Flusberg, Chapter 4, this volume). Tapping into this arena is necessary not only for diagnostic purposes but also to guide parents and professionals regarding where to begin in terms of helping the child learn to adjust his or her language to reflect changing social contexts.

There is no battery of tests available specifically for this purpose— clearly, this is an area in need of development—but there are tests and other resources available that do provide useful clinical information about the child's social understanding (as well as language skills). One such tool is the Test of Problem Solving—Revised (TOPS-R; Zachman, Huisingh, Barrett, Orman, & LoGiudice, 1994), which is recommended by many speech therapists, even though it is not considered to be a formal speech/language assessment measure. The TOPS-R is designed to assess language-based critical thinking skills; questions focus on a wide range of skills, such as clarifying, analyzing, and generating solutions and affective thinking. The TOPS-R provides an approximate age-equivalence level of a child's social reasoning skills. Fourteen large black-and-white photographs depict children in various social scenarios (e.g., a classroom, a doctor's office). The child is asked to describe what is happening in each picture. Children with AS often focus on single elements within the social scenario rather than responding to the overall scene, and/or they fail to utilize the information provided by the examiner to facilitate understanding of the scenario. Further testing may be indicated after the results on the TOPS-R are obtained, to investigate whether a child's difficulties are due to language comprehension, language expression, memory, attention, or other cognitive or social–emotional factors.

The Test of Language Competence (TLC; Wiig & Secord, 1989) is also a normed test that assesses a variety of abstract language skills, including the ability to make logical inferences from verbal information and comprehend the subtleties of language (e.g., understanding ambiguous words and sentences). Additional tests include the Test of Pragmatic Language (Phelps-Terasaki & Phelps-Gunn, 1992), a formal test suitable for children ages 6–17 years. Results may need to be interpreted cautiously, since children often perform much better in a clinical situation than in everyday, real-life situations. Ideally, observing the child in his or her natural environments (e.g., at home and at school) provides the most ecologically valid type of assessment.

Throughout the speech and language assessment, the experienced speech pathologist closely examines several qualitative aspects of the child's style of communication known to be associated with AS, including difficulties with topic initiation and maintenance, changing topics, seeking clarification, perseverative behaviors, verbosity, literalness, use of unusual or very sophisticated language, pedantic tendencies, abnormal prosody (i.e., patterns of stress and intonation), and repetitive questioning. Observations of nonverbal cues that regulate social communication such as facial expressions, eye contact, and body posture, are also highly pertinent.

## Measures of Attention

The Test of Everyday Attention for Children (TEA-Ch; Manly, Robertson, Anderson, & Nimmo-Smith, 1999) is a relatively new test suitable for children with AS between the ages of 6 and 16 years. The TEA-Ch uses a variety of tests that resemble games to assess different types of attention in children and adolescents. The TEA-Ch is appropriate for children diagnosed with problems in attention and those suspected of having attentional difficulties, to more clearly identify particular patterns of attentional problems and to facilitate the development of treatment and/or management programs. Children with AS are sometimes referred for investigation of their attentional problems; an in-depth analysis often reveals that the difficulties involve particular types of attentional abilities, such as selective attention (i.e., the ability to focus on relevant information) and shifting attention (i.e., the ability to stay mentally flexible and to self-monitor). The ability to sustain attention is often relatively intact, in contrast to individuals with ADHD, who have more generalized attentional difficulties (Prior & Ozonoff, 1998).

## Information Processing and Memory Functioning

The Digit Span subtest, forward span, from the Wechsler scales provides one simple measure of auditory–verbal information-processing capacity; the backward component tests working memory capacity, or the ability to "hold" and manipulate information mentally. The Children's Memory Scale (CMS; Cohen, 1997) provides a comprehensive assessment of learning and memory functioning in children and adolescents (ages 5–16). The CMS consists of six subtests that relate to a variety of memory dimensions including verbal learning and memory, visual learning and memory, and attention. The CMS provides valuable information that can help educators circumvent the child's weak areas and capitalize on any strengths in information processing and learning.

## Other Useful Assessments: Tests of Executive Functioning

"Executive functioning" (EF) is an umbrella term used to describe a variety of neuropsychological processes, including the ability to set goals, initiate a plan, inhibit distracting stimuli, monitor performance, and flexibly change from one point of focus to another. EF deficits in children with AS are now well documented in the literature (e.g., Pennington & Ozonoff, 1996). The organizational scores on the Rey–Osterrieth Complex Figure Test (RCFT; Osterrieth, 1944) provide some information about a child's planning abilities and approach to tasks; however, if organization and planning skills are thought to be deficient, more comprehensive assessment is required.

A relatively new instrument, suitable for children with AS (ages 5–18 years), is the Behavior Rating Inventory of Executive Function (BRIEF; Gioia, Isquith, Guy, & Kenworthy, 2000). The BRIEF is relatively quick to administer, and a global executive composite score is derived. The BRIEF was designed to assess problem-solving skills and the capacity for self-control in eight subdomains of EF: Inhibition (the ability to resist distractions), Shift (the ability to switch from one focus to another), Emotional Control (the ability to regulate emotions), Initiate (self-motivation; ability to start a task without prompting), Working Memory (the ability to "hold" information mentally in order to complete tasks), Plan/Organize (the ability to set goals and identify the sequence of steps to achieve the goals), Organization of Materials (the ability to ensure that the materials needed to complete a task are available and well organized), and Monitor (the ability to self-monitor performance while engaged in a task to ensure set goals will be achieved). The BRIEF contains parent and teacher questionnaires designed to assess EF in both home and school environments (Gioia et al., 2000).

The whole process of assessing and diagnosing SLDs needs to be made as therapeutic as possible for the child and family. In written reports focus is best placed on how the child could be assisted to function more adaptively in both home and school environments (rather than emphasizing a multitude of test results per se). The more the recommended treatments or interventions are individually tailored to the child's preferred manner of learning, the better the outcome is likely to be. Incorporating the data from the qualitative observations gathered throughout the assessment is vital to the design of effective interventions. Professionals involved with the child then need to follow up with parents and educators regarding the implementation of the recommended strategies. A follow-up review, possibly 12 months after the assessment, is also desirable, to evaluate the helpfulness of the interventions and ascertain whether any modifications are necessary in response to developmental changes in the child.

The following case studies, taken from a special assessment center, illustrate some of the assessment procedures and analyses used with children with AS and how the data generated can provide the foundation for developing helpful management interventions and facilitating progress in learning.

## CASE STUDIES

### Case Study 1: Jack, Age 8 years

#### Background Information

Jack was formally diagnosed as having AS when he was 8 years of age and in grade 3. Jack's father was a computer consultant, and his mother was involved in home duties. The presenting problems were disruptive behavior, both at home and at school, poor academic progress, and unpredictable mood. Although Jack showed many features of attention-deficit/hyperactivity disorder, including attentional problems and an early history of hyperactivity, he did not meet full criteria for a diagnosis.

Jack's difficulties began when he first started school, where he demonstrated escalating, disruptive behavior in class and academic difficulties, notably in the area of reading. An area of strength throughout primary school was science, while performance in math and general studies was generally commensurate with that of his peers. Jack has shown a particularly strong interest in outer space and is readily able to recite a myriad of facts about black holes, the planets, and related topics. One of the major hindrances to his learning at school is his lack of motivation to complete academic tasks that hold no interest for him or appear "irrelevant" to him. Apart from being bored with much of the curriculum, Jack also has considerable difficulty sitting still, especially when he is having trouble understanding what is being taught. He tends to behave impulsively, and he has a low frustration tolerance, low self-esteem, and particular difficulty with time-management skills.

The developmental history revealed that Jack was born at 38 weeks, weighing a little over 6 pounds, following an easy delivery. He was described as a highly active infant, very determined, but displaying motor clumsiness. He spoke his first words at approximately 3 years of age. Indeed it was concern with this language delay that motivated his parents to consult a speech therapist. The question of autism was raised but not pursued at the time. Apart from suffering from viral meningitis at 4 years of age, Jack has not experienced any major medical problems. However, he showed an aversion to toilet training, and bedwetting persisted until 8 years of age. There were no concerns with his hearing or vision.

Jack's language seemed to explode all of a sudden, after 3 years of age. He used very precise language and tended to be very literal in his understanding. He had difficulty modulating the volume of his voice and talked loudly, often in a monotone. He used repetitive language and had difficulty sustaining a reciprocal conversation with others as he focused on delivering lengthy monologues on favorite topics, oblivious to the responses of his listener. He was capable of making eye contact but often had a flat, deadpan, expressionless look, with little variation in eye gaze.

Jack played on his own and did not relate well to other children. When other children visited his home, he tended to become overly excited, insisting on directing and controlling the play; otherwise, he refused to participate. Visitors provided an opportunity for Jack to attempt to engage them in one of his favorite topics of interest (i.e., space). At school, he did not join in with the games of other children but tended to remain solitary, especially during recess and lunchtime. He was not accepted by his peers and had significant difficulty forming friendships. Jack was indifferent to peer-group pressure, had difficulty cooperating in the classroom in group work activities, and insisted that things be done his way. Jack frequently invaded the personal space of others and showed no empathy toward them. His parents described him as extremely egocentric. When out in public, Jack would make considerable demands; social outings often ended in disaster, due to his tendency to throw tantrums, oblivious of how his behavior impacted others. He did not spontaneously hug any family member in his earlier years but now has learned to accept physical affection from them. It appears that Jack did not spontaneously exhibit joint attention skills, but his parents encouraged him to direct his attention toward sharing pleasurable activities. He showed little in the way of imitation skills or creative, imaginative play activities.

Jack's preference for routines began at an early age and persisted up until the time of assessment (e.g., at 12 months he would only listen to one song being played on the stereo and would scream if he heard a different song). Jack reacted badly to anything that interrupted or altered his routine. He hated his room to be untidy, which it often was, because he collected all kinds of items (e.g., twigs, shells, etc.) that he hoarded in his room. He has shown intense fascination with various subjects since early in life. At 3 years he was asking questions such as "Why are planets round?"

**TABLE 3.1. WISC–III Results (Scaled Scores) for Jack**

| Verbal tests | | Performance tests | |
|---|---|---|---|
| Information | 14 | Picture Completion | 11 |
| Similarities | 14 | Coding | 5 |
| Arithmetic | 10 | Picture Arrangement | 8 |
| Vocabulary | 12 | Block Design | 11 |
| Comprehension | 10 | Object Assembly | 9 |
| Digit Span | 11 | Symbol Search | 9 |
| | | | |
| IQ scores | | Factor scores | |
| Verbal IQ | 112 | Verbal Comprehension | 114 |
| Performance IQ | 93 | Perceptual Organization | 99 |
| Full Scale IQ | 103 | Freedom from Distractibility | 112 |
| | | Processing Speed | 86 |

*Note.* Scaled scores between 8 and 12 are considered to be in the average range. The results are also quoted in percentiles throughout the text, which indicate a child's position relative to other students of the same age. The intellectually deficient range is below the 2nd percentile, the borderline range is from the 2nd to the 9th percentile, the low-average range is from the 9th to the 25th percentile, the average range is from the 25th to the 75th percentile, the high-average range is from the 76th to the 91st percentile, the superior range is from the 91st to the 98th percentile, and the very superior range is above the 98th percentile.

He also shows a history of repetitive activities (e.g., watching the same videos and repeating the dialogue).

Jack was reported to be extremely sensitive to criticism and to respond very badly to even slight corrections. His frustration and anger escalate suddenly, when simple requests are made of him (e.g., told to get dressed). He becomes destructive, smashing his room, swearing, and hitting at family members. He does not have an intuitive understanding of the world around him but responds well to intellectual explanations.

## Neuropsychological Testing at the Age of 13 Years, 2 Months (School Year 8)[2]

Overall, Jack's performance on the WISC-III (see Table 3.1) varied according to the nature of the task. There was a significant difference between his verbal skills (79th percentile) and his nonverbal skills (32nd percentile). His verbal comprehension skills were an area of significant relative strength (82nd percentile) compared with his perceptual organization skills (i.e., his ability to organize visual information; 47th percentile, within the average range for his age). His general knowledge and abstract verbal reasoning

---

[2]The neuropsychological assessment was conducted by Bernice Dodds, neuropsychologist and Director of the Learning Difficulties Centre, Royal Children's Hospital, Melbourne, Australia.

skills were well established, and his word knowledge (i.e., vocabulary) and everyday verbal reasoning skills were age appropriate. In the nonverbal area, Jack showed good attention to visual detail and age-appropriate abstract, visual–spatial, and constructional reasoning.

### Attention, Information-Processing Skills, and Executive Functioning

Jack's auditory–verbal information-processing capacity—that is, attention span—fluctuated from within, to well above, expected levels (he could repeat six digits forward). His working memory capacity was age appropriate (he could repeat five digits backward). On the Wide Range Assessment of Memory and Learning (WRAML; Sheslow & Adams, 1990), Jack's visual information-processing capacity—his ability to "hold" a visual memory trace—was severely impaired and in the deficient range (0.4th percentile). Jack's visual information-processing speed was also significantly below expected levels in the context of high-level attentional and writing demands (as evidenced by his poor result on the Coding subtest of the WISC-III, which required him to process [i.e., remember] and write a series of symbols within a time limit). His copy of a complex visual figure was within expected levels, and his approach to the task was reasonably well planned. His recall of the figure following a time delay was well within expected levels. Jack coped well with competing task demands on the Contingency Naming Test (Taylor, Albo, Phebus, Sachs, & Bierl, 1987), where he was required to name either the color or shape of a stimulus, depending on a number of conditions.

### Memory and Learning for Verbal and Nonverbal Information

Jack's recall of a series of unrelated words was in the low-average range. His memory for more meaningful information (i.e., prose passages) and less meaningful information in the form of unrelated word pairs (e.g., "school–grocery") was in the average range. Jack's overall recall was in the average range; he was able to verify facts related to the stories and to identify target words from a list of distractor items. His immediate visual memory on a dot location, a visual–spatial memory task, was in the average range as was his visual–spatial learning performance. His performance improved with repeated exposure to the dot array, and his recall, following interference and a time delay, was in the high-average range.

### Academic Tasks

*Literacy Skills.* Jack's single-word recognition performance on the Wide Range Achievement Test 3 (WRAT3) was in the low-average range (14th percentile), consistent with an approximate grade 4 level of performance (i.e., four grades behind). His ability to read a series of nonwords (e.g., "gop") was very good and showed strong phonological decoding skills. However, he experienced difficulties recognizing irregular words or words that rely on familiarity (e.g., "cough") and his performance was well below expected levels (< 0.10th percentile).

The results on the Neale Analysis of Reading Ability—Third Edition showed that when reading a short story, Jack's reading accuracy was consistent with an age equivalence of 11 years, 1 month (compared with his age of 13 years, 2 months). Jack's reading comprehension ability was at an approximate age equivalence of 9 years, 2 months. However, he was able to improve this performance significantly (i.e., his reading comprehension was at an age-appropriate level) when he was provided with access to the text and the opportunity for rereading.

*Spelling.* Jack's single-word spelling skills were at a below-average level (10th percentile), consistent with an approximate grade 4 level. He tended to spell words the way they sounded, confirming his difficulties in picturing a word mentally. His sound segmentation skills were excellent, and his misspellings were phonetically correct (e.g., "breaf" for "brief"). This performance was consistent with his good phonological skills in word identification when reading.

*Mathematics.* Jack's ability to perform written mathematical tasks was in the low-average range (23rd percentile), consistent with a grade 6 level of performance. He managed well with simple addition, subtraction, multiplication, and division tasks and exhibited mastery of higher-level regrouping procedures for addition, subtraction, and multiplication. He had a sound knowledge of percentages and fractions but was unsure about decimals. Jack's mental arithmetic performance was in the average range (50th percentile).

*Handwriting.* On the Handwriting Speed Test, Jack performed very slowly and scored within the borderline range (5th percentile).

## Summary and Recommendations for Parents and Teachers

Jack was diagnosed with specific learning difficulties related to literacy; his reading and spelling performances were at least two grade levels, or 2 years below, that of his peers. The test results also indicated a disorder of written expression; Jack demonstrated a slow pace of written output in the context of multiple-task demands, poor handwriting, and extremely poor spelling skills. Jack shows a significant discrepancy between his oral and his written language skills. He readily admits that he finds it very difficult to organize information in the context of written work and tends to get lost in the detail, experiencing difficulty in seeing the broader focus of the work.

Jack has a number of well-developed skills, including general knowledge and verbal reasoning skills, computation skills, word knowledge, general (everyday) reasoning skills, and language-processing skills. In addition, he shows a good capacity to develop his verbal and visual learning over repeated trials. Areas of weakness include impaired visual information-processing skills and severely reduced visual information-processing speed; poor handwriting speed, poor reading accuracy and fluency; poor reading comprehension skills; and poor spelling skills. Jack also reports significant problems with learning multiplication tables.

The effects of these difficulties on Jack's behavior and his capacity to learn within the context of a normal classroom environment (without specialist assistance) are considerable. He experiences difficulty in copying information from the blackboard and loses his place when reading. He also has poor editing skills, giving minimal attention to punctuation and spelling errors. Jack needs a much longer time frame in which to complete assignments that involve researching a topic and selecting the most salient information. Jack's poor spelling skills are likely to deteriorate further when he is composing written work, with its competing attentional demands.

Jack's learning environment needs to be structured to optimize his learning potential and minimize his distractions (e.g., seated near the teacher, close to the blackboard). Jack needs "hands-on," concrete strategies with which to reinforce his learning, particularly in the areas of spelling and reading. He would greatly benefit from participating in a remedial literacy program on a one-to-one basis. To help maintain a positive focus on his work, thereby enhancing his self-esteem, teachers need to apply a little creativity in their formal assessment of Jack's written work, especially in view of his reduced spelling and writing skills. His difficulties in reading comprehension can be assisted by prompting him to pay attention to the title of the book, asking him questions about what he thinks the book is about, identifying when and where the story takes place, providing a list of the characteristics of the main characters, summarizing their role in the story, etc.

Jack's visual processing difficulties suggest that it would be helpful for him to copy work from desk level rather than from the blackboard. The provision of lesson summaries or work sheets is another option. He needs to have access to a written copy of multiplication tables during all set mathematics tasks (including class tests and/or examinations). Given Jack's poor writing skills, he should be encouraged to develop his computer word-processing skills. (This task can be achieved in a fun manner, using one of the commercially available software packages.)

Due to Jack's difficulty with time-management skills, parents and teachers should work together to help structure his time, especially around due dates for assignments. In addition to helping him establish a logical sequence of steps for completion of assignments, illustrating the steps on a visual chart that includes the dates at which each step needs to be completed would be useful. Homework tasks need to be realistic, with an overall goal of facilitating quality, rather than quantity, of work. Considering the multitude of stresses that Jack faces in his daily life, perhaps a reappraisal of the role of homework would be appropriate.

## Case Study 2: Matthew, Age 8 Years

### Background Information

Matthew was referred for assessment at 8 years of age (grade 2) for his long-standing history of difficulties socializing with peers. The outcome of the assessment was a diagnosis of AS. At the time of referral, his parents reported feeling bewildered at Matthew's overriding interest in powerlines, traffic signs, and roads, which he loved to draw repeatedly. They commented on their son's considerable difficulties in organizing his thoughts, and the way in which he becomes confused when attempting to explain two things at once. They also described Matthew as being very egocentric.

The developmental history was unremarkable; the pregnancy and birth were uncomplicated, and Matthew met all milestones roughly within the normal range. He was an affectionate, cuddly infant who enjoyed physical contact with his parents. Matthew's expressive and receptive language skills were within the lower end of the average range for his age. Difficulties were found with spatial concepts (i.e., "middle," "between," etc.) temporal and numerical concepts ("first," "last," etc.) and left–right knowledge and orientation. When instructions become more complex, Matthew's ability to accurately respond declines.

Matthew had some articulation difficulties when younger, and because he used to talk so rapidly, he was not always easy to understand. He used to repeat words and phrases spoken by his parents, and he still uses some "made-up" words (i.e., neologisms) that he was using in early childhood. Matthew has difficulty modulating the volume of his voice; he often speaks too loudly, especially when he is overexcited and wants attention, and sometimes his voice is too soft, particularly when he is confused. He has difficulty remembering a series of instructions and is always interrupting conversations, often talking about whatever is on his mind, which usually has nothing to do with the ongoing conversation.

When younger, Matthew did not show appropriate greeting behavior toward his parents after periods of separation. He tended to overreact to being hurt (e.g., yelling loudly) and did not always come for comfort. He is usually unaware when others are upset or hurt, although he notices when his mother is not feeling well and will ask if she is feeling better. He used to scream when visitors arrived at his home, demanding attention, but now he usually goes off to play by himself. Indeed, he likes to spend a lot of time on his own. Matthew has difficulty talking to other children; he does not relate well to boys but is a little better with girls. His parents have noticed that he seems to regress, "acts the clown," and becomes very child-like in his manner and movements. Matthew plays with a younger boy (6 years) in his neighborhood, engaging in a variety of outdoor activities such as football, bike riding, and running around. He is keen to play "school games," as long as he is in charge of the play, and he becomes very angry when others refuse to do as he requests.

There is little evidence of joint attention skills or imaginative, pretend play. With few exceptions, Matthew has not displayed any imitation skills. When he is playing school, he will mimic his teacher at times, saying, "All eyes on the blackboard," and sometimes he mimics the weatherman on the news. He was not interested in participating in reciprocal simple games when he was younger but was more of an observer. He used to say he was bored and, at times, seemed at a loss as to what to do with himself. Matthew has a history of engaging in repetitive behaviors, including opening and shutting doors and lining up cars in a particular order; he still prefers things to be in order (e.g., colored pencils in the correct color scheme, etc.). When younger, he would stare fixedly at the wheels of his toy trains on their tracks and would scream if the tracks were broken, yelling, "You fix it!." Matthew still enjoys playing with trains, though his play is more elaborated. For example, he uses blocks and string to erect power poles around the train tracks, and he becomes very upset if someone accidentally knocks down one of the power lines. He also has a large collection of cars and street signs that he sets up when making roads.

Matthew's special interests include the weather, in general, tornadoes, in particular, and telegraph poles. He constantly asks questions about the weather, draws pictures on this theme, and borrows books on this topic from the library. He repeatedly watches favorite videos on similar themes and knows exactly what is on each tape, complaining if the tapes are switched off. However, his reactions are much less severe now than they were a few years ago.

Matthew strongly prefers routines and complains loudly when they are altered. He insists on watching the news while eating his dinner—otherwise he throws a major tantrum—and he always insists on having his drawing book and pen with him so that he can draw telegraph lines (an interest that has been present since 2–3 years of age). When traveling in the car, Matthew is particularly attentive to street signs, street lines, and telegraph poles, and informs his parents when he notices where new street lights have been placed.

## School History

From his first entry into the school system, teachers have reported a number of difficulties with Matthew's behavior in class. He has difficulty completing any academic work to a satisfactory standard, and he does not actively participate in classroom activities. Instructions are very difficult for him to follow, and he often needs reassurance that he has accurately understood an instruction. In grade 1, teachers reported that Matthew's difficulty in sequencing his thoughts led him to verbalize confusing ideas, and at times he was teased by his peers when talking in class. He struggles to remember routines and to get things done in their correct order. He is very restless, fidgety, and has difficulty settling down to complete tasks. In the playground he sometimes runs around with other children, but it is not uncommon for him to wander around on his own; occasionally he spends the entire break period talking with a teacher who is on duty. There are concerns about Matthew's obsessive preoccupation with telegraph poles; this topic often appears in class activities such as writing assignments, and it is also his favorite topic of conversation (which, understandably, other children find boring). Matthew is reported to have very low self-esteem, to worry a lot, and to often appear unhappy.

## Neuropsychological Testing at the Age of 7 Years, 10 Months[3]

The results of the general intelligence testing (WISC-III; see Table 3.2) revealed that Matthew's nonverbal skills were significantly better developed than his verbal skills. His perceptual organizational skills (nonverbal) were well within the average range (55th percentile), whereas his verbal comprehension skills fell within the borderline to low-average range (8th percentile). He scored well below average (5th percentile) on the vocabulary test, where he had to verbally express the meanings of commonly used words; similarly, he had difficulty explaining how two words were alike (2nd percentile). His level of general knowledge was below average, and his social reasoning skills were just within the average range. His ability to attend to visual detail, his abstract visual–spatial skills, and his constructional reasoning skills were age-appropriate.

---

[3]The neuropsychological assessment was conducted by neuropsychologist Monica Williams, at the Learning Difficulties Centre, Royal Children's Hospital, Melbourne, Australia.

**TABLE 3.2. WISC–III Results (Scaled Scores) for Matthew**

| Verbal tests | | Performance tests | |
|---|---|---|---|
| Information | 7 | Picture Completion | 12 |
| Similarities | 4 | Coding | 15 |
| Arithmetic | 7 | Picture Arrangement | 8 |
| Vocabulary | 5 | Block Design | 10 |
| Comprehension | 8 | Object Assembly | 11 |
| Digit Span | 8 | Symbol Search | 11 |
| | | | |
| IQ scores | | Factor scores | |
| Verbal IQ | 79 | Verbal Comprehension | 79 |
| Performance IQ | 108 | Perceptual Organization | 102 |
| Full Scale IQ | 92 | Freedom from Distractibility | 87 |
| | | Processing Speed | 117 |

## Attention, Information–Processing Skills, and Executive Functioning

Matthew could remember 3 digits forward (sometimes 4 digits), which placed him below the level of his peers, but he was able to repeat 2 digits backward, which was in the low-average range. Matthew's sentence repetition performance was also in the low-average range (9th percentile). His visual attention span (i.e., his ability to "hold" visual information mentally) was in the borderline to low-average range (9th percentile). His ability to remember and recall meaningful visual–spatial information was in the low-average to average range (25th percentile). His copy of a complex figure was within the normal range, as was his recall of the figure after a time delay.

## Memory and Learning

Matthew's ability to learn a series of unrelated words was in the high-average range (84th percentile), and his recall following a time delay was in the average range. He performed well when required to learn more meaningful prose passages (37th percentile), with his recall scoring in the low-average range. His recognition performance of the same story, given multiple choice options, was in the low-average range.

## Academic Tasks

Matthew's ability to read regular, irregular, and nonwords was good, and his performance fell within the average range. These results indicated that his phonological skills and sight vocabulary were well developed. On the

Neale Analysis of Reading Ability, Matthew's reading accuracy was in the average range (57th percentile), and his reading rate was within the average to high-average range (74th percentile). His comprehension ability was not as good as word recognition but was within the average range (32nd percentile) and consistent with an age equivalence between 5 years, 10 months, and 7 years, 7 months. Both spelling skills (50th percentile) and mathematical performance (39th percentile) were in the average range, consistent with a year 2 level of performance.

## Summary and Recommendations

Matthew's strengths lie in the areas of nonverbal problem solving—he demonstrates good visual–spatial problem-solving skills, and his memory skills for visual material and simple verbal material were sound. Matthew's academic skills in reading, spelling, and mathematics were largely age-appropriate. His major area of weakness is his language-based learning difficulty; he has trouble expressing himself verbally and using language to reason. In brief, Matthew finds it much more difficult to reason and problem solve through verbal means than through nonverbal means. His ability to recall complex verbal material was mildly inefficient, which is most likely linked to the increased language-processing demands. The reported difficulties in sequencing his verbal and written expression also are consistent with his reduced verbal ability. Further areas of difficulty include Matthew's fluctuating auditory–verbal attention span (i.e., his limited capacity to "hold" verbal information mentally) and his borderline visual attention-processing span.

Developing Matthew's language skills is a matter of priority, so consulting with a speech pathologist who has expertise in working with children with AS is highly desirable. Detailed assessment of Matthew's pragmatic skills would need to be conducted. A combination of individual and group therapy sessions is recommended to increase Matthew's basic language skills (including understanding of spatial and temporal concepts) and enhance his ability to express himself verbally. In addition, providing specific interventions designed to assist him in improving his pragmatic language skills (such as how to engage in conversation with peers) is recommended. Because he is likely to misinterpret verbal and nonverbal cues from children, conflict may arise as a result. To address this contingency, he would need to be taught a structured problem-solving approach to resolving any such difficulties.

In addition to the implications for social interaction, Matthew's poor understanding of the meaning of words will diminish his ability to attend to and complete classwork. Combined with the fluctuation in auditory processing and mild weakness in working memory capacity, Matthew could be easily overwhelmed. Suitable strategies for the classroom include gaining Matthew's attention prior to giving an instruction; asking him to repeat the instruction; giving him extra time to respond to questions; encouraging him to say "I don't know" if he can't answer a question (rather than not respond); and monitoring his understanding during class discussion and providing less complex explanations if necessary. As noted, allowing him to copy work from desk level rather than from the blackboard and providing lesson summaries would be helpful.

Matthew would be more likely to succeed in a highly structured environment where predictable routines are established, thereby reducing the mental load and its concomitant stress. He needs (1) help in breaking down tasks into a series of steps and (2) a structured approach to written work. In a large group setting, Matthew will require a high level of individual support and attention in order to follow the verbal information and cope with social situations. Given his difficulties, unhappiness, and low self-esteem, he will require ample praise, encouragement, and reassurance from his teachers to stay motivated. Throughout his school career, close monitoring of Matthew's progress will be necessary and adjustments made to the curriculum to help manage stress.

## Case Study 3: Dylan, Age 9 Years, 5 Months

The school psychologist referred Dylan (grade 4) for his poor social skills and apparent inability to understand other people's points of view. He was given a diagnosis of AS.

### Background Information

The major concern expressed by his parents is Dylan's difficulty forming friendships. Although he often wants to play with other children, other children do not seek his company unless he initiates the contact. Another concern is Dylan's difficulty in recognizing the consequences of his actions; he does not seem to understand how his behavior contributes to conflict, and he does not understand other people's thoughts and feelings. Dylan is talented and capable in some areas (e.g., he has a very good memory), but he lacks the motivation and persistence to apply himself to academic tasks. His parents are worried that this situation will only deteriorate as he grows older. Additional concerns relate to Dylan's difficulties with organization generally, his lack of confidence, and the frustration and conflict he experiences with his siblings.

The developmental history reveals a problem-free pregnancy and delivery. Dylan attained physical milestones within normal limits, although he tended to be on the slow side; for example, he walked at just over 15 months. At 14 months, grommets were inserted in his ears, but there were no concerns about his hearing. He babbled as an infant, spoke single words from 12 months, but was slow to join words together and use sentences. Prior to language development, Dylan communicated his needs by pointing, grabbing his mother, and/or by crying. By 3 years of age, he had not initiated much verbal communication, so his parents took him for a 12-month course of speech therapy. His speech failed to develop as expected, and he underwent more speech therapy when he was in preparatory grade (i.e., first year of school).

At this time he was referred for neuropsychological testing. The primary areas of concern that prompted this referral were concentration and attention problems. The results of this assessment indicated that Dylan's general intelligence was in the average range, with marked variability across subtests. Although his visual–perceptual skills were found to be age-appropriate, he had difficulty processing more complex visual stimuli. Dylan also had difficulty with tasks involving visual–motor coordination. He showed difficulty in adopting a well organized, considered approach to tasks and was unable to persevere when tasks became difficult. He tended to be distractible and impulsive. At the time of this first assessment Dylan's reading skills were below average.

Currently, Dylan has difficulty in remembering a series of instructions. He is always interrupting conversations and often starts talking about whatever is on his mind, oblivious to the responses of others. His speech is typically very pressured, flat, and monotonous; he is long-winded and inclined to interpret language literally.

Dylan was an affectionate, cuddly infant who enjoyed close physical contact. He would often stare into space when sitting in his highchair, and did not always give direct eye contact. At this point in time, he acknowledges visitors but then wanders off to "do his own thing" (e.g., play on the computer) rather than interact with them. Dylan recognizes when another person is hurt and will show concern, but his mother feels that he responds in a mechanical manner, in response to being taught to take notice, not because of any intuitive understanding or concern. There have been times when Dylan has laughed at the misfortune of others. He is happy to participate in joyful occasions with his family, but he shows no understanding of the purpose of a particular celebration, and is more likely to be focused on "what's in it for him."

Dylan's behavior in public is somewhat unpredictable. Although he does have some awareness of what is appropriate and inappropriate behavior, there are times when he can say inappropriate things in public. Dylan has been a fussy eater from the age of 3 and presently has a restricted diet. He has always overreacted to pain, screaming and becoming very distressed at these times. He tends to ignore heat and cold but is oversensitive to certain sounds (e.g., the scraping of a fork). Dylan also tends to be fussy about the texture of his clothing.

Dylan has a couple of children he calls his friends, but they rarely, if ever, contact him. He has tended to play with younger children, especially girls, although one boy of similar age has visited his home (to play computer games). When he is in the company of other children, Dylan likes to act the clown, putting on a show, displaying no shyness or lack of confidence, totally unaware of whether or not others are enjoying his performance. He complains that he is constantly teased and bullied at school and that he has no friends. During the assessment, Dylan said that he would like to have friends but that he had tried everything and "nothing works." When he asks other children to play with him, they say "no" because (according to Dylan) they hate him. He often wanders around the playground by himself during recess and lunchtime.

Dylan has tended to play on his own from a very young age; there is no evidence of pretend or symbolic play in the developmental history, and joint attention skills have been slow to develop. He likes to line up toy cars in a particular way and becomes very upset if this order is disturbed. Despite being encouraged by his parents, Dylan has difficulty playing games with others; he does not seem to understand what he is supposed to do and prefers to go off on his own. His favorite activities include watching television and watching the same videos repeatedly, often reciting lines from his favorite movies. Dylan also enjoys playing computer games, such as Nintendo, and he likes to construct things using his hands (e.g., robotics). He collects various items (e.g., rocks, string, leaves, bark), and although his interests change over time, he often returns to an interest. From about 4 years of age Dylan pretended to be a dog, barking and padding along the floor, though he rarely engages in this behavior now.

### School History

Dylan attended kindergarten at 4 years of age, and no problems were reported. His school history describes disruptive behavior in class, difficulty in completing set tasks, and considerable restlessness and fidgeting. At the time of the present assessment, his teacher reported that he (the teacher) has a good relationship with Dylan as a result of using particular strategies that are highly successful with him. For example, when Dylan becomes angry, rather than risk retaliation, his teacher tends to give him space to calm down. Dylan also responds well to structure and routine. He is coping with academic work and, at times, is very creative, showing sustained attention for activities such as drawing, although he is often distracted and at times appears "as if he's in another world." The teacher is able to bring him back to his work by prompting and asking him what he needs to do next.

Dylan is perceived as different by his peers and presents as very immature and unable to deal with conflict. At times, in his attempts to interact with his classmates, Dylan will behave in annoying ways, such as take objects from them, and he can also become very defensive and verbally aggressive toward them. At times his thinking seems very disorganized.

## Psychological Assessment at the Age of 9 Years, 5 Months

Dylan's nonverbal ability was within the average range (47th percentile), and his verbal ability was in the low-average to average range (23rd percentile). He showed significant relative strength in his ability to organize visual information (i.e., perceptual organization skills, 63rd percentile) compared to his verbal comprehension skills (21st percentile). (See Table 3.3.)

The results of the present assessment are similar to the previous test results conducted 3 years, 5 months earlier; however, there were some differences. For example, Dylan's general knowledge skills were previously in the average range but are now in the below-average range. Dylan was able to answer questions such as "What must you do to make water boil?" and "How many hours are there in a day?" but he was unable to answer questions such as "What month comes after March?" and "How many things make a dozen?" This test result provides some evidence that he is missing out on learning some basic information from his environment. His vocabulary skills were previously below average, whereas his performance now falls within the average range. The results on the nonverbal scale were generally well within the average range; thus Dylan showed age-appropriate abstract visual–spatial and constructional reasoning skills. His previous dif-

**TABLE 3.3. WISC-III Results (Scaled Scores) for Dylan**

| Verbal tests | | Performance tests | |
|---|---|---|---|
| Information | 6 | Picture Completion | 12 |
| Similarities | 5 | Coding | 6 |
| Arithmetic | 9 | Picture Arrangement | 9 |
| Vocabulary | 9 | Block Design | 11 |
| Comprehension | 11 | Object Assembly | 11 |
| Digit Span | 7 | Symbol Search | 10 |
| IQ scores | | Factor scores | |
| Verbal IQ | 89 | Verbal Comprehension | 88 |
| Performance IQ | 99 | Perceptual Organization | 105 |
| Full Scale IQ | 93 | Freedom from Distractibility | 90 |
| | | Processing Speed | 91 |

ficulties with tasks involving visual–motor coordination also were evident in the present assessment (Coding subtest).

Dylan's auditory–verbal information-processing capacity (i.e., attention span) was just below the average range (he could repeat 4 digits forward), and he experienced considerable difficulty "holding" and manipulating this information mentally (he could repeat 2 digits backward). Qualitative observations suggested that Dylan's ability to persevere with difficult tasks has improved, although he is still inclined to give up easily, especially on verbal tasks. Consistent with the previous report, Dylan has difficulty in organizing his approach to tasks (as reported by his current teacher).

### Academic Tasks

Dylan's single-word decoding skills were in the average range (37th percentile), consistent with an approximate grade 3 level of achievement. With unknown words, his preferred strategy was to make a guess, although at times he did attempt to sound out the syllables. His spelling performance was in the borderline to low-average range (13th percentile), consistent with an approximate grade 1 level of achievement. Some of his attempts were phonologically correct but characterized by omissions, missequencing, and sound substitutions (e.g., "drss" for "dress," "amr" for "arm," "tran" for "train"). Dylan performed in the low-average range (23rd percentile) on the Arithmetic test, consistent with an approximate grade 3 level of achievement. He was able to complete some simple addition, subtraction, and multiplication tasks, but did not show evidence of grouping skills.

### Summary and Recommendations

Overall Dylan's results show relative strength in perceptual organization skills compared with verbal comprehension skills. In the academic domain, he is performing somewhat below his peers in reading and mathematics and well below his peers in spelling. His performance in spelling is two grades below his current year level at school, and thus he satisfies criteria for a specific learning difficulty. At this stage, Dylan would benefit from a remedial literacy program to further develop a range of literacy skills. He will also need assistance to develop his written composition skills. His information-processing difficulties in the auditory–verbal domain suggest that he is likely to feel overwhelmed in the classroom. His poor immediate and working memory capacity contribute to difficulties, at times, in sustaining attention. Since he is easily overloaded with new information and has difficulty manipulating information mentally ("in his head"), he may find it difficult to stay on task and he may become distracted. Aids such as checklists and cue sheets would be of assistance. Both home and school environments would need to provide a high degree of structure to help Dylan compensate for a range of organizational difficulties. For example, parents might establish a routine time at home for completion of homework, with set start and finish times, and adult guidance present to assist him in beginning the tasks. On the previous night, organizing all materials to be taken to school (e.g., return of library books, sports clothing, etc.) will also help to reduce stress.

Given Dylan's poor conversational skills, lack of empathy, and inability to understand the rules of social interaction, considerable adult assistance will be necessary to help guide him toward appropriate behavior in social contexts. Social and classroom situations are likely to make him feel anxious and aroused, which may result in unpredictable behavior that ranges from aggressive outbursts to distressed withdrawal. Dylan needs help to understand how his behavior affects others, and he would benefit from learning how to monitor his own behavior. He needs to be exposed to a structured approach to problem solving that utilizes concrete materials (e.g., visual aids such as checklists) to help him learn to handle conflict more adaptively. A social skills group may be particularly helpful in this regard. A peer support program for Dylan is also considered highly desirable, and indeed, is probably the most critical issue to be addressed at the present time, because he is feeling increasingly isolated, lonely, and sad.

## SUMMARY

These three case studies illustrate the high variability of children with AS who also have a range of specific learning difficulties and information-processing inefficiencies. Despite the children's differences in learning styles and in their strengths and weaknesses, there are some common core deficits. The mixture of impairments in attention, information processing, organization and planning; the inability to complete academic tasks satisfactorily, including written composition and homework; disconnectedness from other children and/or inappropriate social advances; as well as pragmatic language difficulties and problem solving difficulties all conspire to render many children with AS at risk of academic failure. The finding that the children invariably suffer from low self-esteem serves to heighten the risk of a poor prognosis at school.

Most children with AS have areas of strength, too, and we know from clinical experience and anecdotal evidence that much can be achieved by harnessing and enhancing these strengths to improve their prospects for school success. Strategies to assist children with their diverse range of diffi-

culties have been cited throughout the case studies. Many more are outlined in later chapters in this volume.

Basic guidelines that underpin more targeted individual strategies (and
can be set up by the child's educators) include the following:

- A highly structured learning environment in which teachers take
  prime responsibility for minimizing distractions
- Using clear, unambiguous language to tell the child what he or she is
  supposed to do (rather than focusing on what the child is doing
  wrong)
- Checking the child's understanding of instructions
- Regular classroom routines (which facilitate the child's ability to pay
  attention to specific instructions)
- Lesson summaries (and a decrease in, or preferably an eradication
  of, material to be copied from the blackboard)
- Visual strategies (e.g., timetables, rules, instructions)
- Clear instructions for projects (i.e., written step-by-step outline of
  the sequence of tasks)
- Opportunities for revision
- Reduced homework requirements (where indicated, especially to re-
  duce stress on child and family)
- Behavior management strategies (particularly useful when obses-
  sional interests dominate and impede learning)
- A collaborative, practical approach between parents and school staff
  to assist with the many organizational demands (particularly important after primary school)
- Consideration of time extensions for completion of set work and assignments (particularly relevant for test/exam situations)
- A nominated mentor (e.g., teacher or other support person) who the
  child can turn to for assistance as required
- Organizing a stress-free zone where the child can go to escape the
  demands of the school environment

It would also be helpful for the children if different approaches for work
completion were more readily accepted by their teachers—for example,
children with very poor handwriting could be assisted by their teachers' approval of computer-assisted generation of work.

Many children with AS will need considerable help in acquiring
problem-solving skills in relation to resolving conflict with peers. Interventions to improve social skills and pragmatic communication skills, especially for those children who crave social acceptance, may need to be
explored outside the school context (depending on the availability of re-

sources) but could be incorporated into peer-support paradigms. It is evident that strengthening children's pragmatic skills will help them interact with the social world (as it is largely mediated via verbal means). There is increasing anecdotal evidence from parents and teachers that social stories can be successfully used to assist children to develop a repertoire of social skills and also improve their social communication skills. Strategies to help foster the often fragile self-esteem of children with AS also need to be included in any positively focused learning program. We know, for instance, that with the assistance of their educators, some children have been encouraged to use their talents and abilities in knowledge areas (e.g., computers, drawing, following maps) to assist their classmates in developing their skills. This approach not only enhances the children's self-esteem but also has the potential of becoming the basis for the development of social relationships.

A fundamental prerequisite for improving outcomes for children with AS in school is a comprehensive assessment (as outlined earlier), which should be integral to the development of any specialized learning program. Naturally, it is important to take into account the unique personality and temperament of each child, as these factors will undoubtedly influence the choice of specific interventions.

## REFERENCES

Cohen, M. J. (1997). *Children's Memory Scale—Manual.* San Antonio, TX: Psychological Corporation.

Connolly, A. J., Nachtman, W., & Pritchett, L. M. (1989). *KeyMath–R: Diagnostic Arithmetic Test.* Circle Pines, MN: American Guidance Service.

Gioia, G. A., Isquith, P. K., Guy, S. C., & Kenworthy, L. (2000). *Behavior Rating Inventory of Executive Function.* Odessa, FL: Psychological Assessment Resources.

Kaufman, A. (1994). *Intelligent testing with the WISC-III.* New York: Wiley.

Klin, A., Sparrow, S. S., Marans, W. D., Carter, A., & Volkmar, F. R. (2000). Assessment issues in children and adolescents with Asperger syndrome. In A. Klin, F. R. Volkmar, & S. S. Sparrow (Eds.), *Asperger syndrome* (pp. 309–339). New York: Guilford Press.

Klin, A., Volkmar, F. R., Sparrow, S. S., Cicchetti, D. V., & Rourke, B. P. (1995). Validity and neuropsychological characterization of Asperger syndrome. *Journal of Child Psychology and Psychiatry, 36,* 1127–1140.

Manjiviona, J., & Prior, M. (1999). Neuropsychological profiles of children with Asperger syndrome and autism. *Autism: The International Journal of Research and Practice, 3*(4), 327–356.

Manly, T., Robertson, I. H., Anderson, V., & Nimmo-Smith, I. (1999). *The Test of Everyday Attention for Children.* London: Thames Valley Test Company.

Neale, M. (1999). *Neale Analysis of Reading Ability—Third Edition.* Camberwell, Australia: Acer Press.

Newcomer, P. L., & Hammill, D. D. (1997). *Test of Language Development—Primary* (3rd ed.). Austin, TX: Pro-Ed.

Osterrieth, P. A. (1944). Le test de copie d'une figure complexe. *Archives de Psychologie, 30,* 206–356.

Pennington, B. F., & Ozonoff, S. (1996). Executive functions and developmental psychopathology. *Journal of Child Psychology and Psychiatry, 37,* 51–87.

Phelps-Terasaki, D., & Phelps-Gunn, T. (1992). *Test of Pragmatic Language.* Austin, TX: Pro-Ed.

Prior, M. (1996). *Understanding specific learning difficulties.* East Sussex, UK: Psychology Press.

Prior, M., & Ozonoff, S. (1998). Psychological factors in autism. In F. R. Volkmar (Ed.), *Autism and pervasive developmental disorders* (pp. 64–108). Cambridge, UK: Cambridge University Press.

Psychological Corporation. (2001). *Wechsler Individual Achievement Test—Second Edition.* San Antonio, TX: Harcourt Brace.

Semel, E., Wiig, E. H., & Secord, W. A. (1995). *Clinical Evaluation of Language Fundamentals—Third Edition.* San Antonio. TX: Psychological Corporation.

Sheslow, D., & Adams, W. (1990). *Wide range assessment of memory and learning.* Wilmington, DE: Wide Range.

Szatmari, P., Tuff, L., Finlayson, A. J., & Bartolucci, G. (1990). Asperger's syndrome and autism: Neurocognitive aspects. *Journal of the American Academy of Child and Adolescent Psychiatry, 29,* 130–136.

Taylor, H. G., Albo, V. C., Phebus, C. K., Sachs, B. R., & Bierl, P. G. (1987). Postirradiation treatment outcomes for children with acute lymphocytic leukemia: Clarification of risks. *Journal of Pediatric Psychology, 12,* 395–411.

Wallen, M., Bonney, M., & Lennox, L. (1996). *The Handwriting Speed Test.* Adelaide, Australia: Helios Art and Book.

Wechsler, D. (1989). *Manual for the Wechsler Preschool and Primary Scale of Intelligence—Revised.* San Antonio, TX: Psychological Corporation.

Wechsler, D. (1991). *Manual for the Wechsler Intelligence Scale for Children—Third Edition.* San Antonio, TX: Psychological Corporation.

Wiig, E. H., & Secord, W. A. (1989). *Test of Language Competence—Expanded Edition.* San Antonio: TX: Psychological Corporation.

Wiig, E. H., Secord, W. A., & Semel, E. (1992). *Clinical Evaluation of Language Fundamentals—PreSchool.* San Antonio, TX: Psychological Corporation.

Wilkinson, G. S. (1993). *Wide Range Achievement Test 3.* Lutz, FL: Psychological Assessment Resources.

Woodcock, R. W., McGrew, K. S.. & Mather, N. (2001). *Woodcock–Johnson Psychoeducational Battery—Third Edition.* Itasca, IL: Riverside.

Zachman, L., Huisingh, R., Barrett, M., Orman, J., & LoGiudice, C. (1994). *Test of Problem Solving—Elementary Revised.* East Moline, IL: Lingui-Systems.

# 4

# Effects of Language and Communicative Deficits on Learning and Behavior

## HELEN TAGER-FLUSBERG

## DIAGNOSTIC CRITERIA FOR ASPERGER SYNDROME

One of the striking aspects of the DSM-IV diagnostic criteria for Asperger syndrome (AS; in the DSM-IV, "Asperger's disorder") is the criterion of the complete absence of any language or communicative impairment. Language is discussed only as an *exclusionary* criterion: "There is no clinically significant general delay in language" (American Psychiatric Association, 1994, p. 77). There is no mention of vocal or speech abnormalities or deficits in social communication or conversation skills. Indeed, according to most diagnostic systems, the main distinction between AS and autism is the degree of language and communication skills. Yet, as Wing (1991) pointed out, Hans Asperger (1944/1991) described numerous symptoms in this domain for all the cases he presented in the original paper that introduced the syndrome now named for him. In this chapter, I review the evidence for the presence of significant language and communication abnormalities in people with AS and consider the implications of such deficits for distinguishing between AS and high-functioning autism (HFA) in future diagnostic classifications of autism spectrum disorders (ASD). In the final section, I discuss how people with AS may use language as a means for acquiring other cognitive and social skills, and the related implications for therapeutic interventions.

## COMMUNICATION IMPAIRMENTS IN ASPERGER'S CASE STUDIES

Asperger (1944/1991) described in detail the developmental history and current behavior patterns of four children—Fritz, Harro, Ernst, and Hellmuth—to illustrate his view that they all shared a common disturbance in "severe and characteristic difficulties of social integration" (p. 37). All the boys showed atypical features of language and communicative functioning. Fritz is described as showing no delays in development; however, he had an abnormal voice quality, spoke very slowly, and used a singsong intonation. He also did not answer questions posed to him, though he sometimes repeated the questions in a stereotypic way, and would make up words or speak "nonsense." Harro also did not respond to questions; instead he "let his talk run single-mindedly along his own tracks" (p. 52). Harro's language developed early, and he had an unusually mature way of expressing himself. His voice and speech rate were also odd, and he tended to tell fantastic stories that became incoherent as they progressed. Ernst and Hellmuth were both delayed in the onset of language. Ernst had speech difficulties early on, but later spoke "like an adult," but in a high, nasal voice that sounded like a caricature of an aristocrat. He spoke incessantly, asking many questions but ignoring those addressed to him. Hellmuth had a pedantic way of speaking. He used unusual words and sounded quite poetic at times. Still, when asked about his daily life, Hellmuth responded in an empty and pompous-sounding way.

All the boys had significant deficits in nonverbal social communication. Their eye gaze patterns were atypical, described as "lost" or unfocused. They showed limited facial expressions, held their faces rigid or immobile, and used few gestures. Their vocal expression was deficient in expressive prosody, which is used to maintain social contact and convey affect. There was some variation in other aspects of language functioning among the boys. Two acquired language on time or even early, while two were delayed. A couple of the boys, Fritz and Hellmuth, had a creative attitude to language, exemplified in their choice of words and linguistic styles. Nevertheless, even the boys who had an adult-like way of speaking had an idiosyncratic approach to communication, ignoring their listeners' difficulty in following conversations. For Hans Asperger, these abnormalities in expression and communication were central to the social deficits that defined the autism he observed in his patients.

# RESEARCH ON COMMUNICATIVE IMPAIRMENTS IN ASPERGER SYNDROME

One difficulty with reviewing the literature on language and communicative abnormalities in AS is that different researchers rely on different criteria for the diagnosis of AS. Many studies that have included participants with HFA are likely to include AS in accordance with a certain diagnostic system; however, the authors do not explicitly differentiate between autism and AS. In this review I focus exclusively on studies that identify their participants as having AS, accepting the authors' definition of the disorder.

## Prosody and Vocal Quality

"Prosodic aspects of language" refer to the properties of the speech signal used to modulate and enhance meaning. There are three levels of prosodic function: grammatical, pragmatic, and affective (Merewether & Alpert, 1990). Grammatical prosody includes cues to the type of utterance (e.g., in the United States, questions end with rising pitch) and different stress patterns used to distinguish different parts of speech (e.g., marking the word *present* with stress on the first syllable, when used as a noun). Pragmatic stress may highlight new information or draw the listener's attention to the significance of the message expressed. Affective prosody conveys the speaker's feelings or attitudes and may include variations in vocal tone and speech rate.

In her overview of communication impairments in people with AS, Twachtman-Cullen (1998) commented on the abnormalities in speech and other prosodic impairments that have been noted by numerous clinicians and researchers. Eisenmajer and his colleagues (1996) compared the clinical behaviors of children with autism and children with AS, using in-depth interviews conducted with their parents. The children with AS were more likely to be described by their parents as having an unusual tone of voice, such as flat or monotonous in quality. The most systematic and direct investigation of prosodic features in AS was conducted by Shriberg and his colleagues (2001). They analyzed speech samples collected during a diagnostic interview, which was conducted with adolescents with autism or AS and adult participants. Using the Autism Diagnostic Observation Schedule (ADOS), the main findings revealed that about one-third of the participants with AS had distorted speech and articulation problems, and two-thirds displayed prosodic abnormalities on grammatical, pragmatic, and/or affective levels. Like Asperger's case studies, the majority of the study participants had loud, high voices with a nasal tone.

One recent study investigated whether adolescents with AS were able to use nonverbal cues, including facial expression, body gestures, and prosody, to interpret the feelings of people acting in videotaped scenes (Koning & Magill-Evans, 2001). The adolescents with AS were significantly worse than controls in interpreting the emotions, and they relied least on prosodic information. These findings suggest that not only are people with AS impaired in expressive prosody, they also have difficulty comprehending prosodic information expressed by others. Together, such deficits contribute significantly to the social and communicative difficulties of people with AS.

## Pedantic Speech

Several investigators have described the speech of people with AS as "pedantic." For example, Wing (1981), who introduced AS to the English-speaking community, commented on the language of people with this syndrome as having a "bookish" quality, exemplified by the use of obscure words. She considered pedantic speech to be one of the main clinical features of this disorder (Burgoine & Wing, 1983).

Only one study has attempted to assess pedantic speech; to do so, the researchers employed a newly devised rating scale composed of several different features that were based on a dictionary definition of the term (Ghazuiddin & Gerstein, 1996). These features included (1) conveying too much information, (2) inappropriate use of formal sentence structure in conversation, (3) monologue speech, (4) sophisticated vocabulary more typical of written than oral language, and (5) a precise, formal speech style. Ghaziuddin and Gerstein (1996) collected audiotaped language samples from 17 participants with AS who were participating in an interview that consisted of a picture description task and a series of open-ended questions. Participants were rated as either pedantic or nonpedantic on the basis of the recordings. Using this rating scale, 13 of the 17 participants—about three-quarters of the group—were judged to be pedantic, though no information was provided about which features were most likely to be present in the pedantic speakers. Further studies need to be conducted to identify the most significant aspects of this speech style and to assess the effects of using this kind of style on social interaction in different contexts.

## Social Discourse

Difficulties in social uses of language, especially in conversations with others and any discourse context, have been widely noted in people with AS (e.g., Klin & Volkmar, 1997; see Landa, 2000, for review). Ghaziuddin and Gerstein (1996) included monologue speech as part of their definition of pedantic speech style, which suggests that people with AS do not generally engage in turn taking during reciprocal conversations with other people, and they may also talk too much. Providing some support for this view, Ramberg, Ehlers, Nyden, Johanssen, and Gillberg (1996) found that children with AS showed impaired turn-taking abilities during dyadic conversations.

Adams and her colleagues (Adams, Green, Gilchrist, & Cox, 2002) compared conversational samples collected from adolescents with AS and a group of age- and IQ-matched children with severe conduct disorder. They carried out a detailed analysis of the conversations elicited while administering the ADOS. Although there were no overall significant group differences in verbosity, the adolescents with AS tended to talk more during conversational contexts that focused on emotional topics. A few participants with AS were extremely verbose. The groups were similar in their ability to respond to questions and comments offered by their conversational partner, but a qualitative analysis of responses revealed that the participants with AS had more pragmatic problems, such as providing an inadequate or tangential response, especially when discussing an unusual event or personal narrative.

Clinicians often report that it is difficult to understand or follow conversations with a person with AS. To investigate this observation systematically, Fine, Bartolucci, Szatmari, and Ginsberg (1994) compared interviews conducted with adolescents with AS, HFA, and conduct disorder (controls). They applied a formal discourse analysis to the transcripts of the interviews and found that the group with AS scored higher than the other groups on measures of unclear reference. Thus the group with AS would refer to individuals without introducing them appropriately, switch reference without clear linguistic marking, and use pronouns with no clear antecedents. These conversational deficits in reference made it harder to understand the adolescents with AS.

## Nonliteral Language and Language in Context

Much of our everyday discourse includes examples of different types of nonliteral language. These include, for example, lies, jokes, sarcasm, idioms, and metaphor. Interpreting these linguistic forms requires the listener to infer the speaker's intended meaning by using a variety of cues, including the social or linguistic context. People with AS are described as being very literal and concrete in their use and interpretation of language, and several studies provide support for this view.

Kerbel and Grunwell (1998) reported that children with AS performed poorly on a task that assessed idiom comprehension; they gave significantly more inappropriate interpretations than age- or language-matched controls. Jolliffe and Baron-Cohen (1999) tested adults with AS on Happé's (1994) strange stories, which contain examples of several different types of nonliteral language, including lies, irony, and figures of speech. The adults with AS performed significantly worse than normal age- and IQ-matched controls, especially in providing context-appropriate interpretations.

In a related study with the same participants, Jolliffe and Baron-Cohen (2000) investigated the ability to process language in context, using two different story tasks. One task required participants to organize a sequence of sentences into a coherent story. In the second task, participants listened to brief stories and were then asked questions, some of the answers to which entailed global inferencing across information provided in the narrative. On both these tasks adults with AS performed more poorly than controls, reflecting their difficulties in processing higher-order aspects of language in context.

Children with AS also have difficulty interpreting language in social contexts. Baron-Cohen and his colleagues (Baron-Cohen, O'Riordan, Stone, Jones, & Plaisted, 1999) devised a task that involved recognizing when someone commits a *faux pas*, defined as saying something inappropriate in a given social context. Children listened to stories and were asked whether someone in the story had said something they should not have said. The children with AS performed significantly worse than matched controls in recognizing the *faux pas*, even though they clearly understood the story and could identify the mental state of the speaker making the inappropriate comment.

## Language Delay

Perhaps the most controversial criterion used to define AS in the ICD-10 and DSM-IV is the requirement that only children who display no delay in acquiring language receive this diagnosis. Indeed, many view this criterion as the primary means for distinguishing between AS and HFA. According to the DSM-IV (American Psychiatric Association, 1994), children receiving the diagnosis of AS must speak their first words before the age of 2 and phrases before 3. There are several problems in implementing this criterion in everyday practice (Siegel, 1996). First, as has been noted by other researchers (e.g., Twachtman-Cullen, 1998), these age limits are extremely generous, given that normative data indicate that, on average, children produce their first word between 10 and 12 months of age and phrases by 18–20 months (cf. Fenson et al., 1994). Second, clinicians and researchers depend on parental report of when their children began to speak, and parents are notoriously poor at retrospective recall, especially as their children get older. Finally, it is interesting to note that using this criterion, two of

Asperger's four case studies (Ernst and Hellmuth) described in the introduction would not have received the diagnosis of AS in today's clinical practice.

Several studies have been conducted to investigate whether there are differences between children who display delayed onset of language and children with no language delay. Most of these studies have explored many different behavioral characteristics; here we focus on whether these groups are different in their current language functioning. Mayes and Calhoun (2001) divided their sample of children with ASD on the basis of those with language delay and those without. The parents of all the children completed a checklist of autism symptoms developed by the authors. No differences were found between the groups on any of the items that tapped expressive language, including Verbal IQ, conversational speech, and atypical speech patterns. Using a different approach, Manjiviona and Prior (1999) compared groups of children who had received a clinical diagnosis of autism or AS on a neuropsychological assessment battery. They also reclassified the children on the basis of whether or not their language was delayed. The children with AS had higher overall IQ scores, due mainly to their Verbal IQ. In contrast, there were no differences between the groups of children with or without delays in the onset of language.

Eisenmajer and his colleagues (1998) compared a large sample of about 100 children clinically diagnosed either with HFA or AS. The parents completed a lengthy interview about their children's developmental history, current symptoms, and behavior, and the children were assessed on a standardized test of receptive vocabulary (the Peabody Picture Vocabulary Test or equivalent). Across both the diagnostic groups, just under half the total sample was delayed in language, and the main analyses compared the children with and without language delay. There were two chief differences in the developmental histories of the two groups: (1) The children who were delayed in language onset did not babble and failed to imitate other people's actions and gestures; (2) the language-delayed children also had lower receptive vocabulary scores but were no different in expressive language symptoms such as echolalia, pronoun reversal errors, or neologisms.

## Summary

Children and adults with AS suffer from a wide range of language and communicative abnormalities. These include deficits in expressive language, such as odd speech and poor use of vocal prosody, pedantic or formal speech style, deficits in conversational discourse, and difficulties in using and understanding nonliteral language. According to several of the studies summarized here, clinical diagnoses of AS are not systematically restricted to those children who showed no delays in acquiring language. The evidence summarized here also suggests that there are few meaningful differences between children with and without language delay.

## ARE THERE DIFFERENCES BETWEEN AUTISM AND ASPERGER SYNDROME IN LANGUAGE AND COMMUNICATION?

This review underscores the presence of a wide variety of language abnormalities in AS, supporting the views expressed by many clinicians and researchers (e.g., Ghaziuddin, Weidmer-Mikhail, & Ghaziuddin, 1998; Gillberg & Ehlers, 1998; Klin & Volkmar, 1995; Siegel, 1996). These findings have led some researchers to question the validity of the Asperger diagnosis (e.g., Schopler, 1996), especially since the only distinction between autism and AS in the DSM-IV or ICD-10 pertains to language onset. In this section we review the literature on the similarities and differences between autism and AS in language impairment in order to assess how clearly these syndromes might be differentiated.

### Pragmatic Problems in Autism

Unlike in AS, a significant proportion of children with autism do not acquire functional language (Lord & Paul, 1997). Many of these nonverbal children are low functioning, which suggests that, at the extremes, there is a clear distinction between autism and AS. At the same time, high-functioning verbal children with autism are much more similar to children with AS, and they experience a broad range of language and pragmatic deficits that parallel those identified in children with AS. For example, autism is associated with abnormalities in vocal expression and prosody (Fay & Schuler, 1980; Lord & Rutter, 1994) and the use of idiosyncratic terms and neologisms (Volden & Lord, 1991), which were also noted by Hans Asperger (1944/1991). Communicative deficits have been widely investigated in different discourse contexts. Children with autism use language in restricted ways, primarily for request making or self-regulation (Loveland, Landry, Hughes, Hall, & McEvoy, 1988; Wetherby & Prutting, 1984), and have difficulty maintaining and expanding an ongoing topic of conversation (Capps, Kehres, & Sigman, 1998; Tager-Flusberg & Anderson, 1991). The ability to tell a story is also quite impaired in children with autism (Loveland & Tunali, 1993; Tager-Flusberg, 1995; Tager-Flusberg & Sullivan, 1995), and they often provide too much or too little information in everyday discourse, making it difficult for listeners to understand them (Paul & Cohen, 1984; Surian, Baron-Cohen, & Van der Lely, 1996). These conversational deficits are viewed as closely linked to the social impairments associated with autism, as they are in AS (Tager-Flusberg, 2000).

## Overlap between Autism and Asperger Diagnoses

Numerous researchers and clinicians have evaluated the similarities between autism and AS. Some have concluded that there are no real distinctions between these diagnostic groups (Gillberg, 1989; Mayes, Calhoun, & Crites, 2001). However, different researchers use different criteria to define AS, which obscures any potential differences between the groups. For example, Gillberg (1989) includes communicative impairments among the criteria for AS; in his view the main difference between autism and AS is the greater motor clumsiness found among people with the Asperger diagnosis (Ehlers & Gillberg, 1993). Several studies have explored the potential overlap between autism and AS, and most conclude that this overlap is very significant (Szatmari, 2000). Leekam, Libby, Wing, Gould, and Gillberg (2000) found that among 200 individuals with an ASD, only three met the ICD-10 criteria for AS, in that they did not have language or communicative impairments. Using the absence of language delay as a diagnostic criterion for AS, Gilchrist and her colleagues found that 80% of adolescents diagnosed with AS met criteria for autism on the Autism Diagnostic Interview—Revised Edition (ADI-R), the most widely used instrument in research investigations for diagnosing autism (Gilchrist et al., 2001). Szatmari, Archer, Fisman, Streiner, and Wilson (1995) obtained similar findings in their study of preschoolers. These latter studies suggest that, despite the absence of significant language delays, children with AS have communicative impairments that meet the same criteria as those found in children with autism.

## Are Communicative Deficits Less Severe
## in Asperger Syndrome?

At a qualitative level, there is little to distinguish between the communicative deficits in autism and AS. Nevertheless, several studies directly compared the pragmatic problems in children with HFA and AS, and several reported that these problems are less severe in AS. For example, Gilchrist and colleagues (2001) reported that adolescents with AS were less impaired in structured dyadic conversation than age- and IQ-matched adolescents with autism. Bishop and Baird (2001) used parent and professional ratings of communication difficulties on the Children's Communication Checklist for several different clinical groups. Composite scores on the checklist were lower for the children with autism compared to the children with AS. Several studies discussed earlier also show this same pattern of less severe problems in participants with AS (e.g., Jolliffe & Baron-Cohen, 1999, 2000).

On the other hand, Ramberg and colleagues (1996) found no differences between their participants with autism and AS, and Eisenmajer and colleagues (1996) reported that their participants with AS were *more* likely than the autism group to have problems with turn taking, use of idiosyncratic words and phrases, and a pedantic speech style with a flat, monotonous vocal tone. Fine and colleagues (1994) also found that their participants with AS were worse than HFA adults on measures of discourse cohesion, especially use of unclear reference.

Given the widely different diagnostic criteria used across studies for differentiating between autism and AS, it is not surprising that no clear pattern of findings has been found. Furthermore, the wide variability and heterogeneity in symptom expression that is found among people with AS and people with autism also contributes to the lack of any clear pattern of severity differences. Across most studies, autism and AS cannot be clearly distinguished from one another at the level of pragmatic impairment. Instead, it seems likely that the *same* symptoms are found in both syndromes, suggesting much greater similarity between them than is suggested by the most widely used classification systems (American Psychiatric Association, 1994).

## Verbal and Linguistic Abilities in Asperger Syndrome

Studies that have compared autism and AS on other aspects of language have yielded a more consistent picture. Outside the domain of pragmatics, research has focused on verbal reasoning skills, as assessed on IQ tests, or vocabulary, syntactic, and higher-order semantic abilities, as assessed on standardized language tests. Across most studies, participants with AS have significantly better language and verbal skills compared to participants with autism. For some clinicians, high Verbal IQ is a defining feature of AS (e.g., Nass & Gutman, 1997). This feature is consistent with findings from several studies using standardized IQ tests, which have found normal Verbal scores among participants with AS (Eisenmajer et al., 1996; Ramberg et al., 1996).

Ghaziuddin and his colleagues (2000) compared children with autism and AS on measures of syntactic complexity that were coded from natural language samples. They found significant differences between the groups in both sentence length and syntactic complexity, with the AS group using more advanced linguistic skills in spontaneous speech. Iwanaga, Kawasaki, and Tsuchida (2000) also found that syntactic comprehension was better in their preschool-age sample of children with AS, as measured by sentence repetition skills and the ability to follow directions in a standardized assessment protocol.

Szatmari and colleagues (1995) conducted the most systematic comparison of language skills in nonretarded preschoolers with autism and AS, using standardized language tests. The groups were differentiated diagnostically on the basis of delays in the onset of language, following DSM-IV criteria. They found that the children with AS performed significantly better than the children with autism on measures of vocabulary, higher-order syntax, and semantics. In contrast, the groups were not different on pragmatic impairments, adaptive scores, or other neuropsychological measures. More recently Szatmari and his colleagues (Szatmari et al., 2000) conducted a 2-year follow-up of these same children and found that, as a group, the children with AS continued to perform better than the children with autism on the language tests, with their scores now firmly in the normal range. However, language scores at this point were better predicted by the children's initial language scores than by their clinical diagnosis. Thus some of the children with a history of language delay had good language test scores by the time they had reached the preschool years. Language test scores, rather than delayed onset, were the only significant predictor of later outcomes for children with ASD. The preschool children with autism diagnoses who had fluent language, as measured on the language tests, were later indistinguishable from the children with AS. Szatmari and colleagues (2000) suggest that verbal abilities are a very important predictor of outcomes but that among children with ASD, there may be some differences in the early developmental timing.

The most consistent difference found between groups of individuals with ASD is in the domain of verbal and linguistic abilities. Szatmari's longitudinal study provided evidence that linguistic skills were important for predicting outcomes in verbal, but not pragmatic, abilities. Furthermore, delayed onset was not a significant predictor of later abilities, and most children who met DSM-IV or ICD-10 criteria for AS also met criteria for autism on diagnostic measures such as the ADI-R.

## Diagnostic Differences between Autism and Asperger Syndrome

The literature on language and communicative impairments in AS suggests that the current DSM/ICD criteria have no clinical or empirical validity. Children with ASD, with and without language delay, are not clearly different from one another, and virtually all individuals with AS have communicative impairments that are strikingly similar to the defining features of classic autism. At the same time, there are important differences between individuals with good structural language abilities and those with impaired language, as illustrated in Szatmari and colleagues' (2000) study. Language abilities predict social and adaptive outcomes and may be highly correlated with measures of other neuropsychological and social cognitive measures (cf. Lord & Paul, 1997; Tager-Flusberg, 2000).

Recently, we investigated language profiles in a large group of verbal children with autism, using a battery of standardized tests (Kjelgaard & Tager-Flusberg, 2001). The children, ages 5–14 years, all met criteria for autism (using the ADI-R and the ADOS). Based on their performance on the language tests, the children were divided into subgroups. About 75% of the children had language scores that were significantly below the mean. These children had distinctive profiles of performance across the language measures, suggesting that they formed a subtype of children with autism and language disorder. About 25% of the children had language scores in the normal range, and their profile of scores was considerably different from what was found for the children with language disorder. Thus, among children meeting a diagnosis of autism, some display normal language abilities. These children are verbally fluent and seem to be the same children who would be classified as AS by other clinicians and researchers.

Across the spectrum of children and adults with pervasive developmental disorders (PDD), there are some with normal cognitive abilities, as measured by IQ tests, and some with normal linguistic skills, as measured by language tests. These abilities vary in a dimensional rather than categorical way, and they are correlated with one another. However, some individuals with normal IQ scores show impaired language, and some with low IQ scores show normal language. The best outcomes for people with ASD are associated with the combination of normal IQ and language. If we are to move toward a reliable and valid way of differentiating between autism and AS, then perhaps these are the criteria that should be used in future classification systems. Many clinicians are already applying these criteria for defining AS in everyday practice, depending more on intuitive judgment of verbal fluency and intact cognitive skills, and less on developmental history of language delay. Diagnostic criteria for AS should include impairments in communication, along with impairments in social reciprocity and circumscribed interests, thereby moving us away from the contradictions that currently exist in both the DSM-IV and ICD-10.

## THE SIGNIFICANCE OF INTACT LINGUISTIC SKILLS FOR LEARNING AND BEHAVIOR

As we have seen, people with AS have good verbal abilities. They acquire rich and varied vocabularies and excellent grammatical skills during the preschool or early school years. Despite these intact language skills, children and adults with AS have impaired communication that adversely affects their social interactions with others, especially peer relationships. Because they often sound so odd, have difficulty understanding language in different contexts, and cannot communicate effectively, people with AS can remain socially isolated and have trouble negotiating the social world at school, work, or in informal settings. Deficits in interpreting nonliteral language may also impact a child's ability to understand written material, especially fictional narratives, and may lead to an avoidance of movies, television, and other media.

Many children with AS can thrive in academic environments, performing well in most, if not all, school subjects. They are able to capitalize on their linguistic ability to acquire basic reading skills, and their social communicative impairments do not affect their learning of other subjects such as mathematics, science, and geography. Language provides the means by which children with AS learn in school and work environments.

There is also evidence that some people with AS use language to acquire some social cognitive skills, which in turn enhance their adaptive functioning in everyday life. For example, Grossman, Klin, Carter, and Volkmar (2000) found that children with AS performed similarly to controls in recognizing facial expressions of emotions when they were paired with neutral or matching verbal labels. They had greater difficulty when the faces were paired with mismatching labels, suggesting that they relied more than the control children on verbal strategies in processing social–affective information. The findings suggest that children with AS can be taught compensatory strategies and that learning to label different emotional expressions—in faces, voices, or body gestures—may be a useful method for teaching social knowledge that is not acquired intuitively. Children with AS need to be taught explicitly the nonverbal social communicative signals that are crucial for everyday functioning in social interactions. The study by Grossman and his colleagues suggest that children with AS can successfully learn these cues via language. Recently Baron-Cohen and his colleagues (1999) developed a computer-based emotions training program, called "Mindreading," for this purpose. The program employs a practical, interactive approach that uses dynamic stimuli across a wide range of emotions to teach emotion-recognition skills (Baron-Cohen, 2002). Future research should focus on the effectiveness of this kind of training, with special reference to how easily (or not) people with AS can transfer the training to improve their social interaction skills in daily life.

Studies on theory of mind, or cognitively based mind-reading abilities, have found that children with AS perform significantly better than children with autism on false-belief and other related tasks (e.g., Eisenmajer et al., 1998; Ozonoff, Rogers, & Pennington, 1991). It has long been known that performance on theory-of-mind tasks is highly correlated with standardized language scores in children with autism (Dahlgren & Trillingsgaard, 1996; Eisenmajer & Prior, 1991; Happé, 1995; Sparrevohn & Howie, 1995;

Tager-Flusberg & Sullivan, 1994). In a recent longitudinal study, using a developmentally sensitive battery of tasks, we found that language was the single best predictor of which children with autism would show the most significant change over 1 year in theory-of-mind abilities (Steele, Joseph, & Tager-Flusberg, in press). More specifically, we found that performance on false-belief tasks was predicted by mastery of grammatical competence, especially with regard to complex embedded sentences (Tager-Flusberg & Joseph, in press). In contrast, false-belief performance did not predict the children's language abilities. In this study, only the children with the most advanced language skills, the majority of whom would be considered by most clinicians as having AS, passed the false-belief tasks. We would suggest that these children used their language and cognitive skills to reason logically through false-belief tasks. In this way, language can be an important bootstrap into social–cognitive understanding for people with AS.

The key to developing interventions for children with AS is to capitalize on their strengths in intellectual ability and language. Linguistic knowledge may be the route to learning about the social world for children with AS. For example, they can be verbally taught about false-belief and other mental states, and how to apply this knowledge in real-world situations. Special attention should be paid to teaching the important cues for how to "compute" the belief states of people, such as attending to other people's desires, intentions, and access to information. Children with AS also need to be taught the lexical terms for mental states, including both emotions and cognitive states, and how they apply in different situations.

As noted earlier, despite their strengths in linguistic knowledge, people with AS continue to experience significant impairments in pragmatics. Again, explicit verbal training, perhaps using role-playing scenarios, could be used to guide the development of more appropriate conversational skills. More attention also should be given to teaching children with AS those aspects of nonliteral language that they find so difficult to grasp. Their social relationships with peers will be significantly influenced by their ability to grasp idiomatic expressions, sarcasm, teasing comments, and lies. As Hans Asperger noted: "to put it bluntly, these individuals are intelligent automatons. Social adaptation has to proceed via the intellect . . . " (1991, p. 58).

## CONCLUSIONS

We began this chapter with a detailed discussion of language and communicative impairments that were identified by Asperger in his seminal paper describing a new syndrome. Many studies conducted over the last two decades have attempted to document the kinds of impairments that characterize individuals who receive the diagnosis of AS, using either clinical judgment or some objective classification system. Across all these studies, it is clear that Asperger's observations of vocal and communicative deficits and unusual speech style have been confirmed. The current official criteria in the DSM-IV and ICD-10 for differentiating between autism and AS on the basis of differences in developmental language history and the absence of communicative deficits are not empirically valid and are no longer tenable.

The one consistent difference found between autism and AS is in the domain of verbal and linguistic abilities. People with AS have superior verbal abilities, and the presence of these abilities has important implications for their ability to do well in some academic learning environments. Some people with AS may use their superior linguistic skills as a means for acquiring affective and cognitive skills that are at the heart of their deficits in social functioning. Future diagnostic systems should consider using this difference in linguistic ability as the basis for differentiating between autism and AS.

## ACKNOWLEDGMENTS

Preparation of this chapter was supported by grants from the National Institutes of Health (PO1 DC 03610 and RO1 NS 38668). I appreciate the help of Alyssa Verbalis and Laura Stetser in writing this chapter.

## REFERENCES

Adams, C., Green, J., Gilchrist, A., & Cox, A. (2002). Conversational behaviour of children with Asperger syndrome and conduct disorder. *Journal of Child Psychology and Psychiatry, 43,* 679–690.

American Psychiatric Association. (1994). *Diagnostic and statistical manual of mental disorders* (4th ed.). Washington, DC: Author.

Asperger, H. (1991). Autistic psychopathy in childhood. In U. Frith (Ed.), *Autism and Asperger syndrome* (pp. 37–91). Cambridge, UK: Cambridge University Press. (Original work published in German 1944)

Baron-Cohen, S. (2002). *Mind reading: The interactive guide to emotions.* Cambridge, UK: Human Emotions Limited.

Baron-Cohen, S., O'Riordan, M., Stone, V., Jones, R., & Plaisted, K. (1999). Recognition of faux pas by normally developing children and children with Asperger syndrome or high-functioning autism. *Journal of Autism and Developmental Disorders, 29,* 407–418.

Bishop, D. V. M., & Baird, G. (2001). Parent and teacher report of pragmatic aspects of communication: Use of the Children's Communication Checklist in a clinical setting. *Developmental Medicine and Child Neurology, 43,* 809–818.

Burgoine, E., & Wing, L. (1983). Identical triplets with Asperger's syndrome. *British Journal of Psychiatry, 143,* 261.

Capps, L., Kehres, J., & Sigman, M. (1998). Conversational abilities among children with autism and children with developmental delays. *Autism, 2*, 325–344.

Dahlgren, S., & Trillingsgaard, A. (1996). Theory of mind in non-retarded children with autism and Asperger's syndrome: A research note. *Journal of Child Psychology and Psychiatry and Allied Disciplines, 37*, 759–763.

Ehlers, S., & Gillberg, C. (1993). The epidemiology of Asperger syndrome. *Journal of Child Psychology and Psychiatry and Allied Disciplines, 34*, 1327–1350.

Eisenmajer, R., & Prior, M. (1991). Cognitive linguistic correlates of "theory of mind" ability in autistic children. *British Journal of Developmental Psychology, 9*, 351–364.

Eisenmajer, R., Prior, M., Leekam, S., Wing, L., Gould, J., Welham, M., & Ong, B. (1996). Comparison of clinical symptoms in autism and Asperger's disorder. *Journal of the American Academy of Child Adolescent Psychiatry, 35*(11), 1523–1531.

Eisenmajer, R., Prior, M., Leekam, S., Wing, L., Ong, B., Gould, J., & Welham, M. (1998). Delayed language onset as a predictor of clinical symptoms in pervasive developmental disorders. *Journal of Autism and Developmental Disorders, 28*, 527–533.

Fay, W. H., & Schuler, A. L. (1980). *Emerging language in autistic children.* Baltimore: University Park Press.

Fenson, L., Dale, P., Reznick, J. S., Bates, E., Thal, D., & Pethick, S. (1994). Variability in early communicative development. *Monographs the Society for Research in Child Development, 59*, v–173.

Fine, J., Bartolucci, G., Szatmari, P., & Ginsberg, G. (1994). Cohesive discourse in pervasive developmental disorders. *Journal of Autism and Developmental Disorders, 24*, 315–330.

Ghaziuddin, M., & Gerstein, L. (1996). Pedantic speaking style differentiates Asperger syndrome from high-functioning autism. *Journal of Autism and Developmental Disorders, 26*, 585–595.

Ghaziuddin, M., Thomas, P., Napier, E., Kearney, G., Tsai, L., Welch, K., & Fraser, W. (2000). Brief report: Brief syntactic analysis in Asperger syndrome: A preliminary study. *Journal of Autism and Developmental Disorders, 30*, 67–70.

Ghaziuddin, M., Weidmer-Mikhail, E., & Ghaziuddin, N. (1998). Comorbidity of Asperger syndrome: A preliminary report. *Journal of Intellectual Disability Research, 42*, 279–283.

Gilchrist, A., Green, J., Cox, A., Burton, D., Rutter, M., & Le Couteur, A. (2001). Development and current functioning in adolescents with Asperger syndrome: A comparative study. *Journal of Child Psychology and Psychiatry, 42*, 227–240.

Gillberg, C. (1989). Asperger syndrome in 23 Swedish children. *Developmental Medicine and Child Neurology, 31*, 520–531.

Gillberg, C., & Ehlers, S. (1998). High-functioning people with autism and Asperger syndrome: A literature review. In E. Schloper, G. Mesibov, & L. Kunce (Eds.), *Asperger syndrome or high-functioning autism?* (pp. 79–106). New York: Plenum Press.

Grossman, J., Klin, A., Carter, A., & Volkmar, F. (2000). Verbal bias in recognition of facial emotions in children with Asperger syndrome. *Journal of Child Psychology and Psychiatry and Allied Disciplines, 41,* 369–379.

Happé, F. (1994). An advanced test of theory of mind: Understanding of story characters' thoughts and feelings by able autistic, mentally handicapped, and normal children and adults. *Journal of Autism and Developmental Disorders, 24,* 129–154.

Happé, F. (1995). The role of age and verbal ability in the theory of mind task performance of subjects with autism. *Child Development, 66,* 843–855.

Iwanaga, R., Kawasaki, C., & Tsuchida, R. (2000) Brief report: Comparison of sensory–motor and cognitive function between autism and Asperger syndrome in preschool children. *Journal of Autism and Developmental Disorders, 30,* 169–174.

Jolliffe, T., & Baron-Cohen, S. (1999). The Strange Stories Test: A replication with high-functioning adults with autism or Asperger syndrome. *Journal of Autism and Developmental Disorders, 29,* 395–406.

Jolliffe, T., & Baron-Cohen, S. (2000). Linguistic processing in high-functioning adults with autism or Asperger's syndrome. Is global coherence impaired? *Psychological Medicine, 30,* 1169–1187.

Kerbel, D., & Grunwell, P. (1998). A study of idiom comprehension in children with semantic–pragmatic difficulties. Part II: Between-groups results and discussion. *International Journal of Language and Communication Disorders, 33,* 23–44.

Kjelgaard, M., & Tager-Flusberg, H. (2001). An investigation of language impairment in autism: Implications for genetic subgroups. *Language and Cognitive Processes, 16,* 287–308.

Klin, A., & Volkmar, F. (1995). Autism and the pervasive developmental disorders. *Child and Adolescent Psychiatric Clinics of North America, 4,* 617–630.

Klin, A., & Volkmar, F. (1997). Asperger's syndrome. In D. J. Cohen & F. R. Volkmar (Eds.), *Handbook of autism and pervasive developmental disorders* (pp. 94–122). New York: Wiley.

Koning, C., & Magill-Evans, J. (2001). Social and language skills in adolescent boys with Asperger syndrome. *Autism, 5*(1), 23–36.

Landa, R. (2000). Social language use in Asperger syndrome and high-functioning autism. In A. Klin, F. R. Volkmar, & S. S. Sparrow (Eds.), *Asperger syndrome* (pp. 125–155). New York: Guilford Press.

Leekam, S., Libby, S., Wing, L., Gould, J., & Gillberg, C. (2000). Comparison of ICD-10 and Gillberg's criteria for Asperger syndrome. *Autism, 4,* 11–28.

Lord, C., & Paul, R. (1997). Language and communication in autism. In D. J. Cohen & F. R. Volkmar (Eds.), *Handbook of autism and pervasive developmental disorders* (2nd ed., pp. 195–225). New York: Wiley.

Lord, C., & Rutter, M. (1994). Autism and pervasive developmental disorders. In M. Rutter, L. Herson, & E. Taylor (Eds.), *Child and adolescent psychiatry: Modern approaches* (3rd ed., pp. 569–593). Oxford, UK: Blackwell.

Loveland, K., Landry, S., Hughes, S., Hall, S., & McEvoy, R. (1988). Speech acts and the pragmatic deficits of autism. *Journal of Speech and Hearing Research, 31,* 593–604.

Loveland, K., & Tunali, B. (1993). Narrative language in autism and the theory of mind hypothesis: A wider perspective. In S. Baron-Cohen, H. Tager-Flusberg, & D. J. Cohen (Eds.), *Understanding other minds: Perspectives from autism.* Oxford, UK: Oxford University Press.

Manjiviona, J., & Prior, M. (1999). Neuropsychological profiles of children with Asperger syndrome and autism. *Autism, 3,* 327–356.

Mayes, S., & Calhoun, S. (2001). Non-significance of early speech delay in children with autism and normal intelligence and implications for DSM-IV Asperger's disorder. *Autism, 5,* 81–94.

Mayes, S., Calhoun, S., & Crites, D. (2001). Does DSM-IV Asperger's disorder exist? *Journal of Abnormal Child Psychology, 29,* 263–271.

Merewether, F. C., & Alpert, M. (1990). The components and neuroanatomic bases of prosody. *Journal of Communication Disorders, 23,* 325–336.

Nass, R., & Gutman, R. (1997). Boys with Asperger's disorder, exceptional verbal intelligence, tics, and clumsiness. *Developmental Medicine and Child Neurology, 39,* 691–695.

Ozonoff, S., Rogers, S. J., & Pennington, B. F. (1991). Asperger's syndrome: Evidence of an empirical distinction from high-functioning autism. *Journal of Child Psychology and Psychiatry, 32,* 1107–1122.

Paul, R., & Cohen, D. J. (1984). Responses to contingent queries in adults with mental retardation and pervasive developmental disorders. *Applied Psycholinguistics, 5,* 349–357.

Ramberg, C., Ehlers, S., Nyden, A., Johansson, M., & Gillberg, C. (1996). Language and pragmatic functions in school-age children on the autism spectrum. *European Journal of Disorders of Communication, 31*(4), 387–413.

Schopler, E. (1996). Are autism and Asperger syndrome (AS) different labels or different disabilities? *Journal of Autism and Developmental Disorders, 26,* 109–110.

Shriberg, L., Paul, R., McSweeney, J., Klin, A., Cohen, D., & Volkmar, F. (2001). Speech and prosody characteristics of adolescents and adults with high-functioning autism and AS. *Journal of Speech, Language, and Hearing Research, 44,* 1097–1115.

Siegel, B. (1996). *The world of the autistic child: Understanding and treating autistic spectrum disorders.* New York: Oxford University Press.

Sparrevohn, R., & Howie, P. (1995). Theory of mind children with autistic disorder: Evidence of developmental progression and the role of verbal ability. *Journal of Child Psychology and Psychiatry, 36,* 249–263.

Steele, S., Joseph, R. M., & Tager-Flusberg, H. (in press). Developmental change in theory of mind abilities in children with autism. *Journal of Autism and Developmental Disorders.*

Surian, L., Baron-Cohen, S., & Van der Lely, H. (1996). Are children with autism deaf to Gricean maxims? *Cognitive Neuropsychiatry, 1,* 55–72.

Szatmari, P. (2000). Perspectives on the classification of Asperger syndrome. In A. Klin, F. R. Volkmar, & S. S. Sparrow (Eds.) *Asperger syndrome* (pp. 403–417). New York: Guilford Press.

Szatmari, P., Archer, L., Fisman, S., Streiner, D., & Wilson, F. (1995). Asperger's syndrome and autism: Differences in behavior, cognition, and adaptive functioning. *Journal of the American Academy of Child and Adolescent Psychiatry,* *34,* 1662–1671.

Szatmari, P., Bryson, S., Streiner, D., Wilson, F., Archer, L., & Ryerse, C. (2000). Two-year outcome of preschool children with autism or Asperger's syndrome. *American Journal of Psychiatry, 157,* 1980–1987.

Tager-Flusberg, H. (1995). "Once upon a ribbit": Stories narrated by autistic children. *British Journal of Developmental Psychology, 13,* 45–59.

Tager-Flusberg, H. (2000). Understanding the language and communicative impairments in autism. In L. M. Glidden (Ed.), *Autism* (pp. 185–205). San Diego, CA: Academic Press.

Tager-Flusberg, H., & Anderson, M. (1991). The development of contingent discourse ability in autistic children. *Journal of Child Psychology and Psychiatry, 32,* 1123–1134.

Tager-Flusberg, H., & Joseph, R. M. (in press). How language facilitates the acquisition of false belief in children with autism. In J. Astington & J. Baird (Eds.), *Why language matters for theory of mind.* Oxford, UK: Oxford University Press.

Tager-Flusberg, H., & Sullivan, K. (1994). Predicting and explaining behavior: A comparison of autistic, mentally retarded and normal children. *Journal of Child Psychology and Psychiatry, 35,* 1059–1075.

Tager-Flusberg, H., & Sullivan, K. (1995). Attributing mental states to story characters: A comparison of narratives produced by autistic and mentally retarded individuals. *Applied Psycholinguistics, 16,* 241–256.

Twachtman-Cullen, D. (1998). Language and communication in high-functioning autism and AS. In E. Schloper, G. Mesibov, & L. Kunce (Eds.), *Asperger syndrome or high-functioning autism?* (pp. 199–225). New York: Plenum Press.

Volden, J., & Lord, C. (1991). Neologisms and idiosyncratic language in autistic speakers. *Journal of Autism and Developmental Disorders, 21,* 109–130.

Wetherby, A., & Prutting, C. (1984). Profiles of communicative and cognitive–social abilities in autistic children. *Journal of Speech and Hearing Research, 27,* 364–377.

Wing, L. (1981). Asperger's syndrome: A clinical account. *Journal of Autism and Developmental Disorders, 9,* 11–29.

Wing, L. (1991). The relationship between Asperger's syndrome and Kanner's autism. In U. Frith (Ed.), *Autism and Asperger syndrome* (pp. 93–121). Cambridge, UK: Cambridge University Press.

# 5

# Understanding Social Difficulties

## MICHAL SHAKED
## NURIT YIRMIYA

Impairments in social relationships constitute one of the main characteristics of high-functioning individuals with autism, or Asperger syndrome (AS). These difficulties confer on the syndrome its autistic (i.e., the "alone") quality (Yirmiya & Sigman, 1991). Social impairments are at the heart of the disorder and, for the individual with AS, have far-reaching consequences in all areas of development and adaptation. A diagnosis of AS may first be considered when the child encounters, and responds to, a new social challenge, such as that presented by playground or classroom interactions (Tantam, 2000). Because of their average or above-average cognitive abilities, individuals with AS are often integrated into mainstream schools and occupational vocations. Social skills are a significant, if not crucial, component in trying to fit in and succeed in such settings, and it is therefore extremely important to help them improve their social skills and social integration in a myriad of life contexts.

## DIAGNOSTIC CRITERIA PERTAINING
## TO SOCIAL DIFFICULTIES

Asperger himself (1944/1991) emphasized poor social adaptation, as well as other features that contribute to social difficulties, such as impairments in nonverbal communication; idiosyncrasies in verbal communication; special interests, including egocentric preoccupations with particular topics; and poor empathy, with a tendency to intellectualize feelings (see Frith's [1991] translation). Since Asperger's initial description, diagnostic features of the syndrome have changed considerably, but social inadequacy remains one of the syndrome's hallmarks, as defined and described by different theorists and clinicians. Wing (1981) detailed difficulties in social interaction, including absence of reciprocal social interaction, difficulties in understanding implicit rules governing social behavior, naive or inappropriate behavior, and lack of empathy. She also mentions that children with AS are often bullied and teased by others. Similarly, Gillberg and Gillberg (1989) described impairments in reciprocal social interaction. According to their diagnostic criteria, an individual with AS must display at least two of the following features: inability to interact with peers, lack of desire to interact with peers, lack of appreciation of social cues, and socially and emotionally inappropriate behavior

Tantam's (1991) account of AS includes difficulty in behaving according to socially accepted conventions and lack of close peer relationships. Szatmari, Bremner, and Nagy (1989) include criteria for solitary behavior in their diagnostic scheme: lack of friends, avoidance of others, lack of interest in making friends, and preference for being alone. They also list criteria identifying impaired social interaction, including approaching others only to have own needs met, clumsy social approach, one-sided responses to peers, difficulty sensing feelings of others, and detachment from others' feelings. Consistent with Asperger's description, other writers nominate criteria pertaining to difficulties in nonverbal communication, odd or idiosyncratic speech, and unusual interests, all of which undoubtedly contributes to difficulties in social integration (see also Ehlers & Gillberg, 1993; Howlin, 2000).

## CLINICAL DESCRIPTION
## OF SOCIAL IMPAIRMENTS

Wing and Gould (1979) described the fundamental difficulty in the social functioning of the individual with autism as a triad of impairments spanning social interaction, reciprocal social communication, and socially oriented imaginative pretend play. Children with high-functioning autism (HFA) and children with AS demonstrate impairments in their relationships with peers, difficulties with participating in reciprocal conversations and using nonverbal communication cues within social exchanges, impaired empathy, lack of joint attention, difficulties in understanding others' thoughts, and a consequent inability to predict others' behavior and respond appropriately (Howlin, 1998; National Research Council, 2001; Yirmiya, Sigman, Kasari, & Mundy, 1992).

## Impairments in Communication

A major part of social interaction relies on the participants' ability to communicate thoughts, feelings, ideas, and desires. According to the DSM-IV descriptive criteria (American Psychiatric Association, 1994), "there is no clinically significant general delay in language" in AS, yet individuals with this syndrome do display impairments in several communicative aspects of language (Twachtman-Cullen, 1998). Early on in their development, young children with autism spectrum disorders (ASD) reveal difficulties in those communicative behaviors that enable individuals to enter into each other's experience of the world (Sigman & Capps, 1997). Eye contact is a central component of communication. During a conversation, people use eye contact for different purposes: when starting an utterance, when acknowledging something, when seeking clarification, emphasizing a point, or when ending an utterance. This range of eye-contact usage is often missing in the conversation of individuals diagnosed with AS (Attwood, 1998). They seem to lack the capacity for using eye contact when listening to another person talking (Tantam, Holmes, & Cordess, 1993), and clinical reports indicate that individuals with AS may find it difficult to concentrate on what is said while making eye contact (see Lawson, Chapter 8, this volume). They also lack the ability to use eye contact to acquire information about the other person's mental state or feelings (Attwood, 1998; Yirmiya, Pilowsky, Solomonica-Levi, & Shulman, 1999). What seems to be impaired is the specific use of social gaze to (1) emphasize certain points in conversation, (2) reciprocate others' attempts at getting their attention, (3) convey shared interests with others, and (4) use others' expressions as an aid for deciphering ambiguous situations (Tantam, 1992).

The conversational style of individuals with AS is best described as egocentric, because they often engage in one-sided, unrelenting monologues about their topic of interest. Their speech tends to be poorly organized, and they have severe difficulties with issues of contingency, reciprocity, pragmatics, and other rules of discourse. Furthermore, individuals with AS have distinct difficulties in picking up and following listeners' cues, such as those indicating lack of interest or attempts to change the topic (Howlin, 1998; Volkmar & Klin, 2000). They find it hard to make conversational adjustments to fit different social contexts or the needs of different listeners. Nonverbal aspects of conversation also are problematic (Koning & Magill-Evans, 2001). They often use inappropriate body language and do not appear to recognize others' intentions, as conveyed through nonverbal cues

(Gross, 1994). They have apparent difficulties with prosody, in both expression of language and extraction of the meanings implicit in the prosody of others' speech (Rumsey, 1992; Twachtman-Cullen, 1998).

Informal observation of language use in individuals with autism and AS suggests that they prefer conversations about facts and information and tend to avoid conversations about social–emotional material (Twachtam-Cullen, 1998)—a tendency that further limits their ability to join in social conversations, as these are often laden with affective elements. Finally, individuals with AS are reported to be literal in both their interpretation and use of language (Rumsey, 1992; Twachtman-Cullen, 1998) and tend to use idiosyncratic words and metaphors (Szatmari et al., 1989; Twachtman-Cullen, 1998), thus making it difficult for others to understand their conversation.

## Understanding Emotions

Individuals with HFA and AS display various difficulties in understanding and expressing complex emotions (Capps, Yirmiya, & Sigman, 1992; Macdonald et al., 1989). In laboratory experiments, individuals with HFA show marked impairments in their capacity to discriminate facial, gestural, and vocal emotional expressions, and to recognize how different expressions are coordinated with each other (Hobson, 1986a, 1986b; Hobson, Outson, & Lee, 1988). They also have difficulties in labeling expressed emotions (videotaped protagonists; Yirmiya et al., 1992) and emotions suggested by facial expression (Davies, Bishop, Manstead, & Tantam, 1994). Further impairments have been found in the task of matching the prosodic and linguistic expressions of different emotions with facial expressions of these emotions (Van Lancker, Cornelius, & Kreiman, 1989). Empathic reactions to others' display of distress are also lacking (Sigman, Kasari, Kwon, & Yirmiya, 1992). Clinical observations show that even when the child understands very clear facial expressions and body language, more subtle cues are often missed (Attwood, 1998; Hobson, 1992). There are difficulties not only in understanding others' emotional expression but also in expressing emotions. Children with AS do not usually display the anticipated range and depth of facial expression (Capps et al., 1992) during conversation or when playing, and their facial features tend to have a somewhat wooden quality.

## Theory of Mind

A major advancement in our understanding of autism and AS has come through research on theory-of-mind abilities in typically developing children, as well as in those with pervasive developmental disorders (PDD;

Yirmiya, Erel, Shaked, & Solomonica-Levi, 1998). This research sheds important light on our understanding of the specific social difficulties displayed by children with AS. Children as young as 4 years have what has been termed a "theory of mind"—that is, they understand that other people have thoughts, beliefs, and desires, and that these influence their behavior (e.g., Astington, Harris, & Olson, 1988; Frye & Moore, 1991). In contrast, children with autism and AS show significant difficulties in their ability to conceptualize and appreciate others' thoughts.

However, theory-of-mind impairments in individuals with AS may be subtle. Several researchers have shown that these individuals have adequate theory-of-mind abilities when tested on relatively simple tasks, such as the classic first- and second-order false-belief tasks (Bowler, 1992; Dahlgren & Trillingsgaard, 1996; Leekam & Prior, 1994; Ozonoff, Rogers, & Pennington, 1991). Yet this ability is reached at a later developmental stage (Frith, 1996; Frith & Happé, 1999; Yirmiya et al., 1998).

Various tasks designed to assess theory-of-mind abilities have revealed mind-reading difficulties in individuals with HFA and AS. Impairments include inability to (1) provide mental-state justifications for story characters' nonliteral utterances (Happé, 1994; Heavey, Phillips, Baron-Cohen, & Rutter, 2000), (2) infer a person's mental state from a photograph of his or her eye region (Baron-Cohen, Jolliffe, Mortimore, & Robertson, 1997), (3) recognize faux pas (Baron-Cohen, O'Riordan, Stone, Jones, & Plaisted, 1999), and (4) answer questions on mental states of characters presented in film excerpts, most of whom experience a socially uncomfortable and unpleasant moment (Heavey et al., 2000). These individuals also show marked difficulties in providing narratives that describe cartoon animations in which geometric shapes enact a social plot (Castelli, Frith, Happé, & Frith, 2002; Klin, 2000). The attribution of mental states is vital in social interaction and communication. In its absence, it would be extremely difficult to understand and predict people's behavior, to cooperate, to lie, to understand humor, and much more (Frith & Happé, 1999). All of these are indeed areas of difficulty for individuals with HFA or AS.

## Social Understanding and Codes of Conduct

Children with AS find it very difficult to understand social situations. This difficulty occurs in simple one-to-one situations in which they are expected, for instance, to hold a conversation or to join in reciprocal games; and it is doubly evident in more complex situations involving more than two participants. They are often described as impaired or lacking in "common sense" (Green, Gilchrist, Burton, & Cox, 2000). Because they are often unaware of tacit rules of social conduct, they are liable to say or do things inadvertently that may offend or annoy others. They may make inappropriate comments on others' looks or behavior or may intrude on other people's privacy by walking into their homes or barging into their conversations. They often give the impression of being rude, inconsiderate, or spoiled (Attwood, 1998).

Trying to teach codes of conduct to children with AS can prove quite taxing. Applying these codes requires an ability to perceive and understand complex and changeable subtle social cues and nuances. Children with AS often do not pick up these subtle differences. When taught certain codes of conduct, they tend to apply them rigidly, without real understanding, and in ways that can get them into new, unforeseen trouble (Attwood, 1998). As a result, they find it extremely difficult to join into the social world at school, with all its complex rules of conduct, social sensitivities, and emphasis on fashion and status.

## Interaction and Play with Other Children

Children with AS frequently do not seem to know how to play with other children. They may seem unmotivated to join in play, preferring to be by themselves or to play with much younger or older children. Often they are not interested in the same activities as other children, nor are they inclined to explain what they are doing in a way that would enable another party to join them. When interrupted in the middle of a solitary game, the child with AS may react abruptly or even aggressively, defending his or her solitary world (Attwood, 1998).

Alternatively, the child may actively attempt to join children his or her own age in play, but the gesture is clumsy and not successful (Prior et al., 1998; Volkmar & Klin, 2000; Wing, 1992). This scenario is especially likely to occur in older children who are beginning to have a sense of their isolation and to feel genuinely motivated to socialize with children their own age. However, their attempts at socializing soon reveal that their social play skills are immature and rigid. Moreover, their ability to monitor others' reactions to their social attempts is limited (Kerbeshian, Burd, & Fisher, 1990). Case studies of adolescents indicate that they experience discomfort and anxiety in social situations and show a limited ability to interact with peers (Berthier, Santamaria, Encabo, & Toosa, 1992; Cesaroni & Garber, 1991; Ghaziuddin, Weidemer-Mikhail, & Ghaziuddin, 1998). Their behavior is usually marked by lack of reciprocity, little appreciation of social cues, and failure to share enjoyment, interests, or achievements with others (Attwood, 2000). In play, children with AS may try to impose or dictate the activity, tolerating social contact only as long as others are willing to play according to their rules (Attwood, 1998).

In school settings there are periods in which interactions among the students are not structured or monitored by teachers. During such times children with AS often find themselves on their own. They can be seen in a secluded area of the playground or in the library, reading about their subjects of interest. Often they are not interested in competitive sports or team games, are unable to join in any real and dynamic imaginative play, and are clumsy and unrewarding in conversations. Consequently, other children do not invite them to join in activities during school hours or outside them, such as parties (Attwood, 1998).

Children with AS find it difficult to form and sustain close relationships and friendships with others (Green et al., 2000). Indeed research indicates that they have immature or unusual definitions of friendship (Bauminger & Kasari, 2000; Botroff, Bartak, Langford, Page, & Tonge, 1995). Because they lack understanding of social rules of conduct, individuals with AS may spoil potential friendships by misjudging the appropriate level of self-disclosure. Furthermore, because they lack an understanding of others' mental states and emotions, they may misjudge others' approaches to them (Attwood, 1998). As a result, they often fail to develop satisfactory close interpersonal contacts. However, some do make valued associations with another child or adolescent who shares their specific interests and proclivities.

## CONSEQUENCES OF SOCIAL DIFFICULTIES

The impairments in social skills described above have significant consequences for social integration. Unfortunately, suitable programs for children and adolescents with AS are still lacking. Programs for children with autism or learning disabilities, in general, are not suitable for the unique needs and assets of individuals with AS (Klin, Volkmar, & Sparrow, 2000). Children with AS are usually placed in mainstream schools (Kadesjo, Gillberg, & Hagberg, 1999; Kasari, Freeman, Bauminger, & Alkin, 1999; Tantam, 2000), often without any additional help (Wing, 1992). Insufficient knowledge and understanding of the syndrome in mainstream schools where children with AS are placed often can lead to misunderstandings that may further aggravate their emotional and behavioral difficulties (Mishna & Muskat, 1998).

In social interaction, children with AS encounter a spate of difficulties, especially during unstructured time. Their lack of social common sense, their difficulties in communicating and understanding emotions and mental states, their eccentricities, rigidities associated with moral dictates and inflexible routines, as well as incessant questions and obsessions (Klin et al.,

2000)—all these lead to, and result in, inappropriate social interactions. Many children and adolescents with AS are conscious of their social difficulties and express distress about their lack of friends (Carrington & Graham, 2001), low self-esteem (Capps, Sigman, & Yirmiya, 1995), concerns about peer interactions outside the classroom setting, and a desire for individual activity to fill, for example, lunchtime periods (Connor, 2001).

Whereas younger children are sometimes indifferent to isolation and content to play by themselves, older children with AS usually become increasingly aware of, and frustrated by, their isolation (Attwood, 1998; Wing, 1992). Some individuals with AS continue coping with this isolation by taking refuge in their special world of idiosyncratic interests, routines, and preoccupations. Others are all too painfully aware of their desire for closeness, as well as of how others view them and why they are socially rejected. This awareness often leads to depression (Tantam, 2000; Wing, 1992). Thus individuals with AS may become more distressed by their condition as they become older.

In addition to rejection and isolation, children with AS often suffer from victimization, including teasing and physical bullying (Green et al., 2000; Little, 2001; Tantam, 2000). Typically developing children are quick to recognize oddity, and their reactions often include bullying (Wing, 1992). Yet another concern is the possible abuse of children with AS by those who recognize their naiveté. Exploitation may involve relatively benign intentions and acts, such as encouraging the child with AS to ask others (children and adults) for, and about, certain things, some of which may be inappropriate socially, or can extend to more serious incidents, such as loaning money or even involvement in crimes (Attwood, 1998; Tantam, 2000).

## INTERVENTIONS DESIGNED TO PROMOTE SOCIAL INTEGRATION

The detailed clinical descriptions given above indicate that social impairments in children with HFA, or AS, are both serious and extensive, ranging over a wide array of skills and situations. Specific intervention programs usually focus on one or two areas of social difficulties in a structured and contained manner. One of the impediments to developing interventions designed to increase social skills and improve social integration in this population is the fact that much of human social behavior occurs beyond the ken of conscious attention and is not easily captured and defined (Wing, 1992). Furthermore, it is important to remember that children's social life in school settings is often neither structured nor well contained. Thus, in addition to specific therapies or interventions, careful consideration must be given throughout the day to supervision and guidance of social encounters.

## General Guidelines for Intervention Programs

Any intervention program must begin with a process of assessing existing skills, defining goals, and designing teaching strategies to achieve these goals. In general, most educational programs and approaches for children with ASD fall into one of two theoretical frameworks: developmental or behavioral. To define general goals, the developmental approach employs a model of typical development. It assesses the child's current functioning in the area under consideration in order to tailor specific goals that are assessed to be in the child's area of proximal development (Vygotsky, 1976)— that is, the set of skills the child appears to be ready to learn next.

In a behavioral approach, the child's current functioning is assessed in terms of behavioral excesses (i.e., an abnormal frequency in the emergence of certain undesirable behaviors) and behavioral deficits (i.e., the absence, or low frequency of, typical skills) (Lovaas, 1987). Behavioral interventions are then designed to increase valued behaviors and decrease undesired ones (National Research Council, 2001). When defining target behaviors for intervention, it is important to acknowledge the interdependence of different areas of functioning. Thus, alongside the identification and definition of target behaviors in social interaction and social communication (e.g., Goldstein, Kaczmarek, Pennington, & Shafer, 1992; Odom & Ogawa, 1992; Strain, 1983), it is important to consider verbal abilities (National Research Council, 2001) and play skills (Nadel & Peze, 1993).

## Intervention Techniques

The various techniques used with this population can be divided into four main groups: (1) adult-directed instruction of specific components of social interactions; (2) child-centered approaches, in which adults follow children's leads, stimulate and continue interactions, and, in general, foster higher-level and longer rounds of interaction; (3) peer strategies, in which either adults or peers prompt and sustain social engagement (National Research Council, 2001); and (4) group therapies, in which adult or peer leaders encourage social interactions and discussions within a group of handicapped children. The choice of strategies should be based on both theoretical considerations and assessment of the individual needs of the child or children involved (National Research Council, 2001). Adult-directed instruction, usually more appropriate for younger children with autism who show a very limited range of social behaviors, may be less relevant for children with HFA or AS. Peer strategies and group interventions are usually advised for these higher-functioning individuals who do show a range of social behaviors, even if inadequate ones, as well as a certain degree of social motivation. Another consideration is the child's cognitive abilities. For instance, interventions that require reading ability or engagement in more abstract discussions of social situations are more advisable for high-functioning children who possess the required developmental skills.

## Peer-Mediated Approach

The focus of this strategy is to increase the social behaviors exhibited by children with disabilities by teaching peers to initiate interaction with them and to respond to their social initiations, thus reinforcing their behavior. In this approach, typically developing peers are taught to initiate and repeat behaviors designed to organize play (e.g., sharing, helping, and praise) and to initiate and maintain communication that fosters interaction (e.g., attending to, commenting on, and acknowledging the behavior of the other). Peers are taught these strategies through role play with adults and practice sessions with other peers, and then are cued by adults to use the strategies with children who have an ASD. A targeted behavior, such as maintaining attention, is subdivided into several steps (e.g., the peer moves in front of the child, looking at him or her and/or the toys, saying his or her name and repeating it when necessary, etc.). Researchers have shown this intervention program to be effective in increasing social interactions and have demonstrated processes of generalization and maintenance of the social skills acquired (e.g., Golstein et al., 1992; Hoyson, Jameison, & Strain, 1984; Laushey & Heflin, 2000). This approach has been extended by teaching peers to participate in both parallel and interactive forms of play with the child, and by teaching the child to initiate strategies as well (Oke & Schreibman, 1990).

## Circle of Friends

The aim of this approach is to facilitate the inclusion of vulnerable children, such as those with AS, into the school community. A group of six to eight peer volunteers is formed to support the individual in a proactive manner. The volunteers meet weekly and have three main tasks: to identify difficulties, to set goals and devise strategies for reaching them, and to offer encouragement and recognition for success and progress. These discussions are helpful to sustain the circle of friends and to promote the volunteers' understanding of issues of social acceptability, in general, and the child's social difficulties, in particular. Volunteers are encouraged to discuss openly the difficulties they encounter with the child's behavior. Benefits for the peer group and staff as well as for the child with AS have been reported using this approach (Greenway, 2000; Howlin, 1998).

## Peer Tutoring Using Incidental Teaching

In this approach normally developing peers are trained to use teaching techniques and turn taking in 5-minute teaching segments with children who have autism (National Research Council, 2001). In one such intervention peers were taught to interact via teaching and reinforcing communicative responses of target children (e.g., labeling desired toys when wishing to play with them). Tutors were arbitrarily rotated among target children, in order to provide the potential for generalization through a range of peers. This intervention demonstrated significant improvement in reciprocal social behaviors and social initiations. Increased reciprocal interactions were maintained after adult supervision and assistance were faded. However, generalization to other free-play periods was found only for one of the three boys, and none showed improvement in interaction during lunch periods. Sociometric ratings obtained before and after interventions showed substantial positive increases in peer ratings (McGee, Almeida, Sulzer-Azaroff, & Feldman, 1992).

## Social Stories

This approach, developed by Carol Gray (Gray, 1998; Gray & Garand, 1993) was designed for working with higher-functioning individuals. It involves creating a story that describes a person, skill, event, concept, or social situation and includes appropriate and relevant actions and expressions. The situation is described in terms of relevant social cues, anticipated actions, and information on what is occurring and why. Such a story often includes information that is obvious to others but overwhelming or confusing to the child with AS.

The stories utilize four types of sentences: descriptive (i.e., objective description of who is involved, what they are doing and why, and where the story takes place), perspective (i.e., explanation of reactions and feelings of others involved), directive (i.e., statement of what one is expected to do or say), and control (i.e., development of strategies to help one remember how to understand similar situations and how to act). The story is created together with the child and incorporates his or her understandings and special interests. Thus the child with AS gradually learns codes of social conduct through intellectual analysis and instruction (Attwood, 1998). Research on the long-term gains of the social stories technique is still limited, but clinical reports tend to be very enthusiastic. Children, teachers, and parents feel that through the stories, individuals with HFA or AS have been able to master many of the situations that previously were totally confusing for them (Attwood, 1998; Gray, 1998).

## Comic Strip Conversations

Comic strip conversations were also developed by Gray (1998). They incorporate simple drawings, symbols, and colors to illustrate relevant details, ideas, and abstract concepts in selected conversations. They are designed to visually illustrate the different levels of communication that occur in a conversation. The technique involves drawing stick figures with speech and thought bubbles and designated colors to represent emotions. In this simple way, segments of conversations are presented in which what each person said, thought, felt, and did is evident. Like the stories, the drawings are made while discussing the situation with the child with AS.

As is the case for social stories, research on the effects of the comic strip conversation technique is limited. Nonetheless, clinical evidence and self-reports tend to identify positive changes in the child's behavior, especially around the topic discussed in the story or conversation (Gray, 1998).

## Interventions Facilitating Understanding and Expression of Emotions

Attwood (1998, 2000) proposes ideas for interventions that help children with HFA or AS to understand and express emotions. He suggests handling one emotion at a time by providing as many illustrations as possible for that emotion. The emotion can be illustrated through drawings of facial expressions, body posture, etc. Different situations giving rise to the same emotion are presented and discussed. The fact that each emotion has a range of expressive intensity is stressed and illustrated. Once a particular emotion and its levels of expression are understood, the same procedures can be used for a contrasting emotion. Unraveling the expression of emotion also can be accomplished through discussion of different situations, the emotions they give rise to, and the appropriate behavioral response they should elicit. Specific attention should be given to exploring possible misinterpretations of the child's body language (e.g., aloof, domineering, etc.) and to the presentation of more appropriate styles of expression.

An alternative approach to teaching children with HFA and AS about emotions is described by Silver and Oakes (2001), who employed computers to teach these children to better recognize and predict emotional responses in others. Pre- and postintervention assessments revealed improvement in the ability to identify and understand facial expressions in photographs, cartoons depicting emotion-laden situations, and nonliteral stories. However, generalization and improvement in real-life situations remain to be assessed.

## Interventions Teaching Theory-of-Mind Skills

To teach specific mental state concepts to children with HFA or AS, a range of techniques has been developed that uses photographs, drawings, and texts (Howlin, Baron-Cohen, & Hadwin, 1999; McGregor, Whiten, & Blackburn, 1998; Ozonoff & Miller, 1995; Swettenham, 1996; Swettenham, Baron-Cohen, Gomez, & Walsh, 1996). These interventions are conducted individually or in groups with children whose verbal age is at least 5 years. All of these interventions have been successful in enhancing children's understanding of the specific mental states addressed but show relatively little generalization to other areas and little improvement in social competence or communicative competence, in general. Several explanations have been offered for this lack of improvement in general social competence. One possibility is that people with autism develop an alternative strategy for passing the tasks taught and thus do not gain any real understanding of mental states presented in the task scenarios (Swettenham, 1996). It is also possible that these interventions manage to teach false-belief tasks, with some degree of understanding for the mental states involved, but still do not teach theory-of-mind abilities, in general (Ozonoff & Miller, 1995). Finally, it is possible that theory-of-mind skills are a necessary but not sufficient social–cognitive capacity for social competence; that is, that there are other social–cognitive skills required to achieve social adaptation (Klin, 2000).

## Social Skills Groups

Social skills groups for children and adolescents with AS provide an opportunity for participants to learn and practice a range of advanced social abilities (e.g., Howlin & Yates, 1999; Marriage, Gordon, & Brand, 1995; Mesibov, 1992; Williams, 1989). The group may comprise children attending the same school or different schools. Prior to the sessions, a profile on the strengths and weaknesses of each participant is prepared. Group meetings include structured learning lessons and social activities. Participants learn the skills necessary for effective social functioning and then practice them in natural social situations (Mesibov, 1992). During the sessions, the group can focus on actual events, in which the person was unsure of alternative actions or comments, and try to come up with alternative behaviors. It is also possible to demonstrate inappropriate social behavior and ask participants to identify the errors. Discussions can focus on specific behaviors, such as communication and body language, with the possible aid of video cameras, which enable participants to view themselves. Role playing, modeling, and other techniques can be used to enhance and generalize behaviors discussed. The group also can discuss situations in which participants are bullied and teased and share information about how to handle these trying circumstances (Attwood, 1998).

Long-term effects of social skills groups for children with autism or AS are not yet well established, and it is not certain whether this technique can change specific skills in natural settings and whether the skills acquired are generalized (Greenway, 2000). Nevertheless, parents, teachers, and participants seem to perceive the groups as valuable (Attwood, 2000). Family members tend to report considerable improvement in such areas as conversational and social skills and self-confidence (Howlin & Yates, 1999).

Aside from its educational purpose, the group has yet another benefit: It offers opportunities for social contacts and activities (Mesibov, 1992). Participants often comment on the benefits of meeting people similar to themselves who share the same experiences (Attwood, 2000). On the other hand, it is often beneficial to include nonhandicapped individuals in the group as well, because they tend to be more responsive and enthusiastic than youngsters with HFA or AS. They also can be taught to watch for, and respond to, certain situations (Mesibov, 1992).

## Group Therapy

A somewhat different approach for group work with individuals with AS is group intervention. In this approach, intervention is conducted along the lines of traditional interpersonal group therapy, with several modifications that address the unique social and cognitive characteristics of children with AS (Mishna & Muskat, 1998). The rationale for this sort of group intervention is to provide children with AS with the opportunity for meeting peers with whom they can interact and share problems and experiences. Adaptations of interpersonal group therapy include, on the one hand, flexibility within the group structure, such as enabling participants to wander around the room, and, on the other hand, explicit prohibition of inappropriate behaviors, such as invading others' physical space.

It has been reported that, although verbal communication was difficult for participants, they were increasingly able to talk with one another and give each other feedback. Group members could share interests and experiences, especially difficult encounters with peers at school. All participants stated they had enjoyed the group, and most participants and their mothers thought it was helpful, even after a 2-year follow-up (Mishna & Muskat, 1998). However, actual change in participants' behaviors or integration has not been discussed.

## Individual Treatment and Counseling

Mesibov (1992) stresses the importance of individual work with high-functioning individuals who have an ASD. Individual counseling in the TEACCH (Treatment and Education of Autistic and Related Communication Handicapped Children) program is cited as one of many techniques for improving adaptation (Schopler, 1990). Individual counseling relationships can provide these children with the structure, guidance, information, and support they need to function more effectively in society. For those working with these individuals, one-on-one counseling offers an important opportunity for entering into the child's unique perspective on, and understanding of, the world. Furthermore, it affords the possibility of establishing a relationship of trust and openness with the child. Once rapport and trust are established, counselors can focus on specific objectives, such as aiding the child in organizing his or her thinking, making sense of different perceptions in complex situations, deciphering hidden cues relating to emotions, etc. Counseling also can provide an opportunity for discussing relationships between events and, especially, the consequences of the child's behaviors. In addition, it can be used to help solve everyday problems through discussion and development of coping strategies (Mesibov, 1992).

Hare (1997) has reported the results of conducting individual therapy, based on cognitive-behavioral techniques with an adult with AS. The focus of the intervention was the patient's depression, due to his awareness of his difference from others and to distorted social–affective modes of thought. Discussions during therapy were based on excerpts from a diary the patient kept, and focused on cognitive and behavioral remedial techniques for dysfunctional assumptions held by the patient. This single study reported improvement on the Beck Depression Inventory. Finally, more traditional forms of psychotherapy with young people with AS are being practiced, with reported success (Ruberman, 2002).

## CONSIDERATION OF SPECIFIC SITUATIONS WITHIN THE SCHOOL SETTING

The interventions mentioned above can be used in different situations to expand social skills in children with HFA or AS, thereby improving their capacity for integration into the school community and helping them to overcome social obstacles they are bound to encounter. In a recent study, Bauminger (2002) reported on an effective cognitive-behavioral intervention program that can be implemented in school settings to improve interpersonal problem solving, affective knowledge, and social interaction of children with HFA. It is important to evaluate the child's specific school environment and devise ways whereby the school setting can adjust to the child's needs and further enable social and emotional growth. As stressed throughout this chapter, one of the most difficult and demanding tasks for children with HFA or AS is integration within the school setting. It may be relatively easy to learn and employ social skills strategies with adults interested in understanding and helping the child, but it is much more difficult to adjust to peers who have other interests, and who can be quite thoughtless, if not even cruel, in their interactions with others (Howlin, 1998).

It is of utmost importance for the teacher and others in the school setting to be informed about the nature of AS and the social difficulties it entails. Such information should prevent both inappropriate expectations of performance based on the child's cognitive abilities and misinterpretation of the child's behavior as deliberate or malevolent (Attwood, 2000).

Attwood (1998) and Howlin (1998) have written comprehensive guidebooks for parents and teachers that offer guidelines for teachers on promoting adequate social behavior in the classroom. These include (1) using other children as cues to indicate what must be done; (2) encouraging cooperative work, in which small groups of children work together as a team on various classroom activities; (3) explaining and modeling the possibility of seeking help from peers as an alternative to the teacher; (4) modeling how normally developing peers should relate to the child; and (5) encouraging prospective friendships by identifying and furthering interaction with a restricted number of children who show motivation for helping the child. Hopefully, these children will support the child with AS in bullying situations, will include him or her in games, will act as his or her advocates in the classroom, and will remind or instruct the child on what to do or say in different situations.

Teachers also are encouraged to find ways in which the child's special skills can be used to foster social interactions or to increase his or her acceptance within the classroom. It is important to provide supervision during recess in the playground. Supervisors should encourage the inclusion of the child in games when this is desired, or enable and respect his or her need for solitude. Finally, the use of teacher aides should be considered even for those high-functioning individuals who presumably can meet curriculum demands in mainstream schools. Aid should focus on different social skills, which, of course, are not taught as specific components of the school curriculum.

## CONCLUSION

The social difficulties encountered by children with HFA or AS present serious challenges for therapists, teachers, and other professionals working with these children, especially in the school setting. The multitude of therapeutic interventions described in this chapter attests to the fact that professionals working in the field of autism are making an extensive effort to meet this challenge. Many intervention programs, some of which were specifically designed for children with HFA and AS, have been implemented, and research on their effectiveness is now accumulating.

As stressed throughout this chapter, one of the main difficulties in assessing intervention programs is their specificity of focus. In many cases, questions concerning generalizability of gains to other areas relating to social understanding and behavior and to improvement in general day-to-day functioning have not been addressed. A second issue that needs more in-depth evaluation is the short- and long-term effects, in terms of social, emotional and cognitive gains, of mainstreaming these children. However, as we become better acquainted with the syndrome's specific and subtle difficulties, and as more individuals with HFA and AS are able to share their experiences and understandings of social encounters, especially in mainstream education, we will hopefully be better equipped to adjust techniques to their specific needs.

## REFERENCES

American Psychiatric Association. (1994). *Diagnostic and statistical manual of mental disorders* (4th ed.). Washington, DC: Author.

Asperger, H. (1991). Autistic psychopathy in childhood. In U. Frith (Ed.), *Autism and Asperger syndrome* (pp. 37–91). Cambridge, UK: Cambridge University Press. (Original work published in German 1944)

Astington, J. W., Harris, P. L., & Olson, D. R. (Eds.). (1988). *Developing theories of mind*. New York: Cambridge University Press.

Attwood, T. (1998). *Asperger syndrome: A guide for parents and professionals*. Philadelphia: Jessica Kingsley.

Attwood, T. (2000). Strategies for improving the social integration of children with Asperger syndrome. *Autism, 4*, 85–100.

Baron-Cohen, S., Jolliffe, T., Mortimore, C., & Robertson, M. (1997). Another advanced test of theory of mind: Evidence from very high functioning adults with autism or Asperger syndrome. *Journal of Child Psychology and Psychiatry, 38*, 813–822.

Baron-Cohen, S., O'Riordan, M., Stone, V., Jones, R., & Plaisted, K. (1999). Recognition of faux-pas by normally developing children and children with Asperger syndrome or high-functioning autism. *Journal of Autism and Developmental Disorders, 29*, 407–418.

Bauminger, N. (2002). The facilitation of social–emotional understanding and social interaction in high-functioning children with autism. *Journal of Autism and Developmental Disorders, 32*, 283–298.

Bauminger, N., & Kasari, C. (2000). Loneliness and friendship in high-functioning children with autism. *Child Development, 71*, 447–456.

Berthier, M. L., Santamaria, J., Encabo, H., & Toosa, E. S. (1992). Recurrent hypersomnia in two adolescent males with Asperger's syndrome. *Journal of the American Academy of Child and Adolescent Psychiatry, 31,* 735–738.

Botroff, V., Bartak, L., Langford, P., Page, M., & Tonge, B. (1995, July). *Social cognitive skills and implications for social skills training in adolescents with autism.* Paper presented at the 1995 National Autism Conference, Greensboro, NC.

Bowler, D. (1992). "Theory of mind" in Asperger's syndrome. *Journal of Child Psychology and Psychiatry, 33,* 877–893.

Capps, L., Sigman, M., & Yirmiya, N. (1995). Self-competence and emotional understanding in high-functioning children with autism. *Development and Psychopathology, 7,* 137–149.

Capps, L., Yirmiya, N., & Sigman, M. (1992). Understanding of simple and complex emotions in non-retarded children with autism. *Journal of Child Psychology and Psychiatry, 33,* 1169–1182.

Carrington, S., & Graham, L. (2001). Perceptions of school by two teenage boys with Asperger syndrome and their mothers: A qualitative study. *Autism, 5,* 37–48.

Castelli, F., Frith, C., Happé, F., & Frith, U. (2002). Autism, Asperger syndrome and brain mechanisms for the attribution of mental states to animated shapes. *Brain, 125,* 1–11.

Cesaroni, L., & Garber, M. (1991). Exploring the experience of autism through firsthand accounts. *Journal of Autism and Developmental Disorders, 21,* 303–313.

Connor, M. (2001). Asperger syndrome (autistic spectrum disorder) and the self-reports of comprehensive school students. *Educational Psychology in Practice, 16,* 285–296.

Dahlgren, S. O., & Trillingsgaard, A. (1996). Theory of mind in nonretarded children with autism and Asperger's syndrome: A research note. *Journal of Child Psychology and Psychiatry, 37,* 759–763.

Davies, S., Bishop, D., Manstead, A. S. R., & Tantam, D. (1994). Face perception in children with autism and Asperger syndrome. *Journal of Child Psychology and Psychiatry, 35,* 1033–1057.

Ehlers, S., & Gillberg, C. (1993). The epidemiology of Asperger syndrome: A total population study. *Journal of Child Psychology and Psychiatry, 34,* 1327–1350.

Frith, U. (1991). *Autism and Asperger syndrome.* Cambridge, UK: Cambridge University Press.

Frith, U. (1996). Social communication and its disorder in autism and Asperger syndrome. *Journal of Psychopharmacology, 10,* 48–53.

Frith, U., & Happé, F. (1999). Theory of mind and self-consciousness: What is it like to be autistic? *Mind and Cognition, 14,* 1–22.

Frye, D., & Moore, C. (1991). *Children's theories of mind: Mental states and social understanding.* Hillsdale, NJ: Erlbaum.

Ghaziuddin, M., Weidemer-Mikhail, E., & Ghaziuddin, N. (1998). Comorbidity of Asperger syndrome: A preliminary report. *Journal of Intellectual Disability Research, 42,* 279–283.

Gillberg, I. C., & Gillberg, C. (1989). Asperger syndrome: Some epidemiological considerations. *Journal of Child Psychology and Psychiatry, 30,* 631–638.

Goldstein, H. L., Kaczmarek, R., Pennington, R., & Shafer, K. (1992). Peer-mediated intervention: Attending to, commenting on, and acknowledging the behavior of preschoolers with autism. *Journal of Applied Behavior Analysis, 25*, 289–305.

Gray, C. A. (1998). Social stories and comic strip conversations with students with Asperger syndrome and high-functioning autism. In E. Schopler, G. Mesibov, & L. J. Kunce (Eds.), *Asperger syndrome or high-functioning autism?* (pp. 167–198). New York: Plenum Press.

Gray, C. A., & Garand, J. (1993). Social stories: Improving responses of individuals with autism with accurate social information. *Focus on Autistic Behavior, 8*, 1–10.

Green, J., Gilchrist, A., Burton, D., & Cox, A. (2000). Social and psychiatric functioning in adolescents with Asperger syndrome compared with conduct disorders. *Journal of Autism and Developmental Disorders, 30*, 279–293.

Greenway, C. (2000). Autism and Asperger syndrome: Strategies to promote prosocial behavior. *Educational Psychology in Practice, 16*, 469–486.

Gross, J. (1994). Asperger syndrome: A label worth having? *Educational Psychology, 10*, 104–110.

Happé, F. (1994). An advanced test of theory of mind: Understanding of story characters' thoughts and feelings by able autistic, mentally handicapped, and normal children and adults. *Journal of Autism and Developmental Disorders, 24*, 129–154.

Hare, D. J. (1997). The use of cognitive-behavioral therapy with people with Asperger syndrome: A case study. *Autism, 1*, 215–225.

Heavey, L., Phillips, W., Baron-Cohen, S., & Rutter, M. (2000). The awkward moments test: A naturalistic measure of social understanding in autism. *Journal of Autism and Developmental Disorders, 30*, 225–236.

Hobson, R. P. (1986a). The autistic child's appraisal of expressions of emotion. *Journal of Child Psychology and Psychiatry, 27*, 321–342.

Hobson, R. P. (1986b). The autistic child's appraisal of expressions of emotion: A further study. *Journal of Child Psychology and Psychiatry, 27*, 671–680.

Hobson, R. P. (1992). Social perception in high-level autism. In E. Schopler & G. B. Mesibov (Eds.), *High-functioning individuals with autism* (pp. 157–184). New York: Plenum Press.

Hobson, R. P., Ouston, J., & Lee, A. (1988). Emotion recognition in autism: Coordinating faces and voices. *Psychological Medicine, 18*, 911–923.

Howlin, P. (1998). *Children with autism and Asperger syndrome: A guide for practitioners and carers.* Chichester, UK: Wiley.

Howlin, P. (2000). Assessment instruments for Asperger syndrome. *Child Psychology and Psychiatry Review, 5*, 120–129.

Howlin, P. Baron-Cohen, S., & Hadwin, J. (1999). *Teaching children with autism to mindread: A practical guide.* Chichester, UK: Wiley.

Howlin, P., & Yates, P. (1999). The potential effectiveness of social skills groups for adults with autism. *Autism, 3*, 299–307.

Hoyson, M. B., Jameison, B., & Strain, P. S. (1984). Individualized group instruction of normally developing children and autistic-like children: The LEAP curriculum model. *Journal of the Division of Early Childhood, 8*, 157–172.

Kadesjo, B., Gillberg, C., & Hagberg, B. (1999). Brief report: Autism and Asperger syndrome in seven-year-old children: A total population study. *Journal of Autism and Developmental Disorders, 29,* 297–305.

Kasari, C., Freeman, S. F. N., Bauminger, N., & Alkin, M.C. (1999). Parental perspectives on inclusion: Effects of autism and Down syndrome. *Journal of Autism and Developmental Disorders, 29,* 327–331.

Kerbeshian, J., Burd, L., & Fisher, W. (1990). Asperger's syndrome: To be or not to be? *British Journal of Psychiatry, 156,* 721–725.

Klin, A. (2000). Attributing social meaning to ambiguous visual stimuli in higher functioning autism and Asperger syndrome: The social attribution task. *Journal of Child Psychology and Psychiatry, 41,* 831–846.

Klin, A, Volkmar, F. R., & Sparrow, S. S. (2000). Introduction. In A. Klin, F. R. Volkmar, & S. S. Sparrow (Eds.), *Asperger syndrome* (pp. 1–21). New York: Guilford Press.

Koning, C., & Magill-Evans, J. (2001). Social and language skills in adolescent boys with Asperger syndrome. *Autism, 5,* 23–36.

Laushey, K. M., & Heflin, L. J. (2000). Enhancing social skills of kindergarten children with autism through the training of multiple peers as tutors. *Journal of Autism and Developmental Disorders, 30,* 183–193.

Leekam, S. R., & Prior, M. (1994). Can autistic children distinguish lies from jokes?: A second look at second-order belief attribution. *Journal of Child Psychology and Psychiatry, 35,* 901–915.

Little, L. (2001). Peer victimization of children with Asperger spectrum disorders. *Journal of the American Academy of Child and Adolescent Psychiatry, 40,* 995–996.

Lovaas, I. O. (1987). Behavioral treatment and normal educational and intellectual functioning in young autistic children. *Journal of Consulting and Clinical Psychology, 55,* 3–9.

Macdonald, H., Rutter, M., Howlin, P., Rios, P., Le Couteur, A., Evered, C., & Folstein, S. (1989). Recognition and expression of emotional cues by autistic and normal adults. *Journal of Child Psychology and Psychiatry, 30,* 865–877.

Marriage, K., Gordon, V., & Brand, L. (1995). A social skills group for boys with Asperger's syndrome. *Australian and New Zealand Journal of Psychiatry, 29,* 58–62.

McGee, G. G., Almeida, M. C., Sulzer-Azaroff, B., & Feldman, R. S. (1992). Promoting reciprocal interactions via peer incidental teaching. *Journal of Applied Behavior Analysis, 25,* 117–126.

McGregor, E., Whiten, A., & Blackburn, P. (1998). Transfer of the picture-in-the-head analogy to natural contexts to aid false belief understanding in autism. *Autism, 2,* 367–387.

Mesibov, G. B. (1992). Treatment issues with high-functioning adolescents and adults with autism. In E. Schopler & G. B. Mesibov (Eds.), *High-functioning individuals with autism* (pp. 143–156). New York: Plenum Press.

Mishna, F., & Muskat, B. (1998). Group therapy for boys with features of Asperger syndrome and concurrent learning disabilities: Finding a peer group. *Journal of Child and Adolescent Group Therapy, 8,* 97–114.

Nadel, J., & Peze, A. (1993). What makes immediate imitation communicative in toddlers and autistic children? In J. Nadel & L. Camaioni (Eds.). *New perspectives in early communication development* (pp. 139–156). London: Routledge.

National Research Council. (2001). *Educating children with autism.* Washington, DC: National Academy Press.

Odom, S. L., & Ogawa, I. (1992). Direct observation of young children's social interaction with peers: A review of methodology. *Behavioral Assessment, 14,* 443–464.

Oke, N. J., & Schreibman, L. (1990). Training social initiations to a high-functioning autistic child: Assessment of a collateral behavior change and generalization in a case study. *Journal of Autism and Developmental Disorders, 20,* 479–497.

Ozonoff, S., & Miller, J. N. (1995). Teaching theory of mind: A new approach to social skills training for individuals with autism. *Journal of Autism and Developmental Disorders, 25,* 415–433.

Ozonoff, S., Rogers, S. J., & Pennington, B. F. (1991). Asperger syndrome: Evidence of an empirical distinction from high-functioning autism. *Journal of Child Psychology and Psychiatry, 32,* 1107–1122.

Prior, M., Leekam, S., Ong, B., Eisenmajer, R., Wing, L., Gould, J., & Dowe, D. (1998). Are there subgroups within the autistic spectrum? A cluster analysis of a group of children with autistic spectrum disorder. *Journal of Child Psychology and Psychiatry, 39,* 893–902.

Ruberman, L. (2002). Psychotherapy of children with Pervasive Developmental Disorders. *American Journal of Psychotherapy, 56,* 262–273.

Rumsey, J. M. (1992). Neuropsychological studies of high-level autism. In E. Schopler & G. B. Mesibov (Eds.), *High-functioning individuals with autism* (pp. 41–46). New York: Plenum Press.

Schopler, E. (1990). Principles for directing both educational treatment and research. In C. Gillberg (Ed.), *Diagnosis and treatment of autism* (pp. 167–183). New York: Plenum Press.

Sigman, M., & Capps, L. (1997). *Children with autism: A developmental perspective.* Cambridge, MA: Harvard University Press.

Sigman, M. D., Kasari, C., Kwon, J., & Yirmiya, N. (1992). Responses to the negative emotions of others by autistic, mentally retarded, and normal children. *Child Development, 63,* 796–807.

Silver, M., & Oakes, P. (2001). Evaluation of a new computer intervention to teach people with autism or Asperger syndrome to recognize and predict emotions in others. *Autism, 5,* 299–316.

Strain, P. S. (1983). Identification of social skill curriculum targets for severely handicapped children in mainstreamed preschools. *Applied Research in Mental Retardation, 4,* 369–382.

Swettenham, J. (1996). Can children with autism be taught to understand false belief using computers? *Journal of Child Psychology and Psychiatry, 37,* 157–165.

Swettenham, J., Baron-Cohen, S., Gomez, J., & Walsh, S. (1996). What's inside someone's head? Conceiving of the mind as a camera helps children with autism acquire an alternative to a theory of mind. *Cognitive Neuropsychiatry, 1,* 73–88.

Szatmari, P., Bremner, R., & Nagy, J. N. (1989). Asperger syndrome: A review of clinical features. *Canadian Journal of Psychiatry, 34*, 554–560.

Tantam, D. (1991). Asperger syndrome in adulthood. In U. Frith (Ed.), *Autism and Asperger syndrome* (pp. 147–183). Cambridge, UK: Cambridge University Press.

Tantam, D. (1992). Characterizing the fundamental social handicap in autism. *Acta Paedopsychiatrica, 55*, 83–91.

Tantam, D. (2000). Psychological disorder in adolescents and adults with Asperger syndrome. *Autism, 4*, 47–62.

Tantam, D., Holmes, D., & Cordess, C. (1993). Nonverbal expression in autism of Asperger type. *Journal of Autism and Developmental Disorders, 23*, 111–133.

Twachtman-Cullen, D. (1998). Language and communication in high-functioning autism and Asperger syndrome. In E. Schopler, G. B. Mesibov, & L. J. Kunce (Eds.), *Asperger syndrome or high-functioning autism?* (pp. 199–226). New York: Plenum Press.

Van Lancker, D. R., Cornelius, C., & Kreiman, J. (1989). Recognition of emotional–prosodic meanings in speech by autistic, schizophrenic, and normal children. *Developmental Neuropsychology, 5*, 207–226.

Volkmar, F. R., & Klin, A. (2000). Diagnostic issues in Asperger syndrome. In A. Klin, F. R. Volkmar, & S. S. Sparrow (Eds.), *Asperger syndrome* (pp. 25–71). New York: Guilford Press.

Vygotsky, L. S. (1976). Play and its role in the mental development of the child. In J. Bruner, A. Jolly, & S. Sylvia (Eds.), *Play: Its role in development and evolution* (pp. 537–554). Middlesex, UK: Penguin.

Williams, T. I. (1989). A social skills group for autistic children. *Journal of Autism and Developmental Disorders, 19*, 143–155.

Wing, L. (1981). Asperger syndrome: A clinical account. *Psychological Medicine, 11*, 115–129.

Wing, L. (1992). Manifestations of social problems. In E. Schopler & G. B. Mesibov (Eds.), *High-functioning individuals with autism* (pp. 129–142). New York: Plenum Press.

Wing, L., & Gould, J. (1979). Severe impairments of social interaction and associated abnormalities in children: Epidemiology and classification. *Journal of Autism and Developmental Disorders, 9*, 11–29.

Yirmiya, N., Erel, O., Shaked, M., & Solomonica-Levi, D. (1998). Meta-analyses comparing theory of mind abilities of individuals with autism, individuals with mental retardation, and normally developing individuals. *Psychological Bulletin, 124*, 283–307.

Yirmiya, N., Pilowsky, T., Solomonica-Levi, D., & Shulman, C. (1999). Brief report: Gaze behavior and theory of mind abilities in individuals with autism, Down syndrome, and mental retardation of unknown etiology. *Journal of Autism and Developmental Disorders, 29*, 333–341.

Yirmiya, N., & Sigman, M. (1991). High-functioning individuals with autism: Diagnosis, empirical findings, and theoretical issues. *Clinical Psychology Review, 11*, 669–684.

Yirmiya, N., Sigman, M., Kasari, C., & Mundy, P. (1992). Empathy and cognition in high-functioning children with autism. *Child Development, 63*, 150–160.

# 6

## Understanding and Managing Circumscribed Interests

TONY ATTWOOD

In 1944, Hans Asperger provided the first precise description of the circumscribed interests that are a fascinating characteristic of autism. The following description is as accurate today as it was nearly 60 years ago:

> We know an autistic child who has a particular interest in the natural sciences. His observations show an unusual eye for the essential. He orders his facts into a system and forms his own theories even if they are occasionally abstruse. Hardly any of this he heard or read, and he always refers to his own experience. There is also a child who is a "chemist." He uses all his money for experiments which often horrify his family and even steals to fund them. Some children have even more specialized interests, for instance, only experiments which create noise and smells. Another autistic boy was obsessed with poisons. He had a most unusual knowledge in this area and possessed a large collection of poisons, some quite naively concocted by himself. He came to us because he had stolen a substantial quantity of cyanide from the locked chemistry store at his school. Another, again, was preoccupied by numbers. Complex calculations were naturally easy for him without being taught. Another autistic child had specialized technological interests and knew an incredible amount about complex machinery. He acquired this knowledge through constant questioning, which was impossible to fend off, and also to a great degree through his own observations. He came to be preoccupied with fantastic inventions, such as spaceships and the like, and here one observes how remote from reality autistic interests are. (Asperger, 1944/1991, p. 72)

Almost 60 years later, we remain in the preliminary stages of describing and defining the characteristics of Asperger syndrome (AS). One of the characteristics about which we have the least clinical knowledge and research data is the presence of a circumscribed interest. Included in the diagnostic criteria for AS in the DSM-IV (American Psychiatric Association, 2000, p. 77) is Criterion B:

> Restricted repetitive and stereotyped patterns of behavior, interests, and activities, as manifested by at least one of the following:
> (1) encompassing preoccupation with one or more stereotyped and restricted patterns of interest that is abnormal either in intensity or focus
> (2) apparently inflexible adherence to specific, nonfunctional routines or rituals
> (3) stereotyped and repetitive motor mannerisms (e.g., hand or finger flapping or twisting, or complex whole-body movements)
> (4) persistent preoccupation with parts of objects

The text adds that autistic disorder also includes restricted, repetitive, and stereotyped interests and activities that are often characterized by the presence of motor mannerisms, preoccupation with parts of objects, rituals, and marked distress in change, but in AS, these behaviors are primarily observed in the all-encompassing pursuit of a circumscribed interest involving a topic to which the individual devotes inordinate amounts of time, amassing information and facts. The interests and activities are pursued with great intensity, often to the exclusion of other activities. The presence of circumscribed interests appears to be a dominant characteristic, occurring in over 90% of children and adults with AS (Bashe & Kirby, 2001; Kerbeshian, Burd, & Fisher, 1990; Tantam, 1991). This characteristic is also remarkably stable over time (Piven, Harper, Palmer, & Arndt, 1996). However, we have yet to describe adequately the nature of the interests and how they may change over time, or the consequences and function of the interests, or strategies to reduce or utilize them.

## THE DEVELOPMENT AND NATURE OF CIRCUMSCRIBED INTERESTS

The person with AS has a natural affinity for the physical, rather than mental, world, which is reflected in his or her choice of interests. Whereas other children are busy exploring their social world, children with AS are fully occupied by exploring objects, machines, animals, and concepts about those areas. The benefits of the interest can be considerable for individuals with AS. They may have natural abilities in determining the function of objects and an interest in the forces that physically influence life, such as the weather, geography, and the patterns or formulae of life determined by history, taxonomies, and mathematics. The autobiographies of adults with AS often describe their perception of chaos and unpredictability in their daily lives. They seek predictability and patterns, and these are more readily available in the physical world.

Circumscribed interests can develop as early as age 2–3 years (Bashe & Kirby, 2001). As described in the above diagnostic criteria, these interests may commence with a preoccupation with parts of objects, such as spinning the wheels of toy cars or manipulating electrical switches. The next stage may be a fascination with a specific category of objects and accumulating as many examples as possible. Sometimes the collections comprise items acquired by typical children, such as stones and bottle tops, but some can be quite eccentric, such as toilet brushes and yellow pencils. These children eagerly seek any opportunity to gain new additions to their collection, and much of their free time is spent on the search for a new example or "trophy." The attachment to the objects can be remarkably intense, eliciting considerable distress if one is missing and visible delight when it is found. The "affection" for the objects can appear to be more intense than affection for family members.

The research literature on theory-of-mind skills has established that such children have considerable difficulty understanding and responding to the thoughts and feelings of others. The social and interpersonal world is confusing, but the world of objects and machinery is easier to understand and more reliable than people; objects do not change their mind or become distracted or emotional. My sister-in-law, Penelope, has AS. In her autobiography (unpublished), she wrote: "It's easy to bestow love onto objects rather than people because although they can't love back they can't rebuke either. It is a very safe form of idolization where no one can get hurt."

The child's play can become somewhat eccentric, such as pretending to be the favored object. One child who would rock from side to side in the playground explained that he was pretending to be car wiper blades. Another child would go to his bedroom; soon thereafter his grandmother would hear unusual noises coming from that location. Her grandson would frequently crash into the furniture and bounce between the walls of his bedroom. He explained that he was pretending to play soccer, but the play was unusual in that he was pretending to be the *ball*, not the player. Another child, preparing for a special costume day at school, persuaded his mother to make the costume he most wanted to wear. Whereas most children dressed as a character from a film or children's story, or an animal, he went to school dressed as a washing machine, his circumscribed interest.

The essential components of the circumscribed interest are the accumulation of desired objects and learning how the physical world works (Baron-Cohen & Wheelwright, 1999). These may be followed by a fascination with information regarding a topic or concept, such as transportation systems, animals, or electronics. Some of the circumscribed interests are developmentally appropriate and typical of their peers, such as an interest in Thomas the Tank Engine, dinosaurs, castles, and computer games, whereas other interests may be unusual—such as drain covers, vacuum cleaners, or alarm systems. The reason for the interest is usually idiosyncratic, and not that the topic is popular with peers or the "currency" between friends.

These children's near encyclopedic knowledge can be astonishing; they may be perceived as "little professors," eager to read about their interest, ask adults questions related to the interest, and instruct their peers about the interest in a manner that resembles a teacher rather than a peer. Sometimes children with AS convey the impression of being potential geniuses, and their extensive knowledge and enthusiasm for the topic can lead to a "halo" effect. However, teachers note that, although their attention span and attention to detail when engaged in their circumscribed interest is impressive, the same degree of motivation, attention, and ability is conspicuously absent when other classroom activities are the focus, especially the activities that would be of interest to their peers.

The focus of the interest invariably changes, but at a time dictated by the child, when it is replaced by another circumscribed interest that is the choice of the child, not a parent. The complexity and number of interests vary according to the child's developmental level and intellectual capacity. Over time there is a progression to multiple and more abstract or complex interests, such as periods of history, specific countries, or cultures. A recent survey of the circumscribed interests of children with AS established that many develop two or more simultaneous interests, and that the number of simultaneous interests increases with maturity: 17% of adults within the sample of 142 had six or more such interests (Bashe & Kirby, 2001).

Clinical experience suggests that there may be a difference in the categories of interests favored by boys and girls with AS. The girls may develop an intense interest in dolls, animals, and fiction. Again, some of the interests are age- and gender-appropriate but unusual in their intensity. The interest in dolls can lead to a huge collection but a preference to play with dolls alone rather than with a peer. The doll play may include detailed reenactments of scenes from television and the child's daily life. The interest in animals can be so consuming that the child attempts to act like the animal; for example, if the interest is horses, the child may want to sleep in a stable. The interest in fiction can include collecting, and reading many times, the novels of a favorite author, and an interest in classical literature such as Shakespeare's plays and the stories of Charles Dickens. This focus is unrelated to any desire to achieve success at school in English literature;

rather, it stems from a genuine interest in the great authors and their literature.

In the teenage years the interests can evolve to include electronics and computers, fantasy literature, science fiction, and sometimes a fascination with a particular person. All of these mirror the interests of their peers but the intensity and focus, again, are unusual. Some children with AS may demonstrate a natural ability in understanding computer languages, graphics, and advanced computer programming skills. The interest in fantasy literature and fantasy figures and figurines can be so intense that the adolescent develops his or her own role-play games or remarkably detailed drawing skills based on the circumscribed interest. There may be a fascination with a particular character—whether mythical, historical, or real. When such an interest is focused on a real person, the behavior can be interpreted as a teenage "crush," but the intensity also can lead to problems with apparent stalking, harassment, and the misinterpretation of intentions. In the adult years, individuals with AS are more likely to read about their interest than talk about it, and the interest can become a hobby or source of employment. These adults may be regarded as experts in a specialized subject within a hobby or interest group, or they may be employed to provide information or advice on their interest.

One of the common characteristics that threads throughout the development of circumscribed interests is a lack of appreciation for the perspective and priorities of others, especially peers. Children, adolescents, and adults with AS do not appear to recognize whether the topic is appropriate to the context, or to respond to the subtle signals of others' boredom. Although the enthusiasm for the topic can be endearing and the knowledge extraordinary, the delivery of the information can be experienced as annoying and intrusive by other people. There can be a tendency for those with AS to be pedantic, often providing far more information on the topic than is necessary or appropriate. The desire for completion means that once the topic is raised in the conversation, all relevant information on it must be explained and described.

Some of the interests would not usually be expected for children with AS. There can be an interest in sports, which would not be anticipated when one considers their motor clumsiness. However, sports-related interests may focus more on statistics and sporting records than participation in the sport itself. There are exceptions, of course; some children with AS develop an interest in solitary (rather than team) games and in sports that rely on solitary practice, accuracy, timing, and stoicism (e.g., golf, swimming, snooker, rock climbing, marathon running). The single-minded determination and intensity of practice, of which individuals with AS are capable, can lead to outstanding success.

Much of the knowledge acquisition associated with the chosen interest is self-directed and self-taught. Whereas the young child may ask adults many questions, and the older child may read about his or her interest, both engage in solitary and intuitive problem-solving activity. As the information regarding the interest increases, there is a need to develop a cataloguing system. The system has to be logical but can be unconventional. For example, Gisela and Chris shared an interest in classical music and combined their record collection when they married. Chris has AS, a condition not shared by his wife. He completed the cataloguing and sorting of the combined record collection based on the birth date of the composer rather than alphabetical order (Slater-Walker & Slater-Walker, 2002). The enjoyment of the interest includes both the accumulation of information and the identification of a pattern or taxonomy, and the development of a cataloguing system.

When the interest is focused in the creative arts, amazing abilities in drawing, painting, sculpture, music, or poetry may emerge. The attention to detail, realism, and use of color, shape, notes, or words can be quite extraordinary. The artworks are usually focused on a particular interest, for example, oil paintings of steam trains. There may be rare qualities, such as singing with perfect pitch, or a remarkable ability to communicate emotions in musical compositions and performances (which appears to be such a contrast to the difficulties the person has with empathy and the communication of emotions in his or her interpersonal and social life).

## MULTIDIMENSIONAL VIEWPOINTS

### Parents' and Teachers' Perspectives

There are many sides to a story. From the perspective of the parents of the child with AS, the circumscribed interest entails a number of problems, given the almost insatiable thirst for access to the interest displayed by these children. A survey of parents found that they frequently (1) had to make special trips to replace or purchase an item related to the circumscribed interest, (2) were late for appointments for reasons due to the particular interest, (3) drove out of their way or scheduled vacations to accommodate access to the interest, or (4) prematurely left a social gathering or public place because they were unable to negotiate access to the interest for their child (Bashe & Kirby, 2001). The intensity and duration of time involved in the interest can have additional consequences. The play date arranged by the parents might collapse as the child dominates the play with a conspicuous lack of reciprocity in the chosen activities or conversation.

At school, the monologue style of speech can appear eccentric, opening the child to teasing and bullying from other children who do not have the tolerance levels of adults. The interest then becomes a barrier to social inclusion.

Teachers often express concern that the interests interfere with the child's inclusion in social exchanges and the attention he or she gives to other activities. In addition, the amount of time devoted to pursuing the interest may preclude the learning of new skills (Klin, Carter, & Sparrow, 1997; South, Klin, & Volkmar, 1997). Other students may perceive the child with AS as overbearing, pedantic, self-centered, and rude. The child's unrelenting enthusiasm for the circumscribed interest can lead to a social "myopia" such that they do not notice other students' boredom or frustration.

## Perspective of the Person with Asperger Syndrome

Individuals with AS may be oblivious to the feelings and concerns of others with regard to their particular interest. Unfortunately, the determination to maintain access to the interest can lead to problems within the family and society. Bringing about access to the interest may occur without careful planning with regard to the consequences. For example, one child whose passion was trains would undertake journeys without considering how to return and without informing his parents of his trip and destination.

Denial of access to the source material can cause the person with AS to be in conflict with the law. For example, one young man, fascinated by the lottery forms in the local newsstand, would spend several hours a day in the shop filling in his chosen numbers, although he did not have the financial resources to submit the forms. The owner of the newsstand was not sympathetic, and the young man was banned from the shop. Several days later there was a break-in at the shop. No money or cigarettes were stolen, just the stock of lottery forms. The police apprehended their prime suspect, who was filling in the forms at his home. Being thwarted in gaining access also can lead to anger. In his autobiography, Luke Jackson (2002) describes, "I feel an overwhelming excitement in me that I cannot describe. I just have to talk about it and the irritation of being stopped can easily develop into raging fury" (p. 44).

An interest in computer programming and the Internet can lead to a fascination with computer hacking. The intention is to solve an intellectual problem, not necessarily to achieve financial gain, engage in espionage, or seek retribution as a disgruntled employee. An interest in firearms and a tendency not to reflect on the consequences of what might be said in "the heat of the moment" can lead to a school suspension for threats that others perceive as likely to be enacted. The person's financial planning also can be affected by the disproportionate amount of income spent on the interest. Those with AS are usually very concerned that others obey the law, but they can be tempted themselves to commit criminal offenses to obtain money to achieve access to their circumscribed interest.

## The Clinician's Perspective

The presence of a circumscribed interest can be of value to the clinician. During a diagnostic assessment, the child or adult with AS often interacts with the clinician in a guarded manner, thinking before giving a response and evincing tension and nervousness, unsure of the "script" in a new situation with someone he or she does not know well. However, his or her persona can change quite dramatically when the topic of his or her particular interest is broached. The person may visibly relax, showing enthusiasm and energy as well as a delight in impressing the clinician with the specialized knowledge. The nature of the interest also can be of clinical value. A change of preoccupation to a morbid or macabre topic such as death may indicate a clinical depression, and an interest in weapons, the martial arts, and revenge may point to bullying at school.

The intensity of the interest can become so compelling that the interest is no longer an activity of intellectual value and pleasure but evidence of an obsessive–compulsive disorder, in which gaining access is both irresistible and unwanted (Baron-Cohen, 1989). In his autobiography Luke Jackson (2002) commented: "I cannot begin to explain the feeling if something wasn't performed. This was when I felt like my whole body was going to burst" (p. 56). The circumscribed interest also can be associated with a delusional disorder (Kurita, 1999), as may be the case, for example, if the interest is fantasy literature and superheroes, and the person with AS acts as if he or she were the hero in an attempt to be successful and respected in social situations with peers. An interest in the supernatural during adolescence may be considered as indicative of schizophrenia.

## Society's Perspective

When considering the causes and functions of the circumscribed interests, it is important to consider not only the benefits to the person with AS, but also the benefits to society. There have been suggestions that successful individuals in the sciences and arts have personalities that resemble the profile of abilities associated with AS (Ledgin, 2002; Paradiz, 2002). Hans Asperger (1979) noted:

> It seems that for success in science or art, a dash of autism is essential. For success, the necessary ingredient may be an ability to turn away from the everyday world, from the simply practical, an ability to re-think a subject with originality so as to create in new untrodden ways, with all abilities canalized into the one specialty.

Or as Temple Grandin has said, "If the world was left to you socialites, we would still be in caves talking to each other."

## THEORIES OF CIRCUMSCRIBED INTERESTS

### Information-Processing Deficit

A recent psychological theory developed by Frith and Happé (1994) may help to explain some aspects of the circumscribed interest phenomenon. They suggest that those with an autistic spectrum disorder (ASD) such as AS have a different system of information processing. These individuals focus on the details of their environment rather than the gestalt or "big picture." Indeed, they may get "lost" in the detail. The person may not perceive the wider context or meaning due to problems with what Frith and Happé term "central coherence." The circumscribed interests are an attempt to achieve an elusive coherence. Once they discover the taxonomy of the interest (e.g., the different types of insects, the Periodic Table, or their own cataloguing system), they attain an understanding and predictability that is extremely satisfying. The interests can be an attempt to make order out of perceived chaos. An interest in trains could be attributed to a fascination with order (the cars are linked in a line) and predictability of outcome (the train must follow the tracks). An interest in symmetry or patterns is also mirrored in the parallel track and sleepers or ties.

Luke Jackson (2002) writes: "I would say that collecting something is a pretty harmless way of feeling secure and no one should stop anyone from doing so. Organizing something is a wonderful way of shaking off the feeling of chaos that comes from living in such a disorganized world" (p. 50). Carolyn, a client, explains in an e-mail: "Facts are important to us because they secure us in what is otherwise a very unstable world. Hard, cold facts give us comfort and security."

The difficulties children with AS encounter with advanced theory-of-mind skills and empathy suggest that those patterns of life, especially the codes of social conduct that are determined by thoughts and feelings rather than the mechanics of the physical world, appear to be illogical, unpredictable, and bewildering to them. Their success in assimilating and comprehending aspects of the physical world contrasts sharply with their confusion in the interpersonal world, explaining their retreat into the circumscribed interest and why their priority may be to pursue that interest rather than socialize with their peers.

If a person is not a good conversationalist, unsure of the cues for the topic of conversation and occasionally at a loss for words, he or she will feel a surge of confidence and verbal fluency if the "conversation" turns toward his or her circumscribed interest. If someone asks him or her a question, he or she will probably know the answer and thereby impress others with their knowledge. My discussions with children and adults with AS reveal that they place great value on intelligence in comparison to other personal attributes. They often view a conversation as a means of exchanging factual information rather than a means of encouraging social cohesion. The child may end a conversation, satisfied that he or she has conveyed knowledge and impressed listeners with his or her intellectual capacity. This type of delivery may impress teachers and adults, but it rarely impresses peers. However, if the circumscribed interest is valued by their peers, such as knowledge of Pokemon characters or computers, the interest can lead to sincere respect and admiration.

The determination to acquire knowledge regarding the interest may also explain other aspects of these individuals' interaction patterns with their peers. In the pursuit of knowledge, their preference will be to interact with adults, who can provide the specialized knowledge and explanations they seek, as well as to read and access information from a computer and the Internet. Other children often know very little about their particular interest; hence children's company has limited value in their quest for knowledge.

For adolescents and adults with AS, the search for the pattern or rules of life can include a fascination not only for the laws of science but the rules of law, leading to a career as an estate or contract lawyer, and religious laws, leading to an interest in the Bible and fundamentalist religions. This context also provides access to a peer group that shares the same beliefs and a community that promotes similar values. However, care must be taken that, as a consequence of their social vulnerability, these individuals are not unwittingly recruited into extremist organizations. Such events are prone to occur when the circumscribed interest is politics or religion and the person expresses and acts upon his or her "black-and-white" views. On the other hand, the pursuit of knowledge on a specified topic can lead to a successful career as, for example, an academic. I had a discussion with a professor with AS who said, "The best thing about academia is that we get paid to talk about our favorite topic, and students take notes and feed back our words of wisdom at exams."

## Impaired Executive Function

One of the characteristics of the circumscribed interest shown by the person with AS is repetition, suggesting a lack of flexibility in thinking (a "one-track mind") and invariance. Being "locked into" or perseverating on an activity could be indicative of impaired executive function (Hughes, Russel, & Robbins, 1993; Ozonoff, Pennington, & Rogers, 1991; Turner, 1997). According to Turner (1997, 1999), one of the roles of the executive system, which is a function of the frontal lobes of the brain, is to regulate and control volitional acts, including the ability to generate and inhibit actions and thoughts—that is, the cognitive control of the start and stop of behavior. The circumscribed interest could be an example of perseverative behavior and the term "stuck in set" (Turner, 1997). When individuals with

AS start to think or talk about their interest, they have great difficulty shifting their attention and there is a need for completion. Discussions about their particular interests often include reference to not being able to remove the thought from their mind, and parents and teachers report that they have great difficulty interrupting or distracting them when they are totally absorbed in the interest.

## SOURCE OF ENJOYMENT
## AND ANXIETY REDUCTION

A recent survey of people with AS examined the role circumscribed interests play in their lives (Bashe & Kirby, 2001). Genuine enjoyment, security, comfort and relaxation, and the facilitation or avoidance of social interaction were the most common categories of response. For adults, finding a rare specimen of the interest could be described as an intensely pleasurable experience—in contrast to a lack of pleasure in the more usual interpersonal activities of daily life.

The interest can be a source of humor. Grace has a fantasy world and draws imaginary machines with idiosyncratic names, such as the "Turbo Fan Cuddle Cubicle" and the "Glinker Flinker Macho Machine." Neologisms and imaginary worlds are a cognitive feature of AS and Grace incorporates her interest in her fears and pleasures. She has a hatred of corduroy trousers and therefore invented the "corduroytrousersnatcher." Her puns or jokes are based on her interest and are not intended to be humorous to others as shared enjoyment (Werth, Perkins, & Boucher, 2001).

The interest is not only a source of enjoyment but also a means of reducing anxiety. Research studies suggest that two-thirds of adolescents with AS concern their parents or clinicians because of the presence of a mood disorder, particularly a depressive disorder and/or an anxiety disorder (Ghaziuddin, Wieder-Mikhail, & Ghaziuddin, 1998; Gillot, Furniss, & Walter, 2001; Green, Gilchrist, Burton, & Cox, 2000; Kim, Szatmari, Bryson, Streiner, & Wilson, 2000; Tantam, 2000b; Tonge, Brereton, Gray, & Einfeld, 1999). The person with AS may have relatively fewer pleasures, so that the circumscribed interest is the "silver lining" to a somewhat gloomy life—a natural antidepressant. The DSM-IV diagnostic criteria refer to the presence of repetitive mannerisms. In the general population, rituals and repetition are used to reduce anxiety (e.g., worry beads, twirling hair around finger, the superstitious ritual of "knocking on wood"). Two important characteristics of circumscribed interests are their ritual and repetition. An adolescent with AS had a consuming interest in Japanese culture and performed the elaborate and ritualized Japanese tea ceremony whenever she felt anxious.

In behavioral terms, the soothing aspects of the repetitive action, thought, or interest become a form of negative reinforcement. It is interesting that the degree of motivation for, and duration of time spent on, the interest is proportional to the degree of stress (Bashe & Kirby, 2001). The more the person experiences stress in the form of change, failure, or low self-esteem, the more the interest becomes obtrusive, dominant, or bizarre. If the person has few means of enjoyment and relaxation, what may have started as a source of pleasure and tranquility, under conditions of stress, can become the kind of compulsive act that characterizes an obsessive–compulsive disorder.

## TRIGGERS TO THE DEVELOPMENT OF A CIRCUMSCRIBED INTEREST

We are only just beginning to understand what triggers the development of a particular circumscribed interest. They may commence in association or response to the experience of fear or pleasure. Lisa Pyles, in her biography of her son who has AS, writes that the interest can help the child control his or his fears (Pyles, 2000). Her son's interest in witches was his way of coping with his fear of them. Several parents have described how an initial source or focus of fear can develop into a circumscribed interest. A fear of the toilet can evolve into a fascination with plumbing, an acute auditory sensitivity to the noise of a vacuum cleaner can lead to a fascination with the different types of vacuum cleaners and how they work, a fear of thunder become an interest in the weather. The child's intelligent and practical way of reducing his or her fear is to learn about the cause of their anxiety. Unfortunately, due to the nature of AS, receiving compassion and affection from others may not be as effective an antidote to anxiety as occurs with other children. For these children, knowledge can be a powerful antidote to anxiety, and their way of understanding and conquering their fear can be to use their cognitive skills.

Some interests are triggered by situations associated with a pleasurable experience. The interest is commemorative, linked to a memory of a happier or simpler time (Tantam, 2000a). One of my sister-in-law, Penelope's, early interests was trains. In her brief autobiography (unpublished), she wrote:

> Most of the happier times were during vacations, which is why I love ships and trains (the only times when we would experience these things). These occasions were more secure and stable for me.

A parallel interest to the trains and ships also developed as an imaginary "escape" and an opportunity for pleasurable thoughts. She wrote:

> When I was about 7, I probably saw something in a book, which fascinated me and still does. Because it was like nothing I had ever seen before and totally unrelated and far removed from our world and our culture. That was Scandinavia and its people. Because of its foreignness it was totally alien and opposite of anyone and anything known to me. That was my escape, a dream world where nothing would remind me of daily life and all it had to throw at me. The people from this wonderful place look totally unlike any people in the "real world." Looking at these faces, I could not be reminded of anyone who might have humiliated, frightened, or rebuked me. The bottom line is, I was turning my back on real life and its ability to hurt, and escaping.

Penelope developed a circumscribed interest in Scandinavia and the Vikings to an extent that she insisted her mother make her a Viking outfit, and as an 8-year-old she wandered around her home village in England pretending to be a Viking. Fortunately, her reading about the Vikings did not result in attempts to burn farms and steal cattle!

## REDUCING OR UTILIZING
## THE CIRCUMSCRIBED INTEREST

Whereas the motivation for children with AS is to increase their access to their interest, perhaps at the expense of other activities, the motivation for parents and teachers is to reduce the duration of the access to enable these children to engage in a wider range of activities. Reducing access is particularly important when the interest appears to exclude social interaction with family members at home and peers at school, or affects the completion of homework assignments. What strategies can be used to reduce the time spent engaged in the interest? Should some interests be ended, or can they serve a constructive purpose?

### Controlled Access

The problem may not be the activity itself but the duration and dominance over other interests. Some success can be achieved by limiting the time allotted, using a clock or timer. When the time period is over, the activity must cease. The person can be actively encouraged to pursue other interests, as well as reassured that another time for his or her chosen interest is scheduled. It is important to keep the alternative activity out of sight of the resource material for the interest. The temptation to continue the activity will be quite strong, so the new activity is best located in another room or outside. The replacement activity also needs to be something the person enjoys, even if it is not as enjoyable as the circumscribed interest. The approach is to ration access and to actively encourage a wider range of interests.

The controlled access program can allocate specific social or "quality" time for pursuing the interest as a social activity. A parent or teacher makes a schedule of regular times to explore the interest with the child. The adult ensures that they do not get distracted, and both parties typically view the experience as enjoyable. I have found that such sessions can be an opportunity to improve my own knowledge of such interesting topics as the *Guinness Book of World Records*, the *Titanic*, and weather systems. I am then able to talk with some authority to other children with AS I meet who share the same interest. The conversation can become more reciprocal if the adults explain what they are interested in, and they can then spend time exploring each other's interests.

## Unacceptable Interests

If the interest is potentially dangerous, illegal, or likely to be misinterpreted, steps can be taken to terminate it, although clinical experience suggests that this is not an easy task. One must explain why the interest is not acceptable, perhaps using the "Social Stories and Comic Strip Conversations" developed by Gray (1998). The stories and pictures include an acknowledgment of the child's perspective but also the perspectives of family members, other adults, the community, relevant legislation, and possible consequences. An appeal is made to the intellectual vanity and self-image of the child in that the logical, mature, and wise decision is to modify the focus of the interest. For example, an interest in poisons can be modified to an interest in the digestive system and the benefits of different diets. The alternative is to terminate pursuit of the interest. A replacement interest that is mutually acceptable can be actively sought and encouraged. However, the choice must be based on the child's character, previous types of interests, and the function of those interests. If the interest is weapons and retaliation for being bullied at school, then steps must be taken to end the bullying as the source of a particular preoccupation.

## Constructive Application

### Motivation and Learning

Children are usually motivated to please their parent or teacher, to impress the other children, or to imitate or be included in the activities of their peers. These conventional desires or forms of motivation are not as powerful for children with AS. In contrast, they have significant motivation and attention span when involved with their circumscribed interest. The strategy is to incorporate the interest into the undesired activity or to use it as a reward. For example, if the young child has an interest in Thomas the Tank Engine, there is a wide range of merchandise available that incorporates the engines in reading books for different reading ages, mathematical activities, and writing and drawing. If the young child is interested in geography, and flags in particular, he or she could count flags rather than the conventional items being counted by their peers in the classroom or for homework. Indeed, one of the problems encountered by parents is the child's lack of motivation for doing homework. If the homework assignment involves an aspect of his or her circumscribed interest, there are fewer issues with the completion of homework assignments (Hinton & Kern, 1999).

Another alternative is to use the interest as a reward. Completion of allocated tasks in class results in free time to pursue the circumscribed interest. For example, if the child completes the 10 sums within 10 minutes, he or she earns 10 minutes on the class computer to pursue the interest. Access to the interest is a remarkably potent reward (Mercier, Mottron, & Belleville, 2000). For older children, an interest in science can lead to knowledge of scientific methodology and success in science and mathematics competitions. This strategy does require teachers to be more flexible in the presentation of the class tasks, the curriculum, and the reward systems. However, the benefits can be extraordinary for these children, who thereby widen their knowledge base, demonstrate their intellectual ability to their teacher, parents, and peers, and attain prizes and certificates of achievement. Some parents have used the removal of access to the interest as a punishment for tasks not completed or misbehavior. Although this strategy can be an effective component of a home-based behavior management program, it could become a trigger to aggressive behavior if the child cannot tolerate reduced access.

Gagnon (2001) has developed the concept of "power cards." The strategy uses the interest to motivate and facilitate learning in other areas, be they academic or social in nature, and can be used in the classroom and at home. A card the size of a business or trading card is created that provides an explanation and, if pertinent, advice that incorporates pictures of scenes or characters associated with the circumscribed interest. The text is written much as a Social Story (Gray 1998). For example, one girl was notorious for making direct and sometimes offensive personal comments about, or to, her peers (she might loudly comment, "You have bad breath"). She needed to learn to inhibit such comments or to say them in a more tactful way. Because she had a great interest in the popular singer Britney Spears, a power card was created with a picture of Britney and a text that included Britney's "advice" to her on what to say to the other children in her class. The inclusion of the interest can focus the child's attention, and the recommendations are more likely to be remembered and used by him or her.

## Employment

Some interests can become a source of income and employment. One teenager with AS has an amazing knowledge of fishing, especially the different types of fish and fishing equipment. His high school offered a vocational experience at the end of the school year, whereby each student was assigned to an employment situation for a day, for work experience. The teachers discussed what work experience would be appropriate for this teenager. Eventually the suggestion was made that he work for a day at the local fishing tackle shop. He went for the day—and never returned to school; he was employed by the end of the day, as the shop owner recognized that his knowledge and enthusiasm would make him a valued employee. An interest in the weather could lead to employment as a meteorologist; an interest in maps, a job as a taxi driver or truck driver; an interest in different cultures and languages, a job as a tour guide or translator. Parents may consider private schooling or tutoring to develop those interests that could become a source of income or employment. Temple Grandin has advocated that those with autism and AS develop a level of expertise such that others seek their knowledge, rather than having to acquire the social ability to gain entry into employment. A work portfolio containing examples of their abilities and knowledge can compensate for their difficulties in the social skills required in a job interview.

## Part of a Cognitive-Behavioral Therapy Program

Clinical experience indicates that individuals with AS primarily use physical acts to regulate and manage emotion. Damaging property and engaging in excessive solitude and pursuit of their circumscribed interest can require intervention. I have developed several modifications to cognitive-behavioral therapy (CBT) to accommodate the unusual profile of cognitive and social skills demonstrated by people with AS (Attwood, 2003). One of the modifications is the use of a metaphorical "toolbox" that contains a variety of tools to "repair" an emotion. One part of this program focuses on enabling and encouraging the person with AS and his or her family to detect the early warning signs of emotional distress and to have available a wider variety of emotional repair tools. One of the tools can be access to the circumscribed interest as an emotional restorative. Thus access to the interest is not exclusively achieved by a schedule of controlled availability or as a form of reward, but actively used in specific situations to manage emotions. When distraction, consolation, and conversation are unsuccessful, one option may be to encourage time engaged in the circumscribed interest. If the interest calms the person, then it may have a constructive application.

The interest also can be incorporated into the cognitive restructuring component of the CBT program. For example, one client had a dual diagnosis of AS and a specific phobia—fear of contamination by bacteria. His circumscribed interest was the television program "Dr. Who," a time traveler. A therapy activity was designed whereby the client was encouraged to imagine himself as Dr. Who, marooned on a planet with an invisible monster that creates and thrives on fear. I, as a clinical psychologist, could be imagined as a scientist who has studied the behavior of the monster. Working as a team, the two of us, as Dr. Who and the scientist, developed strategies to overcome the monster and escape from the planet. This theme was typical of many of the television adventures of Dr. Who, and provided a role and conceptualization that was appealing to the client.

In the affective education component of CBT, designed to improve the client's knowledge of emotions and how they affect thoughts, feelings, and behavior, the circumscribed interest can again be used as a metaphor. For example a client with an interest in the weather was able to develop a "barometer" to forecast changes in mood, express thoughts and emotions as weather features (e.g., confusion described as fog), and explain her state of being in the terms of a weather report.

### A Means of Making Friends

Research on children with autism suggests that including the circumscribed interest in an activity can increase willingness to participate and enhance the development of appropriate social skills with peers (Baker, Koegel, & Koegel, 1998) and siblings (Baker, 2000). Can the circumscribed interest facilitate friendships with children with AS? One of the common replies of children and adults to the question "What makes a good friend?" is the reply "We like the same things." Shared interests can form the foundation of friendship. I know one child with AS who has a remarkable interest in, and knowledge of, ants. His classmates tolerated his enthusiasm and monologues on ants, but he was not a popular choice as a companion. In therapy and at school, he was learning a range of friendship skills, such as how to engage in reciprocal conversation skills, waiting, sharing, giving compliments, and demonstrating empathy. He engaged these new skills through intellectual effort and planning, and, not surprisingly, his behaviors were perceived by others as somewhat contrived and artificial. He had few genuine friends.

By chance, another child with AS, who also has an interest in ants, lived near him. A meeting was arranged, whose outcome amazed their parents and teachers. They became companions on ant-finding expeditions, conducted a joint ant study, and regularly contacted each other to share their latest ant-related discoveries. Observation of their interactions revealed a natural fluency and quality to their social skills. They waited patiently, listened attentively, showed empathy, and gave compliments at a level not observed with their peers.

Parents can consider doing some well-planned social engineering, using the child's circumscribed interest to encourage prospective friendships. Local parent support groups usually include the names and addresses of group members but may also identify the circumscribed interests of the members' children to facilitate the engineering of an arranged, but potentially successful, friendship. However, I have noted that when the shared interest ends for one partner, the friendship also may end. Adults with AS can meet like-minded individuals and prospective friends at special clubs and gatherings, such as a train spotters club or a Star Trek Convention.

The interest itself can be used to facilitate friendship with those who do not have AS, though problems also accompany the effort. For example, Penelope, who has an outstanding ability in art, wrote: "Longing to make friends [at school], when someone complimented a drawing I had done, I started giving people drawings until someone accused me of bragging—a rebuke I never forgot. I was only trying to win friendship." Computer abilities are usually popular with peers, and the child with AS may experience great delight in being sought after for advice, to repair a computer "crash," or to develop a new computer program or graphic. The special ability can provide a rare moment of feeling genuinely needed and valued by others. A small group of friends may form at school, based on a common interest in, say, computers, and within this group the person with AS can make genuine friends. Sometimes the friendship based on a common interest develops beyond the platonic stage and becomes a more significant relationship. My conversations with partners of adults with AS often include reference to how the partner's circumscribed interests were initially viewed as endearing and an attractive quality. This opinion can change when the adult with AS has to decide his or her priorities as a partner or parent. The same partners can later complain that they spend too much time and resources on the interest.

A special interest in fiction can provide an opportunity for the child with AS to learn about characters' thoughts and feelings and the social consequences of certain actions. In adolescence this interest may develop into a fascination with television "soap operas." This activity also provides a "safe" vantage point from which to observe and absorb knowledge on interpersonal relationships. However, if the role models and story lines are overdramatized and inappropriate, they will not be helpful "rehearsals" for the person with AS in real-life situations. As an adult, an intense interest in books may lead to reading popular psychology books that provide practical and much-needed advice on relationships. For example, Liane Holliday-

Willey has AS; her interests and abilities in literature have not only been the basis of her academic career but reading books on normal child development has enabled her to better understand her own children (Holliday-Willey, 2001).

Children with AS usually have to be taught to recognize the relevant cues and responses to ensure that a conversation is reciprocal and inclusive. They can be taught to "spot the message"—that is, to recognize signs of boredom, embarrassment, or annoyance in the listener. They may have to be reminded to check in regularly with the other person, looking for nods of approval and signs of jointly focused attention. In addition, they need to learn to seek information about how the conversation is going from the other perspective when they are unsure about the signals. Comments or questions such as "I hope that this isn't boring you" or "What are your thoughts and opinions on this?" are handy tools on such occasions. Sometimes parents or teachers create a "secret sign" with the child with AS, to cue him or her to respond to the subtle signals from the other child and to incorporate his or her friend's knowledge and suggestions or switch the topic to the other child's interests. The child with AS may also need to be given explicit information on who may or may not be an appropriate person with whom to engage in a conversation about his or her interest. The concept of "concentric circles" can be described: Within certain inner circles, such as the family, relatives, and close friends circles, the topic could be appropriate, but when engaging in a conversation with someone the child with AS does not know well, to be more aware of the person and context. These children also seem to have a different perception of time when talking about their interest, and they need to learn to monitor how long they have dominated the conversation with their particular interest. Time goes faster when you are having fun!

## SUMMARY

The circumscribed interest is a distinct and enduring characteristic of AS. The intensity and focus of this interest usually distinguishes children with AS from their peers. The nature and number of interests change over time, and specific triggers may precipitate a new interest. The functions of these interests range from expressing intellectual curiosity regarding the physical world to providing a source of pleasure. Parents are often concerned by how they have had to adapt their personal and family life to accommodate their child's access to the interest. However, strategies that reduce the time spent engaged in the interest or eliminate inappropriate interests are available. The interest can be either a barrier or bridge to social contact; in either case, it can also be used constructively at school and in therapy. The interests can be perceived as a problem—and will then remain a barrier—or as a talent—and will then become a bridge. Some interests can even become a source of personal success and employment.

## REFERENCES

American Psychiatric Association. (2000). *Diagnostic and statistical manual of mental disorders* (4th ed., text rev.). Washington, DC: Author.

Asperger, H. (1979). Problems of infantile autism. *Communication: Journal of the National Autistic Society, 14,* 45–52.

Asperger, H. (1991). Autistic psychopathy in childhood. In U. Frith (Ed.), *Autism and Asperger's syndrome* (pp. 37–91). Cambridge, UK: Cambridge University Press. (Original work published in German 1944)

Attwood, T. (2003). Frameworks for behavioral interventions. In A. Klin & F. Volkmar (Eds.), *Child and adolescent psychiatric clinics of North America: Asperger syndrome* (pp. 65–86). Philadelphia: Elsevier Science.

Baker, M. (2000). Incorporating the thematic ritualistic behaviors of children with autism into games: Increasing social play interactions with siblings. *Journal of Positive Behavior Interventions, 2,* 66–84.

Baker, M., Koegel, R., & Koegel, L. K. (1998). Increasing the social behavior of young children with autism using their obsessive interests. *Journal of the Association for Persons with Severe Handicaps, 23,* 300–309.

Baron-Cohen, S. (1989). Do autistic children have obsessions and compulsions? *British Journal of Clinical Psychology, 28,* 193–200.

Baron-Cohen, S., & Wheelwright, S. (1999). "Obsessions" in children with autism or Asperger syndrome: Content analysis in terms of core domains of cognition. *British Journal of Psychiatry, 175,* 484–490.

Bashe, P., & Kirby, B. L. (2001). *The oasis guide to Asperger syndrome.* New York: Crown.

Frith, U., & Happé, F. (1994). Autism: Beyond "theory of mind." *Cognition, 50,* 115–132.

Gagnon, E. (2001). *Power cards: Using special interests to motivate children and youth with Asperger syndrome and autism.* Kansas City, KS: Autism Asperger Publishing.

Ghaziuddin, M., Wieder-Mikhail, W., & Ghaziuddin, N. (1998). Comorbidity of Asperger syndrome: A preliminary report. *Journal of Intellectual Disability Research, 42,* 279–283.

Gillot, A., Furniss, F., & Walter, A. (2001). Anxiety in high-functioning children with autism. *Autism, 5,* 277–286.

Gray, C. (1998). Social stories and comic strip conversations with students with Asperger syndrome and high-functioning autism. In E. Schopler, G. B. Mesibov, & L. J. Kunce (Eds.), *Asperger syndrome or high-functioning autism?* (pp. 167–198). New York: Plenum Press.

Green, J., Gilchrist, A., Burton, D., & Cox, A. (2000). Social and psychiatric functioning in adolescents with Asperger disorder compared with conduct disorder. *Journal of Autism and Developmental Disorders, 30,* 279–293.

Hinton, M., & Kern, L. (1999). Increasing homework completion by incorporating student interests. *Journal of Positive Behavior Interventions, 1,* 231–234.

Holliday-Willey, L. (2001). *Asperger syndrome in the family.* London: Jessica Kingsley.

Hughes, C., Russell, J., & Robbins, T. W. (1993). Evidence for executive dysfunction in autism. *Neuropsychologia, 32,* 477–492.

Jackson, L. (2002). *Freaks, geeks and Asperger syndrome: A user guide to adolescence.* London: Jessica Kingsley.

Kerbeshian, J., Burd, L., & Fisher, W. (1990). Asperger's syndrome: To be or not to be? *British Journal of Psychiatry, 156,* 721–725.

Kim, J. A., Szatmari, P., Bryson, S. E., Streiner, D. L., & Wilson, F. (2000). The prevalence of anxiety and mood problems among children with autism and Asperger disorder. *Autism, 4,* 117–132.

Klin, A., Carter, A., & Sparrow, S. S. (1997). Psychological assessment of children with autism. In D. J. Cohen & F. R. Volkmar (Eds.), *Handbook of autism and pervasive developmental disorders* (2nd ed., pp. 418–427). New York: Wiley.

Kurita, H. (1999). Brief report: Delusional disorder in a male adolescent with high-functioning PDDNOS. *Journal of Autism and Developmental Disorders, 29,* 419–423.

Ledgin, N. (2002). *Asperger's and self-esteem: Insight and hope through famous role models.* Arlington, TX: Future Horizons.

Mercier, C., Mottron, L., & Belleville, S. (2000). Psychosocial study on restricted interest in high-functioning persons with pervasive developmental disorders. *Autism, 4,* 496–425.

Ozonoff, S., Pennington, B. F., & Rogers, S. J. (1991). Executive function deficits in high-functioning autistic individuals: Relationship to theory of mind. *Journal of Child Psychology and Psychiatry, 32,* 1081–1105.

Paradiz, V. (2002). *Elijah's cup: A family's journey into the community and culture of high-functioning autism and Asperger's syndrome.* New York: Free Press.

Piven, J., Harper, J., Palmer, P., & Arndt, S. (1996). Course of behavioral change in autism: A retrospective study of high-IQ adolescents and adults. *Journal of the American Academy of Child and Adolescent Psychiatry, 35,* 523–529.

Pyles, L. (2000). *Hitch hiking through Asperger syndrome.* London: Jessica Kingsley.

Slater-Walker, G., & Slater-Walker, C. (2002) *An Asperger marriage.* London: Jessica Kingsley.

South, M., Klin, A., & Volkmar, F. R. (1997, April). *Circumscribed interests in higher functioning autism and Asperger syndrome.* Poster presented at the 1997 biannual meeting of the Society for Research in Child Development, Washington, DC.

Tantam, D. (1991). Asperger syndrome in adulthood. In V. Frith (Ed.), *Autism and Asperger syndrome* (pp. 147–183). Cambridge, UK: Cambridge University Press.

Tantam, D. (2000a). Adolescence and adulthood of individuals with Asperger syndrome. In A. Klin, F. R. Volkmar, & S. S. Sparrow (Eds.), *Asperger syndrome* (pp. 367–399). New York: Guilford Press.

Tantam, D. (2000b). Psychological disorder in adolescents and adults with Asperger disorder. *Autism, 4,* 47–62.

Tonge, B., Brereton, A., Gray, K., & Einfeld, S. (1999). Behavioural and emotional disturbance in high-functioning autism and Asperger disorder. *Autism, 3,* 117–130.

Turner, M. (1997). Towards an executive dysfunction account of repetitive behaviour in autism. In J. Russell (Ed.), *Autism as an executive disorder* (pp. 57–100). Oxford: Oxford University Press.

Turner, M. (1999). Annotation: Repetitive behavior. *Autism: A Review of Psychological Research, 1,* 839–849.

Werth, A., Perkins, M., & Boucher, J. (2001). "Here's the weavery looming up": Verbal humour with high-functioning autism. *Autism, 5*(2), 111–125.

# 7

## Assessment and Treatment of Comorbid Emotional and Behavior Problems

DIGBY TANTAM

Infants and children with Asperger syndrome (AS) are infants and children first, and AS sufferers second. They, like other infants and children, have their own particular temperaments and are shaped by their particular experiences. Crises and transitions are times of particular stress for children with AS, as they are in all children. Both learning and behavior may be affected by this stress, sometimes leading to a temporary problem and sometimes to a longer-lasting regression. Childhood trauma has been "rediscovered" in the last 20 years, first in children without other developmental problems and, more recently, in children with learning difficulties. The effects of trauma on children with AS is less well researched, but what is known is reviewed in this chapter.

Like other children, those with AS construct the world in which they live. Unlike most children, who do so within the limits set by the co-constructed world of the family and their peers, those with AS are less enmeshed in a jointly constructed world but live in a world of their own making. This solitariness can give the ideas and perspectives of people with AS an originality that is valuable and praiseworthy. It can also have the opposite effect and make people with AS seem strange or even scary. Indeed, fear of people with AS may lead to their victimization. Much of this chapter addresses the individual reactions that people with AS have to their disorder, to other people, and to their own—often very rich—inner worlds.

The reactions of a person with AS are highly individual because, as noted, a person with AS is not molded by socialization to the same degree as people who do not have AS. For the same reason, people with AS are less likely to have an identity ascribed to them. This means that many children and adolescents with AS are searching for an identity; the chapter ends with some considerations of the pitfalls of that process.

My primary perspective in this chapter is on the needs of the person with AS and his or her family, and this focus influences how I formulate these concerns. Teachers also are concerned about their students. There may be some circumstances in which the needs of other children may have to be put ahead of the needs of the child with AS. Educational psychologists, head teachers, and social workers all manage scarce resources. What they give to one child may have to be taken from another, less needy, child. Their concerns, like those of teachers, are not solely with the person with AS. In reality, this multiple focus is often also true for clinical psychologists, doctors, and other health professionals who may have waiting lists, and for parents who may have other children who need their attention—and of course, they themselves have needs, too. But parents and professionals also have an advocacy role in which they must put the needs of the person with AS first, and champion those needs without thinking of the needs of others who are competing for the same resources. Which perspective one takes—the needs of the group or the needs of the individual—will affect whose concerns are paramount.

## ASSESSMENT CONSIDERATIONS

Because AS is a *developmental* disorder, it is essential that assessment takes developmental considerations into account. Because it is a *neuro*developmental disorder, it is associated with other neurodevelopmental conditions. Finally, because it is often a *hereditary* disorder, it is associated with other hereditary conditions. It is therefore important that any assessment of behavioral and learning cover these distinct difficulties. Differential assessment is especially important in later childhood, adolescence, and adulthood, when behavior and learning may be more affected by the emotional complications of having AS than by the underlying neurodevelopmental impairment.

Assessment is simplified by following a systematic assessment procedure. I have suggested (Tantam, 2002) that psychological treatment is most appropriately based on an assessment of the concerns chosen and that intervention presented by the patient and carers have a palatable emotional flavor and be consistent with the values of the patient and his or her caregivers. This scheme, which was developed for psychotherapy, can be usefully adapted to the assessment of people with AS, with one important modification: It is usually the concern of someone else that leads to a problem being identified, rather than the concern of the person with AS. This is not to say that the person with AS will not *be* concerned; in fact, I assume that, on every occasion a person with AS gives others cause for concern, the person him- or herself has a concern, too.

## COGNITIVE DEFICITS

The cognitive revolution in the social sciences has been accompanied by a decisive shift from psychoanalytic theories of autism as an emotional disorder of some kind to cognitive theories of the disorder. What is meant by this is becoming clearer as functional neuroimaging technology takes a hold on cognitive psychology. Cognitive disorders such as autism are disorders of large-scale neuronal networks that integrate lower-level functions into higher-level and more complex competencies. Object perception, face perception, visuospatial orientation, attention, executive function—all of these are examples of higher-order cognitive functions. Many of these neural networks involve the frontal lobes and adjacent structures of the brain. It is not surprising that several different networks, and therefore several different integrative functions, are often affected in one person. It is important to note that these networks are not necessarily, possibly not even typically, affected by brain damage. There is evidence that the brains of a proportion of people with autism and AS are larger than average, that this structural characteristic is hereditary, that it is particularly demonstrable in middle childhood (Aylward, Minshew, Field, Sparks, & Singh, 2002; Fidler, Bailey, & Smalley, 2000; Fombonne, Rogé, Claverie, Courty, & Frémolle, 1999), and that having a large brain increases the risk of AS in cerebromegaly (Naqvi, Cole, & Graham, 2000; Tantam, Evered, & Hersov, 1990). What seems more likely to be the cause of the problem is a failure of cell death during uterine development, so that neurons with connections that do not assist processing survive alongside neurons that do assist processing. Some have speculated that this dysfunction is one reason why people with AS seem particularly good at detail, and relatively impaired at integrating and abstracting; detail benefits from *numbers* of neurons, whereas the whole picture benefits from *connections* between neurons.

### Catastrophic Reactions

The core cognitive difficulties in AS are discussed more fully in Chapters 3 and 4 of this book. I have mentioned them here for two reasons: The first is that many people with AS are told by others, and often believe, that they have brain damage. It is important to address this misperception, not least because people with AS are often *more* able to perform in some areas than people without AS. Another reason for mentioning cognitive difficulty is that one of the commonest causes of behavior problems is what neurologists call "catastrophic reactions"—the extreme emotional or behavioral responses that can be elicited by failing at a task. These reactions are common in people who have disorders affecting their frontal lobes, such as Alzheimer's disease. In the case of the person with Alzheimer's disease, it is not an impossible task that provokes a catastrophic reaction but often an everyday problems, such as trying to find spectacles that he or she has just put down and now cannot recognize.

In younger children catastrophic reactions are more common during periods of high social interaction, such as getting up in the morning, getting out of the house, breaks at school, after first coming home in the evening, and at bedtime. They are more likely to occur when a person is already aroused, for example, during a new or unexpected situation or because of teasing or bullying by others. Catastrophic reactions also may occur in early childhood, when they are usually referred to as temper tantrums. Some temper tantrums are learned, but others may be due to the immaturity of the child's frontal lobes and the consequent difficulties the child experiences with executive tasks such as choosing between, or switching from, one activity or/to another. Examples of catastrophic reactions in people with AS are shown in Table 7.1.

The best treatment for catastrophic reactions is to avoid them. This cannot always be achieved, but careful assessment of a person's cognitive profile in relation to the situations that the person may have to respond to *can* prevent many of them.

One challenge that has received considerable attention from therapists is the sensory load that some situations can create. The underlying hypothesis is that novel, high-amplitude, and multiple stimuli add to the sensory load and processing breaks down, leading to catastrophic reactions. The theory is attributed to an occupational therapist, Jean Ayres (*http://*

---

**TABLE 7.1. Examples of Catastrophic Reactions**

- Screaming, shouting, swearing
- Overactivity, disruption of others' activities
- Breaking things
- Biting, scratching, hitting others, if restrained
- Biting, scratching, hair pulling, hitting self
- Running away

---

*www.sensoryint.com/ja.html*), and it has been applied by occupational therapists in recent years. The hypothesis receives support from the autobiographical experience of Temple Grandin (Grandin & Scariano, 1986). Many people with AS seem to be particularly sensitive to stimulation, sometimes developing aversions or phobias. Loud or high-pitched noises, scratchy materials, strong lighting, or contrast between dark and light (as in printed text or some soft foods) are just some of the stimuli that people with AS may find aversive (or sometimes attractive; see Lawson, Chapter 9, this volume). Variants of sensory integration include the auditory integration training of Bérard (1993), based on his observation of what he termed hyper- and hypoacusis in children with developmental disorders. Clinical experience seems to bear out the extreme sensitivity of some children with AS to certain sounds, and possibly to other stimuli.

A man with AS attacked a baby in a supermarket because, he said, the sound of her crying was at a pitch that he could not stand (Mawson, Grounds, & Tantam, 1985). This man also had an aversion to the sound of brass band music, and he had smashed furniture on one occasion when it was played on the radio. Other people with AS whom I have known become distressed at the sound of vacuum clearers, ice cream vans, or certain musical tunes. Hyperesthesia is another problem. For example, food fads may be determined by a dislike of certain food textures or the wish to avoid the conjunction of some foods that are hot and some that are cold. Vestibular and olfactory stimulation rarely seem to cause the same problems. Children with AS often resort to stereotyped movement for comfort, and these movements often involve repetitive vestibular stimulation. By contrast, people with AS may show hypalgesia, with an underreaction to pain, although this diminished responsivity may be associated with an increased reaction to injury.

The commonest catastrophic reactions do not occur as a result of particular stimuli but of nonspecific overstimulation. Noisy environments, bright lights, people encroaching on personal space are all potential causes. Catastrophic reactions are more likely when a person with AS is hungry or tired. Repeated studies have failed to support the value of exclusion diets in people with AS, but some parents continue to report dramatic improvements. One possible reason for this reported improvement might be related to simple blood-sugar levels: A large intake of sugar may lead to the overproduction of insulin and a consequent drop in blood sugar 30–60 minutes later, triggering a catastrophic reaction, because the hypoglycemia may produce an effect similar to starvation. Constipation and retention of urine also may increase the chance of a catastrophic reaction.

Catastrophic reactions are indiscriminate; their sole "purpose" is to secure escape from the cognitive overload as quickly as possible. I therefore differentiate them from behavioral problems that may occur when a person reacts with anxiety, shame, anger, or frustration to another person or people. The reaction in these cases is directed at the person, and there is usually a goal. I consider these extreme emotional reactions in the section on psychiatric disorders.

A reaction that begins as a catastrophic one may be repeated in a more controlled, and more calculated, manner, if the person with AS discovers that this emergency response also elicits a desirable response from others in addition to providing an escape. The distinction between catastrophic reactions and extreme emotional reactions is not a hard and fast one.

## How Should Others Respond to a Catastrophic Reaction?

The first consideration is safety, both the safety of the person with AS and the safety of bystanders. Professionals or carers should make a quick assessment to determine whether they need to *do* anything. Since the best response to a catastrophic reaction is to reduce the level of stimulation, it is often best, if safety considerations allow, to withdraw from the person, giving him or her emotional and physical "room." Confrontation or containment increase stimulation loads and should be used only if safety considerations demand the measure. Nor should any attempt be made to talk the affected person "out of" his or her reaction. Talking comes later, after calm has been restored. Carers should try to maintain a calm demeanor and avoid becoming angry or distressed, if possible. Exogenous stimulation, like loud music or shouting, should be reduced whenever possible.

## ASSOCIATED COGNITIVE DEFICITS

Some cognitive deficits are so much a part of AS that it is unclear whether or not they should be considered to be associated or core deficits. Motor delay and clumsiness are commonly seen in people with AS, and the pattern is indistinguishable from children who have an isolated developmental dyspraxia (Green et al., 2002). It seems likely that dyspraxia and AS are either genetically or etiologically linked. Dyslexia, too, is genetically linked to AS (Folstein & Rutter, 1988).

Tics and involuntary vocalizations may occur in children with AS, and some have these problems to a degree that meets criteria for Tourette syndrome. These children are particularly likely to have empathy and attentional problems (Houghton et al., 1999; Kadesjoe & Gillberg, 2000). A subgroup of children with attention-deficit/hyperactivity disorder (ADHD) has been reported to have executive disorders (Houghton et al., 1999; Kadesjoe & Gillberg, 2000), impaired ability in interpreting facial expressions (Cadesky, Mota, & Schachar, 2000), and language disorders (Javorsky, 1996). Children with AS presenting to psychiatrists have an increased likelihood of also having ADHD (Ghaziuddin, Weidmer-Mikhail, & Ghaziuddin, 1998).

Epidemiological studies are still lacking, but the results of case series suggest that there are particular associations between these various disorders, and that children with AS, particularly those with marked empathy disorders, should be carefully reviewed for signs of ADHD, Tourette syndrome, and dysexecutive syndrome. Clinical indicators of the latter syndrome are an inability to switch rapidly between tasks, difficulty in reorganizing a series or list according to new information or difficulties in switching to another strategy when one problem-solving strategy fails, and problems in planning.

Overactivity is common in younger people with AS and may be a particular problem at night. Many children with autistic spectrum disorders (ASD) seem to catnap at night, possibly because of an abnormality in the initiation of rapid eye movement (REM) sleep (Godbout, Bergeron, Limoges, Stip, & Mottron, 2000). Children may get up many times during the night, waking their parents and causing substantial family stress. In normal subjects, a reduction of nighttime REM sleep leads to attentional disorders during the day, and it is possible that there is a relationship in children with AS, too.

Children with AS may show hyperattention, becoming fixed on objects or activities that interest them, to the exclusion of all else, which also can be a source of friction, for example, if parents are busy trying to get the family organized for an outing. It reflects a deeper attentional problem, namely, that people with AS do not automatically assimilate other people's attentional patterns. Other-directed gaze provides a simple example. When we look at another person, normally we look at his or her eyes, at the pupils, rarely veering off to areas of the face near the eyes. Presumably this direct gaze pattern is learned from observation. In contrast, people with AS may look at another person's eyelids, bridge of the nose, eyebrows, but not into his or her eyes.

## ADHD

Unusual deployment of attention is a core problem of AS and there is an overlap with ADHD. ADHD has two components, as currently formulated: an overactivity/impulsivity component and an attentional/executive component. Parents sometimes complain that children with AS are overactive, but this problem usually disappears in middle childhood and is less common in AS than it is in other ASDs. Impulsivity is much rarer in people with AS, and when it does occur, it should raise the possibility of comorbid ADHD, particularly if it is associated with persistent overactivity. Impulsivity in AS may lead to destructive play and reckless actions.

The attentional/executive component of ADHD probably encompasses two distinct difficulties. Executive disorder, or "dysexecutive syndrome," occurs in dementia, schizophrenia, and possibly as a separate developmental disorder. Its main symptom is a failure to decompose a complex task into a sequence of subtasks or multiple tasks, and to be able to carry out the sequence or switch from one multiple task to another and back again in the right order. It is considered in more detail below.

The attentional symptoms of ADHD reflect the greater distractibility of people with this disorder. Clinical experience shows that novel auditory or visual stimuli are more likely to catch their attention, compared to people without ADHD, and existing objects of attention are less likely to hold attention. Processing is hurried, and often flawed, producing difficulties in conversation and in the classroom.

How does this profile compare with people who have AS? Like other people with ASD, people with AS glance for shorter periods, but more frequently, at other people's eyes (O'Connor & Hermelin, 1967; Tantam, Holmes, & Cordess, 1993) than is usual. This pattern may give an appearance of inattention and oddity; people with AS give the same length of glance to people as they do to objects, unless they are objects of special interest to which, as already noted, they may give a much longer look. People without AS normally give longer glances to people than to objects. People with ADHD give shorter glances to both objects and people, compared to people without ADHD. Clinical experience suggests that there are a minority of people with AS who also show this glance pattern, indicating that some people with AS do also suffer from ADHD. Clinical experience also suggests that the subgroup with AS and ADHD has relatively greater problems interpreting nonverbal cues than in nonverbal expression, placing them in the "atypical AS" group. Children with ADHD who also have deficits in face processing (Cadesky et al., 2000; Carter et al., 2000; Handen, Johnson, & Lubetsky, 2000) may overlap with this subgroup of children with AS.

No single hypothesis accounts for these attentional problems. It has been argued that they are due to a failure to inhibit distractors or to an intolerance of delay in reward (Sonuga-Barke, 2002). Clinical experience suggests that, in AS, they also may be due to an inability to deal with complexity. One reason for including distractibility and dysexecutive symptoms in the ADHD diagnostic criteria in the DSM-IV and the ICD-10 (National Institutes of Health, 2000) is that executive problems also may be linked to distractibility. Many people with AS are reported to "learn in their own way" and to succeed without apparently paying attention in the classroom. It is certainly difficult for people with AS to pay attention in the classroom because they do not know *on* what to *focus*. Children with AS, for example, may copy everything that the teacher writes on the blackboard without seeing the points behind what is written; or they may describe looking at the blackboard and seeing only a lot of writing without being able to see where in all that writing they should be looking at any particular moment. It seems likely that the child with AS who succeeds in learning often does so by working things out in his or her own time.

Knowing where to look requires short-term memory. If I look at the board, and then look at my book, and then look up again, I need to have remembered where I was looking last time and go on from there. If I do not retain these place markers in what is nowadays called working memory, I constantly have to begin tasks anew. For example, if I pay attention as someone whispers to me, I will lose what I was thinking if I do not have enough working memory. Or, say, I intended to pack my books, but just then I realized I would have to fetch one from the sitting room. I might come back to the bedroom, having lost my place in the ongoing task of packing the books and end up going to school without them—if, that is, I do not have enough working memory to hold this and other place markers.

Assessment of short-term memory should therefore be included in any assessment of a person with AS. Short-term working memory deficit provides a satisfying explanation of why some people with AS have difficulties in remembering lists, or why their performance of linked tasks may become so easily disrupted. Verbal memory store also explains why people with AS may have problems with multitasking. Parents often observe that if they ask their child a question when the child is absorbed in some other task, a near catastrophic reaction erupts. This level of reactivity can be explained by the child's inability to hold the details of the first task in short-term memory while attending to the second task.

Short-term working memory disorders are linked to dyslexia and may account for the difficulty experienced by some people with AS in processing complex sentences, containing subordinate clauses that need unpacking, with details from each clause being stacked in memory until the end of the sentence has been reached, when all the data can be assembled and the sentence can be understood. (The previous sentence is an example of a sentence with several nested clauses. It was composed to demonstrate how cognitive load is increased by complex syntax.)

Bleepers to remind a person of the next step of a task, diaries, and notepads are all aids that supplement short-term memory and can help with dysexecutive syndrome. Dealing with attentional problems is more difficult. Psychological strategies have usually been based on a behavior modification paradigm, and have not been conspicuously successful. Applying holding techniques with younger children involves some element of attention training, since children are held until they engage with the mother's gaze. Although some parents report benefit from these techniques, many also report that they are very distressing for both mother and child, and some parents have told me that they believe the emotional cost was greater than the attentional benefit.

## Medication

Medication remains the most commonly used treatment for attentional disorder and for hyperactivity. Antidepressants have been used, although their efficacy remains less than fully proven. The most commonly used class of drugs are the amphetamines or stimulants; methylphenidate (Ritalin) is the most commonly used, though it is no more effective than amphetamine but produces less euphoria, probably because it is more slowly absorbed and converted into active metabolites. It does have a euphoriant effect if used intranasally. It has been assumed, with little supportive evidence, that the lack of a "buzz" means that it has less abuse potential. However, this assumption is belied by the sale of methylphenidate "on the street." Methylphenidate increases dopamine in the brain and may therefore increase tics in Tourette syndrome.

Methylphenidate, like amphetamine, does increase the attention span of normal individuals as well as those with ADHD (Carey & Diller, 2001), but professionals continue to disagree about its efficacy in ADHD (Schachter, Pham, King, Langford, & Moher, 2002). One reason for this disagreement may be that the criteria for ADHD apply to a sizeable number of children, including children whose attentional problems are due to anxiety or stress. Methylphenidate may worsen anxiety (Vance & Luk, 1998) and so these children may actually get worse on this medication. My own and other's (Handen, Johnson, & Lubetsky, 2000) clinical experience is that a small group of children with AS and ADHD does benefit from methylphenidate, and a much larger group, with symptoms of restlessness and distractibility, does not benefit.

The long-term side effects of methylphenidate are not known. There is a theoretical danger that its long-term use may increase the risk of depression, but there are also risks in ADHD itself, such as an increased susceptibility to substance misuse, which methylphenidate might reduce. Since about half the children with ADHD remit spontaneously in the early teens, the decision to medicate is a complex one, best initiated only by a clinician who is experienced in ADHD assessment and management. Furthermore, its effects should be carefully monitored, it should be continued only if there is unequivocal benefit, and treatment should be reevaluated in adolescence.

## PSYCHIATRIC DISORDERS

It has already been noted that anxiety and major depression, which are themselves genetically linked, are more common in children with AS than in the general population of children (Kim, Szatmari, Bryson, Streiner, & Wilson, 2000). A disposition to anxiety and lack of confidence may affect children's social interactions from an early age, resulting in shyness or timidity that may prevent them from asking questions in class, concentrating on instruction, or even going to school at all.

Adolescence is a time of increased risk of deliberate self-harm, particularly of the kind called "attempted suicide" in which adolescents seek escape. Deliberate self-harm of this kind is, in my experience, less common in adolescents with AS. Deliberate self-harm also may be repetitive, apparently aimed at relieving tension through infliction of pain or tissue damage. The repetitive nature of this type of self-harm, which is sometimes seen in people with AS (although less so than in more severely affected people with autism), has suggested a link to obsessive–compulsive disorder, and SSRIs such as paroxetine are often prescribed. My experience is that this medication has little effect and that psychological treatment is preferable.

Phobic symptoms may occur in people with AS, including social phobia, in which there is performance anxiety, fearful anticipation of social situations, and a fear of making mistakes or being judged by others. But the extreme self-awareness often associated with social phobia—for example, the fear of blushing or shaking—is rare in people with AS. Social phobias may develop at the onset of adolescence, resulting in school avoidance and eventual social withdrawal and the abandonment of all studies.

People with AS become more aware of their differences in adolescence. This intensified awareness may turn into preoccupations that become so intense that they interfere with their studies. Youngsters with AS may spend more and more time worrying about this newly perceived difference, ruminating about past occasions when they felt misunderstood, or making idealistic plans for the future, often based on their own special interests. A sensitivity to criticism may develop; the person with AS may withdraw into special interests, and become increasingly unaware of their impact on other people in the household.

Bipolar disorder is more common in people with AS, and in their family members, than in the general population. Onset is rare before late adolescence. It is more likely that mania will be misdiagnosed as schizophrenia in people with AS because the previous lack of socialization is taken to be evidence of schizoid personality disorder. Rapid cycling disorder, in which there is an alternation between high and low moods over weeks rather than months, also may occur in people with AS, although the condition is probably overdiagnosed. Treatment is along similar lines to treatment of bipolar adults, although people with AS may be more reluctant to take regular blood tests, which are required for some of the drugs used in this condition.

There has been a persistent linkage between AS and a diagnosis of schizophrenia, sometimes at an early age. Many people with AS have unusual visual experiences (e.g., seeing falling lights or shapes in their visual fields), and some have unusual beliefs which do seem similar to the acute or positive symptoms of schizophrenia. It should not be assumed that these symptoms will progress. Acute psychotic episodes may occur in people with AS, but they are short-lived and emerge in response to anxiety. The so-called first-rank symptoms of schizophrenia may be present during these brief episodes, but they are not predictive of a long-term illness or of social deterioration. The psychotic symptoms respond to antipsychotic medication in the usual way.

## EPILEPSY

Epilepsy is more common in people with AS, affecting perhaps as many as one in every five; possibly slightly less than in autism, but still a substantially increased risk compared to the general population. The epilepsy may begin in infancy, though rarely, in which case the epilepsy itself may be implicated in the development of AS; usually it begins later in childhood, sometimes in adolescence. Absence attacks (i.e., cessation of mental activity without loss of motor control) may occur before the development of seizures and may disrupt learning. Complex seizures may be associated with automatic behavior that occasionally causes behavioral problems. All types of seizures may lead to accident and potential harm, and medication is essential.

Unfortunately, medication may affect cognitive function and therefore learning. Since antiepileptic drugs do seem to affect different people in different ways, the best way of minimizing side effects is to try to find the right drug and then to keep the dose at the minimum necessary to control symptoms. Different types of seizure respond to different drugs, and are constantly being developed, so it is best to initiate drug treatment in a specialist center with experience in the range of drugs. Seizures can be provoked by emotional factors, by hunger, fatigue, illness, or other physical changes, or by missing doses. Counseling and support of children with epilepsy are therefore an important element of treatment, and one that can reduce the doses of drugs needed for epilepsy control.

## TRANSITION, CRISIS, AND TRAUMA

Adapting to change is a particular difficulty for people with AS, and major changes, such as going to school for the first time, changing schools, or leaving school, can provoke anxiety, behavioral problems, and regression. Many parents and carers recognize this possibility and talk through what is likely to happen with their child. Preparatory visits to school, getting to know the new teacher, and moving to a new school with other familiar children can all reduce the shock. The shock can be greater if several changes are combined. Moving to a residential school may be particularly stressful, partly because the child has to give up regular contact with parents or family members, but also due to the loss of a familiar environment and routine.

People with AS may not overtly grieve in these circumstances—or, indeed, following any other losses—but they may cling to such routines as are still left. Many times I have been told by shocked parents that, on the day that one of them was being taken to the hospital with an acute illness, their son or daughter with AS could only ask, "What's going to happen for dinner?" This lack of feeling is deceptive. The expression of grief, and other emotional reactions, has to be learned through acculturation—a process that may pass by people with AS. However, they may feel loss, even if they cannot express it. Acute loss results in anxiety, which leads to a need to cling to old routines. Wanting to reestablish some routine may be the reason a child would ask about dinner, or some other everyday concern. Prolonged loss leads to social withdrawal. A person with AS may stand out in the new environment, given his or her combination of social withdrawal and odd routines. If the transition has involved moving into new accommodation, then bullying or teasing may begin in this vulnerable period and, once begun, may be difficult to reverse.

Life changes may not be as sudden as transitions, but similar factors may operate. In later childhood and adolescence, social withdrawal may be gradual but reinforced by a belief that the world is a bad place. Adolescents with AS may spend their time engaging in their special interests, in routines, and in ruminations about past episodes. The interests of younger children often have links with this experience of marginalization, too. They may be compensatory, for example, watching wrestling videos over and over, and identifying with the apparently invulnerable wrestlers who are the object of such veneration. Or the interests may involve a reenactment of the kind of victimization that the child experiences.

Traumatic transitions or crises, in which the change or transition coincides with some emotional trauma, may lead to a regression that is long term. There have been no studies of sexual or physical abuse in children with AS, but people with AS do often find themselves in sexual situations in which they seem to others to be exploited. Exploitation is subjective. Sometimes people with AS who are putting themselves at risk sexually, or who have very one-sided relationships in which others seem to benefit more than them, express pleasure or satisfaction with the relationships. At other times, they do not speak of them, and seem to give them little importance. But in some of these cases there is a discernible deterioration in the mood or behavior of the person with AS, which indicates that he or she is being exploited and suffering in consequence. People with AS may deny they are being exploited, so a negative answer should not stop further enquiries, although these obviously need to be made sensitively and confidentially. A few people with atypical AS make unwarranted accusations about others, including allegations of abuse, and staff may react in a defensive manner. A move of school or accommodation may be the only way to resolve the situation for the affected person. Formal enquiries may prevent problems in the future but rarely provide emotional resolution in the present.

## REACTIONS TO DIAGNOSIS

### The Person with Asperger Syndrome

How AS affects a person will depend on how he or she reacts to the disorder, and how others react. The consequences of the disorder may not be the only cause for a reaction; it may be the fact that a diagnosis has or has not been made. Parents overwhelmingly wish to receive a diagnosis, which they see as being the key to getting the help that their child needs. But receiving a diagnosis may itself be a problem, in two ways. The commonest is that the parents willingly accept the diagnosis, but the person with AS rejects it. This divergence in views may become a source of conflict, and the child may conclude that the parents want to diminish him or her in some way. In these circumstances, I advise parents to discuss what their son or daughter may think the diagnosis means. It is very common for people to think AS means a mental handicap or learning disability, for example. A frank discussion of what AS is—I always say that it is a disorder of nonverbal communication—is helpful. Sometimes the diagnosis is feared because the child may view it as a prelude to being sent away, or that it will lead to some sort of rejection. In adolescence the greater fear is usually that accepting such a diagnosis means having to accept the loss of the kind of future that the adolescent has seen for him- or herself. There is no simple answer to this problem, except to allow the person to undergo some degree of mourning and not to press him or her to accept the diagnosis until he or she is ready.

An alternative to diagnosis is to discuss problems in functional terms. For example, when a 9-year-old boy comes home, upset, from school, saying that no one wants to spend time with him, it may be best to talk about what happens when other people interact with him, and how the 9-year-old's reactions might affect others. This discussion can take place without specifically saying that the boy has AS. Instead, the problem can be described behaviorally: The child does not always know what to say to other children, or wants to talk only about what interests him, or does not notice when other children are getting bored—and so on.

A rarer situation is using AS as an excuse for a behavior that has become problematic. Occasionally, rituals grow to such proportions that they not only monopolize the time of the person with AS but dictate the household routine as well. This is particularly likely to happen if the rituals take the form of obsessive thoughts or questions that require others' participation or response. A person with AS may become dependent on getting reassurance from a family member that he or she is clean enough, that the CDs are still in the order they were in a few minutes before, or whatever it is that obsesses the person. Once a pattern of reassurance has been set, it may be difficult to break, and the person may use his or her AS as a reason for needing the reassurance, implying that having AS entitles him or her to different treatment from that given to people who do not have it. The best way to deal with this dynamic is to hold firmly in mind that reassurance or participation in rituals actually makes the rituals worse, not better. Any short-term gain that is produced is more than wiped out by the long-term cost. The person with AS is entitled to be protected from being made worse, and is therefore entitled to having reassurance withheld, not provided. Sometimes it is necessary to have a formal agreement about such demands. It might, for example, be agreed that a question will be answered once or even tice, and thereafter the response to the question will be "I have given you the answer."

## Others' Reactions

Professionals place considerable emphasis on family factors in all childhood disorders, and rightly so. However, emphasizing the parents' role in their children's difficulties can have a significant downside, too. Already overburdened parents may simply become more stressed and less able to meet their children's needs. Parents may feel blamed and that services are unwilling to accept any responsibility for providing help. All too often, a professional's lack of clarity about the child's diagnosis is resolved by diagnosing a family problem or by brushing off the problem as the concern of an overinvolved or overanxious parent. Some parents do respond to the needs of a child with AS by physical punishment or control; some may have AS themselves and cannot provide for their child's emotional needs at all; some parents develop marital conflicts because of disagreements about how to deal with a child with AS; and some have their own psychological problems who feels that they, and only they, understand what their child needs.

and the enmeshed parent of professional legend. In my experience, the vast majority of parents show extraordinary patience and determination. Those parents who do fail to handle their children's problems as they would like, often volunteer this information, as long as they trust the professional to recognize the challenge of living with children who have AS. It is rare to find a parent who started out with a disregard for the needs of his or her child, and much more common to find one who has become more and more stressed by what he or she perceives as the tendency of professionals to overlook the problems of the child in favor of blaming the parent.

This excessive preoccupation with parenting styles also has directed professional attention away from peers such as siblings, fellow students at school, and children in the neighborhood. Peer relationships are an important basis for self-esteem. People with AS model themselves, without realizing it, on their peers. This is probably the way that people with AS learn social skills (see below). Studies of childhood trauma have focused on parents as the source, but peer relationships also can inflict adverse emotional effects, either through marginalization or victimization.

Most people with AS experience themselves as being excluded, and very often attribute this exclusion to the badness of other people. They may even experience others as malicious or as deliberately trying to harm them. Usually, though, it is at a less intense level; there is the feeling that society is narrow-minded and sometimes hypocritical. People with AS may identify with marginalized subgroups, such as criminals or people labeled as deviant (or other children at school with problems). Later in life, the sense that society is closed against people with AS can lead to a feeling of futility and giving up; children and adolescents have not usually become so disenchanted, and still protest. Victimization can occur through name calling, derogatory comments, catcalling and jeering, physical manhandling, and deliberate humiliation or injury. Such attacks may be extended to siblings, particularly if those siblings try to defend the person with AS. In severe cases, the victimization is extended to the family at home, with objects left in mailboxes. People with AS may be spat at, have their clothes torn, or be put up to escapades that result in further humiliation or punishment.

Bullying always involves humiliation. In fact, there seems to be a strong relationship between the two, since children who are prone to shame are more likely to be bullied and are more likely to be paralyzed by bullying, so that they cannot take effective steps to combat it. Telling parents about the bullying may only compound the problem. Fathers, particularly, are inclined to say that it is just a matter of fighting back, thereby implying that the failure to resolve the problem is the fault of the bullied child. Teachers do not say this explicitly, but they may imply that bullied children are somehow weak. Attitudes toward bullying in school have changed considerably, but there continue to be schools that claim that they "cannot eradicate" bullying, that it is a natural consequence of "kids being kids." Other schools have been able to enact effective antibullying measures, including a "cultural" change of rejecting rather than admiring the playground tough guy.

## DEALING WITH OTHERS' EMOTIONS

Many people with AS develop a theoretical understanding of what makes other people act as they do. The extent to which this understanding is based on what the person with AS would do personally versus a recognition of other people being different varies. Many mothers have a soft spot for their child with AS and enjoy having conversations about why other people have behaved as they have. When conversations like this can be conducted calmly and thoughtfully, they are remembered by the person with AS and can be applied later. The use of "social stories" is a formalization and extension of this ordinary domestic activity.

However well-constructed the narrative about the social world, there will always be a gap when it comes to dealing with social situations. In kindly people with AS, this gap may be apparent only in the most intense situations or in the closeness of an intimate relationship. The readiness of a person with AS to try to put right any lack of empathy makes up for a lot. The difficulty arises when others want or expect to be understood without having things spelled out letter by letter.

Two common situations in which the empathy gap arises are close friendships or intimate partnerships, and in matters involving discipline. Childhood friendships are typically based on common interests and the absence of friction. Mature friendships begin in adolescence and require deeper commitment and loyalty (Argyle & Henderson, 1984), in which empathizing with someone's unspoken feelings becomes important. Discipline, too, is based on empathy, although in this case what is required is a sensitivity to anger rather than to hurt or distress. Fathers will say of their sons with AS, "He never sees what effect he's having" or "You'd think he'd have noticed that he was really winding us up." Teachers at school find that their cherished signals for warning pupils that their patience is limited fail to work with these students. The child with AS carries on regardless. It is not enough to explain that a person with AS may literally lack the capacity to process facial and other nonverbal expressions of feeling. There is a strong, normative sense that people should simply possess this capacity and when it is not in evidence, it is because a person is cocky or brass-faced. Children with AS may turn with panic to ask parents or others if they have acted correctly or "been good." When a child behaves in this manner, it should not be assumed that he or she has been abused or damaged by someone, even if this level of need for reassurance might suggest an abuse history. People with AS tend to stick with social strategies once they have worked, even if they are much less applicable to the new situations in which they apply them.

As noted, a child also may react catastrophically to an emotional demand, withdrawing or exploding. Such reactions can lead to angry confrontations and sometimes physical fights at home, particularly when fathers believe that they should be able to control their own children. A further reaction, most common in children with a lack of empathy, is outrage or uproar. The child learns that he or she can anticipate or derail emotional demands by disruption. One further advantage of doing something so outrageous or upsetting that everyone gets angry is that it is easy to read extreme anger, and the child consequently is faced with less uncertainty.

Successful parents, teachers, and carers of people with AS learn to avoid criticizing the child or making emotional demands, and to set limits calmly but firmly, justifying them in the interests of the child and not of the family or the school. Many parents discover that they have to talk about things to their child that they would normally expect the child to know without being told. Such a discussion might include putting their own obvious feelings into words, something that normally seems odd or demanding. Telling a person with AS how you feel easily turns into a reproach. But if this undercurrent of reproach can be avoided, and the feedback is exactly that—feedback—then verbalizing feelings can be a way of teaching empathy to someone with AS.

## FRIENDSHIP

Not having a close friend is probably one of the most obvious ways that AS shows itself to others. Not having a friend is not just a cause of loneliness, it is also a stigma. So many people with AS will claim to have friends, even if others do not think that they do. Acquaintances may be taken as friends, so may professionals, or even houseguests. There is nothing silly about this behavior. It simply reflects that people with AS may count as friends people toward whom they feel friendly. People with AS may be oblivious to the sharing or mutuality that is such an important basis for adult friendship for many people. However, they may develop close friendships, especially if someone else takes the initiative. The "someone else" may be a third party who arranges meetings, or a casual friend. People with AS are more likely to be friends with someone much older than themselves who takes responsibility for fostering the friendship. The Internet is rapidly becoming a new source of friends for many people, including those with AS. E-mailing and participating in chat rooms are particularly congenial for many people with

AS, because these mediums allow them to circumvent many of the complexities of nonverbal communication.

## SEXUALITY

Asperger discussed sexuality in the cases that he originally reported, only to dismiss it. People with AS were simply not interested, he thought. Although this is true of some, it is by no means true of all. Children with AS who have been sexually abused may show the precocious development of sexual behavior that is a common consequence of childhood abuse. Outrageous behavior may involve inappropriate sexual touching that, although it is probably not perceived by the child as sexual, is certainly considered a mild sexual assault by others. Some children with AS who also have associated physical conditions such as Sotos syndrome may experience early puberty, and the complications that arise. There is no evidence that physical puberty is delayed in AS, but psychological puberty may be, as Asperger noted. However, this delay is not always the case, and once the adolescent has begun to feel sexual longing, significant behavioral problems may follow.

The commonest issue of this time period is the heightened desire to have friends, because it is friends who will become potential sexual partners. Loneliness and recrimination may be reinforced by the difficulties that almost always arise in finding a partner. If a person with AS lacks social awareness, he or she may be unaware of the conventions that surround sexual behavior, and inappropriate or public masturbation can be a problem. Simple rules such as "You can do that in your own room, when you're on your own and won't be disturbed" usually solve this problem. There may be an increase in time spent in the bathroom at this time, perhaps related to sexually provoked cleaning rituals. My clinical experience is that some naive and needy young men with AS may be seduced by older men, which may lead them into a pattern of seeking sexual contact as a kind of substitute for friendship.

Sexual fetishes are not uncommon in people with AS. The most common that I have come across is an interest in blond hair. This interest may manifest initially in admiring comments about blond-haired people, men and women, progress to touching their hair, and end in being an intrusive and disturbing ritual of having to touch blond hair. Occasionally the person with AS may resent the effect that a person with blond hair has on them and target them for abuse or even attack. As is the case with many other interpersonal rituals in AS, it is easier to prevent a hair fetish than it is to treat it once it has developed. Greeting behavior is particularly susceptible to ritualization, and teachers or parents should look out for any greeting behavior that has an aggressive or inappropriate element. A child with AS who taps people he meets on the shoulder in a familiar and hardly perceptible way at the age of 8 may, at the age of 18, be punching strangers unexpectedly and painfully.

People with AS may become overattached to school staff members. Again this attachment may surface in an apparently harmless way but unless firmly addressed, may develop into jealousy-inspired threats or aggression. Female staff are most often the targets, and their fear and vulnerability may reinforce the behavior, because it is interpreted as a symptom of the potency of the person with AS. The partners of female staff also may be targeted. Staff in this situation often fear being stalked. However, I have rarely come across a situation in which a person with AS has actually stalked someone.

Infatuations should always be taken seriously. However much they appear to be one-sided to others, the person with AS may experience the same intensity of attachment as if the feelings were reciprocated. Many women who have become the object of such one-sided attention are frightened or disgusted and do not want to interact with the person subsequently. My experience is that this aversion can make matters worse.

### CASE EXAMPLE

A young man with AS had begun to stare at a pretty neighbor and then to shout insulting things at her. He had known her for years but avoided her now that she had become a young woman. He told his parents that she was interfering with his thinking, and he was referred to a psychiatrist who diagnosed schizophrenia (the diagnosis of AS had not been made at that point) and put the young man on medication. Fortunately, the medication quickly stopped because of unacceptable side effects. However, the situation did not improve. The young man seemed fascinated by his neighbor and was always looking out of his window trying to catch a glimpse of her. If he did see her, he would keep up a running critical commentary on what she was doing. The parents began to worry that there would be a serious incident. Then the two saw each other in the street and the girl crossed over, approached the young man and said that they had known each other a long time, and that she did not want to be his enemy. She hugged him, and invited him to come to the pub for a chat. He declined, but thereafter he had nothing but praise for the young woman when she was mentioned, and his fascination with her disappeared.

The young woman in the case example seems to have been remarkably compassionate and self-confident. It would be inappropriate to recommend her strategy on every occasion. But the example does show that when a woman avoids, or fails to confront, a man who is infatuated with her, or if she gets angry or tries to reject him, it confers a potency on the man that can, in some circumstances, increase the infatuation. A better approach is to openly address the man's behavior, but from a position of invulnerability and untouchability.

Some young people with AS look back from adolescence to early childhood with nostalgia. This wistful longing can be linked to playing with younger children that may have become sexualized. There is insufficient evidence to know whether this behavior progresses to pedophilia. In the United Kingdom several people with AS have had computers seized by the police because they have accessed child pornography, but this has usually been in the context of accessing other pornography, too. It seems more likely that these people failed to apply a judgment about age rather than selectively accessing pedophilic material.

The greatest risk of sexual assault on children by people with AS comes, in my clinical experience, from older children and adolescents whose social age may not be very different from the children they assault. These assaults may be reenactments of assaults that the perpetrators have experienced themselves from other children, and they rarely lead to any kind of sexual consummation. The reaction of the authorities differs markedly from place to place, country to country. There may be no involvement of the police at all, involvement but no prosecution, or prosecution. Once the case gets into the courts, however, little allowance is given for the presence of AS, and sentencing can be harsh.


## AGGRESSION

Aggression, along with socially inappropriate behavior, poor conversational skills, and academic deficits, is one of the commonest problems identified by parents of the children whom I assess. It is likely that there is an element of selection bias; the actual frequency of aggression in the whole population of children and adolescents with AS is not known. When aggression is a problem, it can have special features that make it difficult to address and resolve. The absence of facial expression in many people with AS can make it hard for others to detect emerging aggression. The normal inhibitory factors of aggression, such as the expression of fear on the faces of victims, may be less effective in people with AS, perhaps because people with AS do not read these signals. Those with AS who have dysexecutive difficulties may be unable to anticipate how other people will view the consequences of their aggression and may therefore act aggressively even in circumstances where it will be greatly to their disadvantage. Perhaps one of the most difficult aspects of the aggression displayed by people with AS is that it may be displaced. People with AS may therefore become aggressive some time after the triggering event, displaying aggression to someone unconnected from the person who triggered their anger in the first place. Targets may be chosen for their lack of ability to retaliate; younger siblings, mothers, or, in residential communities, inexperienced female staff, may be particularly at risk.

Violence may be calculated, but it is rarely self-interested. For example, a man with AS manufactured letter bombs and sent them to judges and other people who were, in his mind, "soft" on family values. His motive seems to have stemmed from a fascination with family law, in conjunction with a sense that a grave injustice had been done to his sister during her divorce proceedings, which had taken place many years before. Impulsive violence is much more common than this kind of calculated violence. It may occur as one component of a catastrophic reaction, in which case careful consideration of its antecedents may enable prevention. People with AS who become aggressive sometimes recognize an aggrieved state, when they feel upset or angry about some particular event, which then leads to a pre-aggressive state when they feel wound up and ready to explode. It is difficult to alter the pre-aggressive state, but helping people with AS recognize the aggrieved state and do something about it can be more successful. People with AS often do not know how to deal with grievance. They may often have had the experience that their grievances have been misunderstood or brushed aside. Advice about to how get other people to pay attention to their grievance and respond appropriately can be surprisingly effective.

Bullying or victimization is a common trigger for aggression, though this association may not be obvious if the aggressive response is displaced onto another target, at another time, and in another situation. A careful search for bullying and an active commitment to remedying it are integral to aggression management.

## Self-Harm

Stereotyped self-harming behavior is rarer in those with AS than it is in people with autism, but it may occur. Adolescents with AS also may harm themselves in similar ways, and in similar situations, to other adolescents, cutting their wrists or taking overdoses in response to frustration or hopelessness.

## Fire Setting

Many people with AS seem to have a fascination with fire, and some may deliberately set fires. Fire setting may be motivated by gain or revenge or because fire setting is perceived to be intrinsically rewarding, as occurs in

pyromania. It is reported that pyromania is often motivated by an interest
in fire fighting, and that pyromaniacs will wait at the scene to join in fire-
fighting efforts. People with AS seem more interested in the fire itself, and
may give little thought to what happens after the fire takes hold. Discussion
of the dangers of fire may help as long as setting a fire is not made to sound
bold or exciting. Many people with AS like the power of fire and the fear
that it induces in people, because they feel that they lack this power themselves. Only a few people with AS who take an unusual interest in fire go
on to set a serious fire, such as a fire in a building. When adolescents set
such fires, it is often under the influence of the disinhibiting effects of being
in a social group, being intoxicated, or both. Adolescents with AS who set
fires, unless they have atypical AS, are more likely to act alone and in cold
blood. The risk of repetition is therefore proportionately greater, and regular supervision must be instituted. Assessment by an experienced professional, such as a forensic psychiatrist or psychologist, should be considered.

## Medication

Aggression may become habitual and, once this happens, drug treatment
may become necessary. Aggression can be a consequence of irritability and
a symptom of depression or of hypomania. If either of these conditions is
present, appropriate medication for the underlying mood disorder may reduce the aggression. Anticonvulsant drugs such as carbamazepine and so-
dium valproate are effective treatments of hypomania and can prevent
mood swings. These drugs also seem to reduce aggression in some people
with AS who do not apparently have a mood disorder. Unless there are
medical contraindications, they should be considered if psychosocial management has failed. Propranolol, a beta blocker, can reduce anxiety and
possibly reduce the risk of catastrophic reactions, but in my experience is
not often of benefit. There continues to be concern that serotonergic antidepressants (i.e., those that increase the availability of 5HT [serotonin] at
synapses) may increase aggression toward the self and others. Paradoxical
agitation may occur with these drugs, and it does seem likely, though rare,
that the aggression is worsened. I have had a few patients in whom this
worsening does seem to happen. Selective serotonin reuptake inhibitors
(SSRIs) should therefore be used with caution.

Past forms of treatment for aggression utilized sedating drugs, either
benzodiazepines or sedative antipsychotics. Benzodiazepines adversely affect learning and may increase disinhibition. Furthermore, there is a risk of
dependency and should therefore be avoided for any but the most short-
term of interventions. Antipsychotics have many serious side effects, including tardive dyskinesia, which may be more of a risk for people with AS.
A more subtle, but possibly more important, complication is that high

doses of antipsychotics may themselves cause disinhibition. This is a different disinhibition from that caused by benzodiazepine, and is more akin to mild confusion. The state is difficult to distinguish from the overaroused states that some people with AS can get into when stressed. When it is treated with an increase in the antispsychotic drug, something of a vicious circle is created. The newer atypical antipsychotics are currently thought to have fewer side effects, but there has been insufficient experience with their long-term effects to be confident about this finding. If antipsychotics must be used, it should be remembered that they are purely symptomatic treatments, and that they need to be reviewed regularly.

## IDENTITY ISSUES

The strongest impression that many children and adolescents with AS create is one of uniqueness. Children with AS may seem oblivious to the anxiety that children normally feel in clinical settings and, coupled with their often pedantic language and overfamiliarity, may give an impression of confidence and precocity. This impression can be very misleading. People with AS feel a lack of personal identity, which can lead them to mimic others, copy their mannerisms, or to even adopt their accent, gait, or turns of phrase. This is not to say that people with AS are good at imitation. It is very hard for someone with AS to invent a part or imagine what someone would say in a new situation. What people with AS *can* do is convey, in their own actions or speech, memories of what someone has done or said. Parents may say that when someone with AS mimics another person, the resemblance is "uncanny." This is because they repeat exactly what the other person said or did without reenacting it.

The most able people with AS may be aware of this imitative aspect about themselves and say that they have always played a role or never been real. One young man I met recently told his mother, several times and in some distress, that he had no personality. Routines can provide a kind of identity scaffolding, which may be one reason people with AS are so reluctant to forego them. One young man liked to go to Disney World, in Orlando, Florida. To cope with all the time he was in England rather than Orlando, he had constructed a Disney World identity based on food fads. For example, he would eat cheese at home but never in Florida. But in Florida he would eat shellfish, which he detested at home.

People with AS often continue to develop socially in their adult life. They do so by developing better methods for dealing with social situations, perhaps aided by the greater tolerance of eccentricity in adulthood). These methods are not learned consciously or even by imitation, but by mimicry. When asked how they solved this or that social dilemma, people with AS may say, "I thought, what had I seen Johnnie do in this situation, and I did that." If a person with AS is close to another person who has a full range of social skills, the association can provide an effective source of social skills.

The downside of this lack of identity is that people with AS seem to copy socially disruptive or outlandish behavior readily, perhaps because it clearly has an impact on others. This pattern is particularly problematic in children who lack empathy and experience themselves as powerless. "Friends" may turn out to be antisocial children who gain satisfaction at seeing the person with AS copying their more outrageous behavior and carrying out their suggestions for committing criminal or antisocial acts, without any concern for their likely consequences.

Beliefs and values constitute a substantial part of identity. People with AS may champion strongly held beliefs and values, but these are often borrowed from others and may change quite suddenly. The beliefs or values may sometimes be racist or sexist, and may cause offense. They also may be liberal and democratic. The origin of these values will often be the family. In this way, as with many others, people with AS hold up a mirror to us in which we see that normality (as people with AS say, "neurotypicality") is not necessarily the superior state we believe it to be.

## REFERENCES

Argyle, M., & Henderson, M. (1984). The rules of friendship. *Journal of Social and Personal Relationships, 1,* 211–237.
Aylward, E. H., Minshew, N. J., Field, K., Sparks, B. F., & Singh, N. (2002). Effects of age on brain volume and head circumference in autism. *Neurology, 59*(2), 175–83.
Bérard, G. (1993). *Hearing equals behavior.* New York: Keats.
Cadesky, E. B., Mota, V. L., & Schachar, R. J. (2000). Beyond words: How do children with ADHD and/or conduct problems process nonverbal information about affect? *Journal of the American Academy of Child and Adolescent Psychiatry, 39,* 1160–1167.
Carey, W., & Diller, L. (2001). Concerns about Ritalin. *Journal of Pediatrics, 139,* 338–340.
Carter, A. S., O'Donnell, D. A., Schultz, R. T., Scahill, L., Leckman, J. F., & Pauls, D. L. (2000). Social and emotional adjustment in children affected with Gilles de la Tourette's syndrome: Associations with ADHD and family functioning. *Journal of Child Psychology and Psychiatry, 41,* 215–223.
Fidler, D. J., Bailey, J. N., & Smalley, S. L. (2000). Macrocephaly in autism and other pervasive developmental disorders. *Developmental Medicine and Child Neurology, 42,* 737–740.
Folstein, S. E., & Rutter, M. L. (1988). Autism: Familial aggregation and genetic implications. *Journal of Autism and Developmental Disorders, 18,* 3–30.

Fombonne, E., Rogé, B., Claverie, J., Courty, S., & Frémolle, J. (1999). Microcephaly and macrocephaly in autism. *Journal of Autism and Developmental Disorders, 29*, 113–119.

Ghaziuddin, M., Weidmer-Mikhail, M., & Ghaziuddin, N. (1998). Comorbidity of Asperger syndrome: A preliminary report. *Journal of Intellectual Disability Research, 42*(Pt. 4), 279–283.

Godbout, R., Bergeron, C., Limoges, E., Stip, E., & Mottron, L. (2000). A laboratory study of sleep in Asperger's syndrome. *Neuroreport, 11*, 127–130.

Grandin, T., & Scariano, M. (1986). *Emergence: Labeled autistic.* Novato, CA: Arena.

Green, D., Baird, G., Barnett, A. L., Henderson, L., Huber, J., & Henderson, S. E. (2002). The severity and nature of motor impairment in Asperger's syndrome: A comparison with specific developmental disorder of motor function. *Journal of Child Psychology and Psychiatry and Allied Disciplines, 43*, 655–668.

Handen, B. L., Johnson, C. R., & Lubetsky, M. (2000). Efficacy of methylphenidate among children with autism and symptoms of attention-deficit hyperactivity disorder. *Journal of Autism and Developmental Disorders, 30*, 245–255.

Houghton, S., Douglas, G., West, J., Whiting, K., Wall, M., Langsford, S., Powell, L., & Carroll, A. (1999). Differential patterns of executive function in children with attention-deficit hyperactivity disorder according to gender and subtype. *Journal of Child Neurology, 14*, 801–805.

Javorsky, J. (1996). An examination of youth with attention-deficit/hyperactivity disorder and language learning disabilities: A clinical study. *Journal of Learning Disabilities, 29*, 247–258.

Kadesjoe, B., & Gillberg, C. (2000). Tourette's disorder: Epidemiology and comorbidity in primary school children. *Journal of the American Academy of Child and Adolescent Psychiatry, 39*, 548–555.

Kim, J. A., Szatmari, P., Bryson, S. E., Streiner, D. L., & Wilson, F. J. (2000). The prevalence of anxiety and mood problems among children with autism and Asperger syndrome. *Autism, 4*, 117–132.

Mawson, D., Grounds, A., & Tantam, D. (1985). Violence and Asperger's syndrome: A case study. *British Journal of Psychiatry, 147*, 566–569.

Naqvi, S., Cole, T., & Graham, J. M. (2000). Cole–Hughes macrocephaly syndrome and associated autistic manifestations. *American Journal of Medical Genetics, 94*, 149–152.

National Institutes of Health. (2000). National Institutes of Health Consensus Development Conference Statement: Diagnosis and treatment of attention-deficit/hyperactivity disorder (ADHD). *Journal of the American Academy of Child and Adolescent Psychiatry, 39*, 182–193.

O'Connor, N., & Hermelin, B. (1967). The selective visual attention of psychotic children. *Journal of Child Psychology and Psychiatry, 8*, 167–179.

Schachter, H., Pham, B., King, J., Langford, S., & Moher, D. (2002). How efficacious and safe is short-term methylphenidate for the treatment of attention-deficit disorder in children and adolescents? A meta-analysis. *Canadian Medical Association Journal, 165*, 1475–1488.

Sonuga-Barke, E. (2002). Dual bio-psychological pathways to ADHD: Some general reflections and a specific proposal [Online]. Available: *http://www.inabis2002.org/symposia_congress/SYMP_04/No_01.htm*

Tantam, D. (2002). *Psychotherapy and counselling in practice.* Cambridge, UK: Cambridge University Press.

Tantam, D., Evered, C., & Hersov, L. (1990). Asperger's syndrome and ligamentous laxity. *Journal of the American Academy of Child And Adolescent Psychiatry, 29,* 892–896.

Tantam, D., Holmes, D., & Cordess, C. (1993). Nonverbal expression in autism of Asperger type. *Journal of Autism and Developmental Disorders, 23,* 111–133.

Vance, A. L., & Luk, E. S. (1998). Attention deficit hyperactivity disorder and anxiety: Is there an association with neurodevelopmental deficits? *Australian and New Zealand Journal of Psychiatry, 32,* 650–657.

# II

Asperger Syndrome
in the Schools

# 8

# Remembering School

## WENDY LAWSON

I don't think that I was very "self-aware" when I was a young child. Life was constantly confusing and scary. Maybe subconsciously I knew I was different from other children. I just knew that we had nothing in common, and I wasn't drawn to seek out their company. For most of the time, I certainly was unaware of others as separate beings. I only called them when I needed them for something! My parents and the rest of the family knew Wendy was different. They accommodated my difference by saying, "Oh, that's just Wendy." As a child I was not assessed for autism spectrum disorder (ASD). Although I believe I always qualified for autism, it wasn't recognized by others until I was much older (Lawson, 1998).

The school office was brown and dull. It was very difficult to know where the walls ended and the door began. For Wendy this kind of setting, with its indistinguishable entries and exits, meant walking into walls and things. "Well, it's what we call 'educationally subnormal,' " the lady said (the words most often used today are "intellectually disabled"). I had my own pictures then of what "subnormal" meant. I imagined being like a submarine beneath the water. Despite this assessment, however, I always went to regular schools.

I grew up in England. My family moved around quite a lot. This meant my going to several different schools, seven in all. In this chapter I attempt to share some of my growing-up experiences and memories of school life. This is reflective, written from my perception of what occurred, what I felt, and what I saw. I will number each school with the number of its place in my experience—hence number-one school was my first school, and so on. Keep in mind that though I grew up England, my experiences in school are like those throughout the world.

## SCHOOL NUMBER ONE

As we left the security of our ancient cottage, Mother took my hand. Mother had spent her own childhood in this village, lived in this house, and gone to the small village school I was about to attend. It comprised a school hall and some outbuildings that were classrooms for a small number of children. I liked the look of this school. It was as ancient as our home.

For special assembly times, the worship time before lessons began, we went to the local Church of England, opposite the school. We had our school meals in the school hall. We also had physical education in the school hall. There was a large brass bell located in the bell tower of the main school building. This bell tolled whenever it needed to tell the school community that something was either about to happen or about to finish. Just like all the other bells in England, the bell kept silent during the two World Wars.

We walked briskly along the lane, and other children and their mothers joined the throng. The procession fed into the playground via the cobbled alleyway. The "teachers" were waiting for us in the playground, and they had lists of names of the children who were to be joining their classes for the first time. A tall lady wearing a red cardigan over a white cotton blouse called my name. Mother said I had to go with her. She said I was to stay with this lady at school. This lady was to be my teacher. Mother took her hand away from mine and joined the exit line of other mothers leaving their children. I was only 4½ years old.

I walked over to the lady in the red cardigan. I think she spoke to me, but I don't remember hearing any of her words. I liked the look of her red cardigan. I reached out to stroke the cardigan but my hand was intercepted. I was led off into one of the buildings. Inside, there were various small chairs and well-used wooden desks. The desks had lids that opened and shut as you lifted them. I liked the desks. At first the teacher didn't seem to mind my wandering around the room and lifting up and closing all the desktops. I did this for some time. Then I moved over to the far side of the room, near one of the large windows, and sat down beneath a desk. Yes, I liked it here. I could watch the shadows from the window move across the room and I could touch the smoothness of the desk corners. During the first month at my first school, I frequently sat under a desk.

The well-worn wooden chair squeaked as all four legs were dragged along the polished stone floor. "Stop that, Wendy," said a voice from somewhere. "Stop what?" my mind replied. I had been told to sit on my chair, so I did. However, I needed to go to the toilet, so I etched my way across the classroom floor toward the doorway . . . while seated upon my chair. Eventually the teacher came and repeated her comment. I was stuck. What should I do now? How could I let her know that I needed the toilet? Too late, I wet myself. More trouble.

The bell rang out for end of class, and all the other children seemed to understand what this meant. I watched as they got up from their chairs and moved quickly away from their desks. They were eager to talk and bustled their way out of the classroom, along the hall and on until they were not there any longer. I sat at my desk. The teacher asked me to go out. "Go out"—I pondered upon these words and tried to work out what she meant. "Mum goes out to the shops," I thought. "Dad goes out to work and sometimes to the pub," my thoughts continued. "Which one does Teacher want me to do?" I wondered. Then teacher spoke again: "Don't you want to go out to play?" Once again, I repeated her words to myself: "Don't you want to go out to play?" It was as if echoing back her sentence was meant to make it easier to work out. . . . But it didn't. She came over, took my hand, and led me out into the playground. I stayed still, just where she left me, until the bell sounded again. One of the children, Jane, came over. She didn't speak, she just clasped my hand into hers and led me back into the classroom. This was not an unfamiliar scene. Why did other children do what they did? How did they know what the words meant? Why was Teacher so often cross with me?

Toward the end of the first month of my first school, I remember being told to sit next to a particular child. I don't remember the child, but I remember that this child was sick and vomited over the desk. This whole event and the commotion that followed terrified me. I had not experienced this kind of upheaval before, and I was so upset that Mother was called to the school to take me home. Being sick over a school desk was not a usual part of school life, and I think this sudden, unexpected action terrified me. Any sudden, unexpected action caused panic for Wendy because I couldn't work out what would follow from it. I could not predict an outcome or understand consequences. Therefore, "change" was always a problem for me. Apparently all future attempts to encourage me back to that school failed. My parents decided, since they were moving house anyway, to wait until after the move to return me to school.

Today I understand so much more about why people say and do the things they do. I still don't always "get it," but most of the time I do. However, school was a nightmare for me. I dreaded having to go because it just didn't make sense to me. Why do people say things like "You have to go to school now?" They rarely seem to put closure into their information. For instance, they don't say, "School will close at the end of today, and then you will come home again." Every day I left my home, my room, not ever knowing if I would return.

## SCHOOL NUMBER TWO

By the time my parents decided to try school and Wendy again, I was 6 years old. We had moved from Bathford, near Bath in the west of England, to Chippenham in Wiltshire, a different county, but still in the west. Number 11 Leighwood was a bungalow (this is the English term for a one-story house). It had a decent backyard and was part of quite a large housing estate. For my fifth birthday Grandma had given me a beautiful tabby kitten, and I called him "Sandy." Sandy seemed very much at home in Chippenham; he liked to spend time sleeping and playing in our large garden hedge. I joined him whenever I could.

One crisp autumn morning Mum dressed me in my school uniform. It was a very gray outfit, and I didn't like it at all. Lowden Road Primary School seemed very busy and very big. Mother and the head teacher talked together for some time, while I was allowed to explore some books that sat on Teacher's desk. The books had bold print and large colourful pictures in them. I liked to turn the pages of books, over and over and over again. It was just so lovely to see how the pages always fell back onto themselves. Time and time again each page left its place as I flicked it and then landed right back again! I never tired of this game. Each and every time it intrigued me. Each and every time was like seeing it happen for the first time. At that age I wasn't interested in what was on the pages of the book, only in the pages themselves and how they moved when I flicked them.

Eventually Teacher asked me some questions. "Are you going to be a good girl Wendy and let Mummy go?" I thought this was rather a strange question because, at the time, I wasn't holding Mother and, therefore, didn't need to let go of her. I didn't answer. "Do you like sausages?" Teacher continued. "We have sausages for lunch today." I wasn't interested in what she was going to have for lunch. I did feel rather uncomfortable, though, as Mother then got up from her chair and said that she was going but that I had to stay. She said she would return later to "pick me up." Mother did carry me still sometimes, but it was usually at my insistence. I wondered why she was so keen to pick me up later, especially as I had not asked her to. Mother left.

It was morning break time and children were playing in the playground. The teacher took my hand and walked me over to a small group of other children. "This is Wendy Bateman," she said. "She's a new girl and I want you to take care of her. Take her into Miss Green's class with you when the bell goes. Miss Green knows that you are bringing Wendy." The children, three girls about 6 years old, nodded and then returned to their skipping game. As two of the girls turned the skipping rope by lifting their hands up and making a small circle with them, the rope was hoisted up into the air, then briefly it landed back again onto the ground. I was fascinated by the way the skipping rope swept the tarmac every time it landed and moved upon it. I stood watching it for some time.

I decided I could make the tarmac playground move beneath my feet, too. I left the three girls to their skipping and ran round and round the playground. I ran so fast that I thought I might not ever be able to stop. It was so exhilarating. I laughed and laughed as the ground moved beneath my feet. I didn't see the teacher coming toward me. I didn't hear her as she called my name. Eventually, she stood in front of me and put her hand out. "Stop! Stop running," she said. "You are in the boys' playground." I didn't understand the intention of her words. . . . I didn't know she meant that I was allowed to run but only in the girls' playground. I understood "stop running." I was to be at that school another 3 years, but I never ran there again.

Memories from days spent at this primary school are vivid but very gray. I often had an upset tummy. I lived with constant fear. I was afraid to go to school, afraid to be at school, and afraid to come home from school. I so often didn't understand what teachers meant when they talked to me. "Wendy, you must wait for your turn," Miss Green would say. I wanted to have the book. I didn't want the other child to have it. I needed to have the book now. I was unsure about "turn taking" for a very long time. I didn't understand the concept.

So much of what transpired between children and other children or between children and teachers was based upon mutual understanding of concepts. It might have been the concept of "time" (reading time, home time, playtime) or of "changing" for physical education, for swimming, for indoors or outdoors. When I heard the words "Wendy, aren't you changed yet?" I only felt scared. What was I to become? What might I change into? What and when might this change occur? Would it be a sudden change? Might it happen when I wasn't looking. . . . I had to be vigilant, and maybe if I ran away from times when people expected me to "change," "the change" might be avoided. If it had been explained to me in other words, such as "Take your day school clothes off here and put your PE school clothes on for PE," I would have understood.

At "playtimes" I spent most of my time walking around the playground on the white lines or standing close to the school fence. I did play games of marbles and flick cards sometimes. Usually, however, joining in with other children's games was too complicated and difficult. "What do I say?" "What do they say?" "What do I do?" "What will they do?" It was all too hard, so I played by myself. Other children teased me and laughed at me. "Oh, here comes the crazy girl," they would say. I think I would have liked to have a friend at primary school, and some children did try to befriend me. Unfortunately, I didn't understand the rules of children's interaction, and I couldn't maintain any potential friendship.

Primary school was full of events for me. Usually these events got me into trouble. "Wendy, you can't have that," Teacher would say. "Yes I can, Miss," I would reply. "You are such a rude girl. Go to Headmistress at once." I wasn't being rude. I was being honest. Of course, I can have it—I am holding it, I *do* have it, therefore I *can* have it. I now know that I was not understanding the teacher's words in the way she had meant them. I didn't understand the concept as she did. For me, if I have something, then that equals "can have." If Teacher had said something like, "Wendy, what you are holding belongs to me. It belongs on my desk. Put it back, please," I would have done so. I might have picked it up again another time, however, unless Teacher had said, "This is always mine, Wendy. You are to leave it on the desk for me and must never have it."

Understanding such concepts as "mine," "yours," "ours," and so on, is very difficult for children with autism. It took many more years before I was to know what these concepts meant. "*Oi*, you, you can't have those— you haven't paid for them," the shop assistant said. "Of course, I haven't, Silly. I don't have any money," I replied.

## SCHOOL NUMBER THREE

I liked this school. I would have liked it even more if the children were not there! Miss Smith was a very nice teacher. I liked the way we were allowed to rest our heads upon our hands as we listened to the story the teacher read. I could always hear and understand better if I wasn't looking at the teacher as he or she spoke to me. With my eyes closed and my face down in my hands upon the desk, it was easier to "imagine" what the story was about. I could visualize the babies beneath the water. I could see their colors and their characters. The more Teacher read, the more involved in the story I became. I took the characters home with me. I spoke to Mother in their watery voices. Sometimes Mother told me to speak in my own voice. I thought this was a strange request, because I was talking with my voice.

As a younger child I hadn't known how to join in with another child's game. By the age of 9, although I had learned how to read, I couldn't transfer my knowledge in appropriate ways. "Do you know that 'myxedema' means you have an underactive thyroid gland, and that without thyroxin, you will become a cretin and then go into a coma and die?" I said as I approached another 9-year-old in the playground. I used my "factual" knowledge to relate to other children who appeared to be of interest to me. This was not a successful strategy and only served to alienate me from other children. Today, I still tend to have one area of interest that dominates my life, but I am somewhat more tactful in how I relate to others. I tend to mix with people who share my interest and avoid those who don't.

## SCHOOL NUMBER FOUR

*Transition*

Autism is: "I like it here, please do let me stay."
Autism is: "I know it here, please don't take me away."
If and when I leave this place to travel to another space,
I need to know it right away. I need to know that I'm OK.
Transition is so fleeting, it leaves not time to stay.
Will I have time to settle, or will I be whisked away?

I know that change can happen.
I know it can take time.
But how can I know what this will mean?
What this will mean for mine.

Transition is about moving, "to where or what" one asks?
This is my very question, from present or the past.
Time for me is all the same,
I know not of its future.
I only know I trust in "now" . . . tomorrow can come, I just
     need to know how.

Transition is an amazing part of everyday life. It is so common that most individuals seem to hardly notice it. For example: There is moving from sleeping to waking, from night to day, from nightclothes to day clothes, from home to car, and so on. However, major transitions, like from pre-school to primary school, primary school to secondary school, high school to college or university, appear to be more noticeable. For children with autism, however, any transition can feel like the end of the world. Successful transition depends upon being able to predict an outcome or, at least, having an understanding of consequences. This is something I'm not good at. For Wendy, "now" is what I know, and I so often cannot imagine "later." In autism, the minor transitions of everyday life can be extremely traumatic.

Transition and autism are like enemies. They are foreign to one another because they represent opposing abilities. Transition says "It's time to move on," and it assumes that one is ready, able, and willing. Autism says "I have to stay here because here is all I know." It assumes that outside of "here," there is *chaos, confusion, and conflict.* In order for any transition to "go well" or even just be tolerated, an individual with autism has to have the three C's just mentioned (chaos, confusion, and conflict) sorted into "*order, understanding, and calm.*"

Moving from primary school to secondary school was a transition that did not go very well for me. At the age of 10 years I became very unwell and spent the following year in hospital with a bone disease called osteomyelitis. After my recovery, I left the hospital and returned home. My family had moved while I was in hospital. I had a new home to go to and a new school.

This school was a bus trip away from home. It was an all girls high school with very strict rules and high academic expectations. My mother had four children, two of whom were younger than me. Having to look after my two younger sisters meant that Mother's time was stretched to the limit (stretched, in this instance, means Mum tried to fit lots of things into her day and it was always difficult to get everything done). The more Mother insisted on my hurrying up, the more time I seemed to need. This kind of pressure just made it even more difficult to focus on, and/or remember, what it was I was supposed to do. Consequently, I often got to school without my reader, PE kit, diary, and such like. Getting myself organized was very difficult for me.

I still find it almost impossible to "forward think." Now, as a grownup, I have my lists of things to do, which makes my life so much easier. I need structure and consistency to support my difficulty with getting organized. I also value the support of my family and friends who assist me in this area. As a child, however, I didn't get this support, and each day was a repeat of the nightmare of the day before.

It might be easy to realize that structure in the classroom is useful. What individuals sometimes fail to recognize, though, is that we also need our "free time" structured. I find it difficult to understand the concept of "free time" as it is. "Wendy, this is your time now, time for you to switch off and relax," says a friend. This is all well and good if one has a concept for "free time" . . . relax . . . switch off! I still find this concept difficult and prefer even my "free time" to be structured. For example, after I awaken, I like to have a cup of coffee. Then I spend some time on my computer. Between 8:00 A.M. and 8:30 A.M. I have some breakfast. Then I have a shower and get dressed for the day. Hopefully, my diary has recorded which events I will be engaged in during my "free time." I believe, for autistic children at school, playtime needs to be structured (Lawson, 2001).

It seemed to me that the older children and teenagers at high school had worked out their own kind of relational rules. They seemed to have themselves sorted into various groups. There was the group who hung around the cloakrooms, the groups who played various ballgames like soccer, netball, and basketball, the smaller groups of two who seemed content to walk around the grounds and talk, and the individuals who seemed always on the outside of any group, trying to join in.

I didn't fit into any of these groups. My interests were not shared by them and, anyway, I couldn't work out how to join any of these groups. During my first year at high school, I walked with a full-length calliper on my leg, and my walking was assisted by a walking stick. I wasn't fast at sports, couldn't coordinate my dressing and undressing for PE, was teased for taking too long to answer any question, and generally lacked the "know-how" of any human interaction. By the time I was 13 years of age, I gave up trying.

For me, adolescence was a very confusing time. I definitely knew at this time that I was different from other teenagers. I remember wanting to "fit in." Initially I tried relating to others through the characters of my favorite TV shows. I even talked with an American accent and told outlandish stories about my accomplishments. But it didn't help to endear people to me.

I was very vulnerable. At one school, number seven school, the class voted me into the position of class captain. They did this so that they could manipulate and control me for their own gains. I was often "set up" and then made a fool of. I was so gullible.

I always took people literally and believed all that was told to me. I was taunted as the "crazy girl" and called many other such names. By the age of 17 I saw no reason to live. Suicide occupied my thoughts a lot. I thought up different ways to kill myself, but, although I did attempt to end my life on three occasions, I was unsuccessful!

Between the ages of 13 and 20 life seemed so bizarre! Because I didn't know how to be appropriate with other people, I was so inappropriate! I would attach myself to an individual and become like his or her shadow. I couldn't connect with life unless I was with the person. My clinginess usually became too much for the "needed" person of the time, and he or she would then stay away from me. I have a lot of painful memories of this time period. Unfortunately, attaching in this way has been a pattern for me, and I either live almost as a hermit, or I overattach myself to some desired "other."

## SCHOOL NUMBER FIVE

My fifth and most progressive school in its time was in Taunton. Entering this school coincided with another move and another location. This next house was in the small village of Norton-Fitz-Warren in Somerset. My parents managed the Railway Hotel that once was a busy public house. This old building does not exist today. I remember the cups and saucers use to rattle every time a train went past.

I did not like this next school. Here the school dinners were different. I liked regular meals. The usual school dinners that I had known previously consisted of meals such as shepherd's pie, beef stew, or sausages and mashed potato. I liked desserts with steamed puddings and custard. At this school they did things differently. For example, they gave children rice instead of potato. They cooked savory pasta and had fruit for dessert. This all seemed very strange to me and caused me to experience depression.

I also encountered horrific bullying at this school. There were several boys who took delight in causing me fear. They would ambush me and make me do things I was not used to. Sometimes they stole my things or would trip me over with their feet. They jeered at me, pushed me, and spoiled my clothes. I remember, as if it were yesterday, these boys' faces. I also remember how they made me feel. Whenever possible, I was unwell and could not go to this school. Fortunately for me, within a year my family moved again, and I was able to go to another school.

I think that bullying children with autism, or any other disability, happens more than we can imagine. I believe that schools can only benefit from having a policy on "bullying," and that this policy and its implementation should be mandatory.

## SCHOOL NUMBER SIX

At the age of 13, my family and I moved from Taunton to Bridgewater. The secondary school in Bridgewater that I attended holds memories very similar to those of my previous schools. I don't remember too much bullying, but I do remember how difficult it was to keep up with my academic studies. "Wendy, what is the answer?" Teacher asked. "Oh, I don't know, Miss, but Andrea knows. She always knows the answer." "I don't think you are attending one bit to what I've said, Wendy. You will stay in after school and do a detention." I often had to stay at school longer than other children. This strategy didn't help me in any way, because I didn't understand what I had done or what I needed to do differently!

I believe that individuals with autism usually find it easier to attend to one thing at a time. Dr. Dinah Murray first wrote about this in 1992; she called it "attention tunneling" or "monotropism." I couldn't have lots of co-active interests and therefore couldn't access and use information collaboratively. It was always difficult to work out the context (emotional, physical, or social), scale (size or importance), and intention of any event or person, especially in a changeable and multiple universe. According to Dinah, the dominant emotions for monotropic individuals much of the time tend to be interest, fear, or unrefined dysphoria. Ecstasy and awe also appear to be emotional states associated with monotropism. Of course any of these emotional states also may occur in polytropic (neurotypical) individuals; however, they tend to shift with the individual situation and not dominate it (Murray, 2001).

I know from my own experience that I can only attend to one thing at one time. This means that eye contact or looking at a person while trying to listen to what he or she is saying is very uncomfortable. I actually think one tends to interfere with the other and make it quite difficult to do the two things at once. For example, I cannot listen to Teacher and take notes. I believe some students with Asperger syndrome (AS) avoid eye contact because it is actually painful. I don't believe it is right to put us through such pain. I have learned now how to look in the general direction of someone's eyebrows, so at least they think I'm looking at them! This seems to satisfy other people and keep me out of trouble. At school, however, I hadn't mastered this and was constantly being told off for "not paying attention."

## SCHOOL NUMBER SEVEN

My last secondary school was in Frome, Somerset. My parents had moved to Tytherington and then into Frome itself. I liked Tytherington, especially before they built the big road that now runs through it. The school bus used to collect us from across the road to our house. I waited at the bus stop but didn't talk to the other children.

*Becoming*

I feel you loving me today
I hear your voice, as it drifts this way.
I'll give you breakfast on the floor,
We'll go for a walk across the moor.
Companion faithful and oh so true,
The love of my life,
It could only be you.

I see you standing across the hall.
I notice your smile against the red wall.
Maybe one day I'll be that tall?
I'd like you to stay and not go away,
But, you don't and you can't,
And you're not here today.

I have all of these feelings that tumble around.
I'm not sure I like them,
Certainly don't want them,
How can I make them go back underground?

They won't go away, I hear your voice say.
You have to sort them, they're here to stay.
But I don't understand them, their voice is too loud.
They make me do things,
Especially in a crowd.

"No, Wendy, not here," your louder voice states.
"That should be in private and not for this place."
What is for private and what is the place?
I wish I could read the look on your face.

I loved my dog, Rusty. She was loyal, faithful, and dependable. I often wonder why people are not more like this. Rusty watched as I left for school and was waiting when I returned home. She didn't ridicule me or make unfair demands upon me, she just loved me for who I was—hers.

There was this girl at school. . . . I thought she was my friend. Sometimes she would stay inside with me at break times. We would play tunes on the piano together. She was very good on the piano. We use to play "Morningtown" ("Rockin, rollin', ridin' . . . out along the bay") a song sung by The Seekers (Reynolds, 1966). I liked how she included me in what she was doing. It wasn't like this when she was with the other children at Youth Group, though. For some reason this changed in company, and she ran with the herd and joined in with teasing me by not attempting to stop the others. This is something I still don't understand.

I did quite well at the seventh school, academically. Even though I was in the "lowest" class, my English teacher encouraged and rewarded me. He said that I had potential and that I should write whenever I felt like it. He liked my writing style and my poetry. I once won a book for coming third in English in his class. It was an encyclopedia about nature and animals. I loved encyclopedias!

## WHAT HELPED ME MOST IN MY EARLY DAYS?

Sometimes I think the thing that helped me most in my early days was my need to understand the world around me. I have an insatiable appetite to "learn" the reason for things. If people couldn't help me, then I explored the books about a topic, or I set myself adventures to discover why things happened. I'm glad that I have an inquiring mind and that, although my development has been delayed, I tend to persist until I achieve my goal.

I found people who admired this in me, and in spite of my egocentricity, they supported me. It only takes one person to believe in you, and you can achieve all sorts of things. If people only see the negative and constantly tell you what you are doing wrong, then your self-esteem plunges. When the teacher told me to stop running . . . I did. If she had ushered me into the right play area and explained to me that I could run there, then I could have laughed again as I observed the ground moving beneath me. . . . I felt that that experience was denied me.

I was fortunate to encounter a couple of people who decided to give me some of their time. I remember I was only 2 years old when I met Jenny, my next-door neighbor. Jenny took me for outings in my pram. She was only 12 at the time. Later Jenny joined my family as a big sister. She always had time for me. When I was 13, I met Lesley, a student nurse, who also had time for me and trusted me to run errands for her. Today, Lesley is one of my closest friends.

I tended to be left to my own devices often. This isn't ideal for children with autism. We benefit more from early intervention and activities that keep us "connected" to life. When life is so very scary all the time, it is easiest to retreat into obsessive behavior rather than face your fears—especially when you don't even understand why you are scared or what it is all about.

People tend to say, "Don't be scared, it's OK," and the like. Well, actually, no, it's *not* OK. I *am* scared, I *don't* understand and I would appreciate, firstly, that this be recognized and, secondly, that this be sorted! I needed to gain the understanding that I am OK. To get this understanding, I needed to have the support of suitable explanations of events, of timing, and of expected outcomes.

Children with autism benefit immensely from visual and/or concrete cues. A timetable that shows expectations and what will happen if things change would be so practical and useful. Communication books that have photographs of everything in everyday life work for us like language. Sometimes I hear people say "Oh, isn't it a shame that [he or she] doesn't talk." This attitude isn't exactly helpful. No, it's not a shame that he or she doesn't talk, but it *is* a shame if he or she doesn't have a communication system because no one has thought about developing one for him or her!

I didn't have access to photographs or pictures to help build my understanding. Maybe this is why I turned to books to help me. I am fortunate to have the disposition that I have. Many more children with autism, however, might not have this self-motivation and are at risk of retreating into their fears, and their confusion, and will show this by their behavior. Giving them the ability to build an understanding can be life giving.

## BEST COPING STRATEGIES
## AS A YOUNGER CHILD

I think that these coping strategies have changed over time. When I was young, I used "being outside and away from demand" to help me cope with life. I loved to go for long walks. It seemed that the further I walked, the more distance I was putting between myself and what I didn't understand! I have lots of obsessions, and these change over time, too. I loved smooth material. Stroking it between my fingers or my legs was very calming. I loved to get absorbed into color or sparkly objects. I also loved spinning objects round and round for ages. Whenever I was upset, I could retreat to one of these activities and find comfort again.

I had my books to explore as well. For a very long time I just collected books and then organized them into piles. At times there wasn't much room for Wendy because the books took up all the space. Although I began to read at the age of 9 years, I didn't connect with the fact that the words in books and the words we use in conversation are the same until I was 13 years old. I still love my books.

At school I coped best by being on my own as much as was possible. I could escape demand by watching the wind blow through the trees and by just staring out of the window. I think these times of respite can be useful and it is important to give children time away from demand.

Nonautistic individuals can take in and process information more easily than we do. They can integrate lots of information coming into their minds from seeing, listening, feeling, thinking, and so on, all at the same time. I don't do this. I see something, process it. I hear something, process it. I feel something, process it. I use one channel at one time, so I take longer to build up a picture of an event. I can still be processing the words the teacher said when all the other children have left the classroom! For me, this might mean becoming overloaded with information from multiple sources very quickly—hence the need to "chill out"! Take it slowly.

## COPING STRATEGIES WHEN I WAS OLDER

Since receiving a diagnosis of AS, I have been able to come to terms with both who I am and what I can do. I avoid social gatherings because they are very confusing and scary. I find it difficult to know how to maintain a conversation, unless it's about a favored topic of mine. I also get overloaded with all the sensory information that comes from people in a social situation—for example: conversational noise, movement of people, clothing, doors, and so on. The only time I enjoy social occasions are when they occur on my terms with friends that I know and trust. I can plan these times, enter and exit when I want to, and I can be myself.

For me there are some good things about being autistic. I can enjoy the quiet and peaceful feeling of my own space. I can focus upon a desired object (e.g., a colored sign, butterfly, bird, or a specific study topic) for hours. This means that being committed to the study of my choice isn't difficult for me. While some students easily become tired, bored, or distracted, I am in my element!

The worst thing about being autistic is my experience of being disconnected from social interaction. Life appears as a video that I can watch but so often not partake in (Lawson,1998).

### What Is Play?

"Wendy, Wendy," I hear the teacher say.
"Wendy, Wendy, please look this way."
"Wendy, Wendy," I hear the children say.
"Wendy, Wendy, please come and play."

I hear the words that come each day.
"What do they mean?" I hear me say.
Words without pictures simply go away.
I turn my head and look instead
at all that glitters; blue, green, and red.

"You'll like it here," Father speaks,
"Come and play with Billy."
Inside my head my brain just freaks,
"How can they be so silly?"

"Why would I want to do this thing?"
My mind can find no reason.
"Please leave me with the sparkly string,
This gives me such a feeling."

## CONCLUSION

I grew up believing that my difficulties in everyday life were because I was not as intelligent as other people. Gaining a diagnosis of ASD has helped me understand who I am, what I do, and why I can and cannot do some things. Coming to terms with "my limitations" has been a hard but very important process.

I still don't like this "uneven ability." I often feel very foolish and cross with myself when I can't seem to understand something that other people seem to know so well. Part of the reason for my need of rules, rituals, and routines is to stave off confusion, chaos, and subsequent terror. For example: Someone might just be speaking to me. However, I experience it as someone projecting into my thinking or conversation, and I feel almost violated! "How dare they interrupt my space and distract me from my course. Didn't they understand that now I would have to start over again, recapture my thoughts or plans, and schedule it all again!" A friend replies: "Well, actually, Wendy, no, they did not. You see, people talk to each other quite often. They don't need to put their thoughts on hold to do this, or even take time to go back to the beginning of their sequence of events after the conversation finishes. They can move from one thing to the other most of the time."

Understanding everyday life requires an understanding of "concepts"—concepts such as right, wrong, time, space, age, education, health, and so on. At school the teacher might say, "OK, recess," most children will interpret this concept of recess and understand it to mean "stop work, pack things away, get your snack, and go out to play." All that from two words!

Most of the time I got into trouble at school because I didn't have a concept for what was being said, done, or expected.

*Lost*

The movement is all around me,
Their lips, their hands their faces.
The words come tumbling like a mighty sea,
With waves and without spaces.

The movement then sides away,
I know it will come another day.
When it does, I'll know what to say.
But it'll be too late,
They'll have moved away.

I feel this rush inside of me.
I move, I want to set it free.
I open my mouth,
The movement is gone.
I know I had some wonderful song.

I wander around as my head spins with sound,
I just need more time inside this square mound.
I'll come through that doorway,
I'll know what to say.
I just need more time, maybe today?

## REFERENCES

Lawson, W. (1998). *Life behind glass.* Sydney, Australia: Southern Cross University Press.
Lawson, W. (2000). *Life behind glass.* London: Jessica Kingsley.
Lawson, W. (2001). *Understanding and working with the spectrum of autism: An insider's view.* London: Jessica Kingsley.
Murrey, D. K. C. (1992). Attention tunnelling and autism. In P. Shattock & G.

Linfoot (Eds.), *Living with autism: The individual, the family, and the professional*. Sunderland, UK: University of Sunderland.

Murray, D. K. C. (2001). Seminar session, ASSID Conference, Melbourne University, Melbourne, Victoria, Australia.

Reynolds, M. (1966). *Morningtown* [Recorded by The Seekers]. London: EMI UK.

## RECOMMENDED FURTHER READING

Jordan, R., & Powell, S. (1995). *Understanding and teaching children with autism*. West Sussex, UK: Wiley.

Lawson, W. (2003). *Build your own life: A self-help guide for individuals with Asperger's syndrome*. London: Jessica Kingsley.

Powell, S., & Jordan, R. (1997). *Autism and learning: A guide to good practice*. London: David Fulton.

# 9

# Challenges Faced by Teachers Working with Students with Asperger Syndrome

## VAL GILL

For over 20 years I have been involved in establishing educational services for, and in the direct teaching of, students with autism spectrum disorders (ASD). I am currently the principal of the Western Autistic School, and was one of the first teachers employed in the early days to establish educational programs for autistic students. As educational specialists working with students with ASD, we have had to remain continually open to developments in both theory and practice, and responsive to the changing needs in this field. The Western Autistic School, founded in 1979, provides two distinct programs. The first is a school-based educational program for students across the spectrum of autism. The other is the provision of an outreach service to schools, community agencies, and professional groups involved with students with ASD. Parent support is another important component of this service.

The school-based program is a short-term intensive program for students ages 4½ to approximately 10 years of age. Students participate in individually planned programs, and transitioning to a mainstream or special school can occur any time within a 1- to 4-year period. Western Autistic School staff work closely with staff at the "receiving schools" to provide ongoing support and to monitor the students' progress.

In recent years there has been a significant increase in the demand for

194

services and support for students with Asperger syndrome (AS), with more and more children receiving a diagnosis and families seeking help. As part of our endeavors to meet this need, we established a Saturday social skills program for children with AS, called the "Saturday Club." This is a very successful program, and we are finding it increasingly difficult to meet the growing requests for placement. We also conduct a regular "respite day" for students with AS who attend their local mainstream schools the remainder of the school week. It is a day for debriefing and letting go of the daily struggle to "fit in." Indicative of the stress these students experience, parents sadly report that, for some students, this is the only day that they are happy to get out of bed.

We also conduct a program for students with AS in a mainstream secondary school. This program operates from a homeroom within the school. The program combines participation in appropriate regular classes with a life skills program that covers a diverse range of activities, including such things as community access and work experience. Specialist teachers support the students and provide a resource service to other secondary schools. Lastly, we provide consultative support to a range of schools working with students with AS.

As a teacher in any educational setting, the probability of becoming responsible for the education of students with high-functioning autism or AS is relatively high. Much material about AS is now available, including discussions of the resulting implications for teaching and learning. I focus here on the "journey of experiences" that results when we, as teachers, take on this responsibility and challenge. As well as professional issues, there are also personal implications that have an impact on us and are an integral part of the journey. New learning and expanded understanding, adaptation, adjustment, fear, heartache, hope, humor, delight, and achievement—all are part of this journey. The very way we think, plan, motivate, discipline, and teach needs to change to match our book knowledge with the "hands on" experience of daily interactions with these challenging students.

Let's explore some of the issues and experiences that have significant impact on teachers working in a range of schools, with a range of students with AS across age groups.

## GAINING UNDERSTANDING

A student with AS is, of course, as individual as any other. He or she brings to the learning environment his or her individual personality, temperament, past experiences, fears, successes, failures, and interests. Add to this complexity the impact of autism on his or her development, and we find an ongoing challenge to get to know the "person within," as distinguished from, and yet affected by, the disability. A student with AS may have a shy, quiet temperament or be volatile and fiery.

Samuel, for example, is a quiet, thoughtful student, forever tying to work out where everyone fits into the scheme of life. "Are there autistic animals?" he once asked. He becomes absorbed in his special interests and uses this involvement as a coping strategy when life becomes too confusing or stressful. He is relatively "easy" to live with, and has never been resistant to intervention and specialist teaching. Matthew, in contrast, is loud, forever complaining, and generally demanding. He blames everybody else for his troubles and, all in all, is a difficult person with whom to work or live. These two teenage students have opposing temperaments and yet share common features of AS.

Our experience has shown that it is extremely useful for mainstream teachers to listen to a general explanation of AS presented by a person experienced in this field. This information assists teachers in two ways: (1) It provides a broad framework within which to develop an understanding that students with AS are not alone with their perspectives on life and, in fact, share common difficulties and behaviors with many others; (2) teachers also realize that they are not alone in trying to understand, and address the needs of, these puzzling and complex students.

Students with AS are enigmas. It can take some time to see beneath the "veneer" and comprehend the impact of autism on their lives. Listening to parents is invaluable in enhancing our understanding.

These students can become "masters of the cover-up." We need to know some students very well to accurately read the subtleties of their behavior and what they are trying to communicate. We need to be in tune at all times, to "listen to their behavior."

One example concerns behavior related to a common feature: fear of failure, which may be expressed by noncompliance or disruptive avoidance activities. These smoke screens are really saying "I don't want to fail, but I believe that I can't do this activity or task." One of our young students with AS was asked to think of a sentence for a video that they were going to make. The student was immediately out of his chair and talking rapidly about an unrelated event. His skilled teacher, reading his behavior correctly, ignored the disruption and responded by saying, "I think I would say _____." He sat down immediately and, using this subtle assistance, successfully completed the task. If the teacher had responded directly to the disruptive behavior, it would have escalated, and the session would have ended in failure.

Don't be fooled by the "model" student with AS. So often this compliant behavior camouflages a high state of anxiety as the student strives to fit in, to be what he or she is not. This "fitting in" effort is a constant struggle. It takes enormous effort for students with AS to understand, behave, and achieve in our typical environment. Something has to "give" eventually; often the safety valve releases at home, and the school angel becomes the home terror. Without understanding, it is so easy for teachers to blame parents for this difficult home behavior, when so often it is a direct consequence of the student's struggle at school. With understanding comes the ability to put support structures in place to assist the students with this struggle, and in so doing, reduce their anxiety and stress levels.

As we develop understanding, we realize that we need to make some changes. Change is not always easy. We are trained in a certain way and have clear ideas, expectations, knowledge, skills, and experience. When confronted with the student with AS, our familiar strategies, skills, and knowledge may be rendered "null and void." We find ourselves needing to retrain. As one teacher said to me, "I'm a very experienced teacher, and I have a significant 'bag of tricks,' but *none* of them is working with this student." The only way to work successfully with these students is to accept the fact that we will need to make changes.

I like the analogy of two pathways. One is our normal pathway, and the other is an ASD pathway. The two rarely intersect. As a result of the disability, the person with ASD is unable to cross the dividing strip to journey with us. It is therefore up to us to bridge the gap and do what we can to assist the person to learn and work in what is a confusing, frustrating, and at times frightening environment to him or her. *The bridge is built through understanding.*

## PERSONAL ISSUES

Our journey with these students may include a roller coaster ride of intense emotions. We may be insulted, abused, or assaulted. We may experience fear, frustration, a sense of failure, or even hopelessness. We may feel protective, heartbroken, and want to save them, and at other times long to be rid of them. There is also humor, fun, enjoyment, sharing, and achievement. Most importantly, there can be a special relationship that develops through understanding and acceptance. We need to dig deep within ourselves to find the resources to accommodate and cope. Once "hooked," the challenge can become a quest to develop and share understanding in an attempt to make a difference in the lives of these students, and in turn, their families.

There also can be a physical aspect to this work. Those of us who have been on the receiving end of a physical episode with one of our more volatile students know the feeling of personal assault. Even though we can intellectualize the reason in some circumstances, our natural response is one of shock and hurt.

When working with students with other disabilities, it is possible, to some extent, to imagine their difficulties and challenges and empathize with them. With AS, it's almost impossible to imagine what it's like to have no intrinsic understanding of people and therefore be unable to form normal relationships. Students with AS further confuse us because of their uneven skill development. We so often hear the bewildered question "They can do this so well, why can't they do that also?" They can often tell us what they should say or do in particular situations and will apologize profusely for their own inappropriate or hurtful behavior, but then keep repeating the same. We then assume that they are doing these things deliberately. The assumption is, if they can talk about the right way to behave, then they must understand this way. This assumption is not necessarily correct. They can learn the rules, talk about them, and even demonstrate a strong sense of justice at times (especially as it relates to themselves), but the intrinsic ability that enables us to understand what underpins social situations and social responses is not available to them. They cannot take into consideration extenuating or changing circumstances. A rule is a rule, no matter what! They operate in black-and-white terms, whereas we are so often in the gray. No wonder we confuse them—and vice versa!

Students with AS can be blunt and naively honest, totally lacking in tact and diplomacy. To survive this approach, we need a good sense of humor. One student commented to a teacher, "It's obvious that you have a weight problem, so I wouldn't lean on that if I were you!" Very caring of him!

At times, certain situations really tug at the heartstrings. Watching these students struggle to fit in and be accepted is one example. Seeing their earnest desire to have friends, and failing in their attempts time and time again, is another. One student, desperate for friends, asked, "Is there a Friends for Us?," referring to the Toys R Us store. A teenage student who wanted a romance said imploringly, "I know that I have obsessions with people, but I really do love Michelle." Watching these students struggle to accept who they are and feel OK about it, seeing their fears and frustrations, brings to mind the prayer of serenity: As teachers we must know and accept what we can change, what we cannot change, and where we can make a difference.

## RELATIONSHIPS

Most of us start this journey assuming that we will develop a similar relationship with this student with AS as we have with other students. I really don't know how to describe the relationship that actually develops. Of course, it is an individual experience, and its nature depends on the level of understanding and acceptance we develop in relation to particular students. It may mean a lot of giving on our parts for little acknowledgment on theirs. Our expectations need to change with the knowledge that this will be a new "relationship experience."

A good relationship for the student means that you are a person in his or her life that is predictable, consistent, and clear. You represent security, understanding, support, and assistance. These students like to learn facts about us and will most certainly remember us. We will have a time slot in their lives. I have consulted with teachers who are very hurt by the fact that a student, with whom they thought they had a wonderful relationship, hardly acknowledges them when no longer in their class. I explain that the teacher was a part of last year's scheme. A new scheme now exists. Nothing personal!

One high school teacher was feeling like quite a failure in her attempts to develop a positive relationship with a student with AS. What really compounded this feeling was the fact that the student had a much better relationship with other teachers. She viewed the unsatisfying situation as a personal failure. When asked what subjects the teachers taught, the reason became obvious to me. She taught English and studies of society, both difficult subjects for this student. The other teachers taught formula-based, data-collecting subjects. In this situation, the cause was subject-based and not related to personal issues at all.

Because AS is a hidden disability, it is easy to slip back into conventional thinking and take issues personally. It seems that we have to keep reminding ourselves that all interactions are affected by this disability and are not deliberate personal attacks. As one mother said to me, "He knows just what to say to tear my heart out." At times, these youngsters know just the right "buttons to push" to achieve a required effect or to manipulate a situation, but this accuracy does not necessarily transfer to the ability to empathize with another and understand the emotional impact of his or her actions on that person.

There are times when these children's apparent hard-heartedness has a deep impact and makes it really difficult to cope with their behavior. The mother of a teenager with AS fainted as a result of illness, and when she came around, her son was leaning over her demanding his dinner. Lack of understanding or fear may have triggered his behavior, or just the fact that his routine was disrupted. Whatever the cause, the hurt experienced by his mother, at that moment, was significant. We can't always put our personal feelings on hold and not be affected by some interactions. This is another reason for the need for ongoing support and the opportunity to share experiences.

One consequence of this journey may be a significant increase in our tolerance levels. One of our teachers had experienced a very trying and

challenging day with one of our more difficult students in a high school setting. The teacher was at the point of exasperation by the end of the school
day. Someone commented on the fact that he looked stressed and tired. The
student who was the cause of the stress looked at him and said, "You
should lighten up a bit—get a life." Luckily this teacher could see the humorous side to this situation and appreciate the irony.

## PROFESSIONAL ISSUES

The journey not only impacts us on a personal level, but also has significant
implications and challenges for us as professionals. Skilled teachers are able
to adapt their teaching techniques, strategies, and subject matter to meet
the needs of individual students. This need for adaptations produces significant challenges in regular schools. Meeting the needs of the student with AS
takes us way beyond these boundaries. Almost everything we think, do,
say, and plan needs to be adapted. These students continually confuse us
and take us out of our comfort zones.

### Communication

Let's look at the very way we communicate and the language we use. Is our
language too complex? Is it clear or is it ambiguous? Are we adding to their
confusion? We need to be specific in whatever we say, because students
with AS have great difficulty in reading between the lines and understanding inferences or covert intent. These students are extremely literal. One of
our teachers could not find her briefcase and asked one of our students
with AS to look in her car to see if it was there. She handed him her car
keys, assuming that if he found the briefcase, he would bring it back with
him. He returned, empty-handed, and told her that her briefcase was, indeed, in her car. We are regularly reminded to communicate clearly and not
make assumptions.

A secondary school student with AS was told that he could be
"snowed under" if he didn't catch up with his work. The teacher wondered
why he kept looking up anxiously toward the sky. A student in the library
was told to "keep his voice down" and proceeded to speak just as loudly—
but from a squat position.

We also need to consider literal interpretation of assignment questions.
One such question, at the conclusion of an assignment, read, "What did
you find the hardest part of this assignment?" The student proceeded to
name the hard metals involved in one of the activities.

How can a student who is so capable in certain areas really misinterpret things this way? These students are often judged as "smart alecks."

When we stop to consider our colorful use of language—the sarcasm, humor, exaggeration, metaphor, etc.—it's no wonder we leave the student with AS feeling confused and anxious.

We therefore need to teach these students that people don't always mean what they say. We need to introduce and teach the idea of joking and playing with words, and give them a way of checking if they are confused—for example, to ask "Is that a joke?" An unexpected outcome of our attempts to teach a group of students with AS about jokes was the development of their own fun version of "play on words." We could not see the humor at all, but the experience provided an enjoyable means of interaction for these students. It was good to see them having fun.

We also need to be mindful of the complexity of our language, especially when giving instructions. We can easily assume that because a student is articulate, he or she will automatically understand what we are saying. We know, from reports of people with autism, that this is not always the case. They may catch only the first part of our instructions or conversation and miss the rest. The amount missed creates great anxiety, which exacerbates the situation. We can relate, in part, to this kind of stress from our own anxious times. We need to keep in mind that, despite good verbal skills, students with AS can find it difficult to verbally express their fears, frustrations, and feelings.

One of our students is terrified of thunder and, in his high state of anxiety, is only able to say things like "The vultures are coming." We need to be attuned, to "listen" for the physical signs of stress or anxiety. Parents are often of great assistance here in reading the subtle changes in their child's behavior that communicate difficulties.

As teachers, we love questions. Questions, however, can be nightmares—in particular, "Why?"—for some students with AS, especially when they are young. Answering this question requires the ability to reason abstractly, reflect on a situation, find an explanation, organize the information, and find the language to respond—all difficult tasks for students with AS.

We need to remember that they don't have access to our rich internal imagery, or the natural ability to be flexible and imaginative in their use of language. Therefore, when we ask a question or pose a problem they have never heard or experienced, they find it extremely difficult to respond. This lack of response becomes another source of anxiety. To assist them, we need to give them a visual scaffold or prompts. I was observing a student with AS in a class of 9-year-olds. She was coping extremely well until the teacher instructed the class to imagine themselves shrinking until they were only an inch tall and write about the difficulties they would experience. I could see the visible signs of anxiety as she returned to her seat. Without some assistance, this exercise was an impossible task for this student.

Talking about possible scenarios and using a simply made one-inch "model" gave her the visual/concrete prompt she needed to successfully complete the task.

Before chastising a student with AS for an inappropriate verbal interaction, check to see where this language file may have originated. We have many examples of students repeating a response in one situation that they have heard someone else use successfully in another social situation. They are then thoroughly confused and frustrated when they find themselves in trouble for repeating the same response. For example, listening to an interaction at home, a student heard one parent respond with "You can say that again." Overhearing a similar interaction between two teachers, in which one was commenting on the fact that she thought she was looking older, the student joined in with, "You can say that again!" One father said to his angry young son with AS, "I can't talk to you until you stop crying." Having caused another child to cry at school, he was told to apologize and repeated, "I can't talk to you until you stop crying." Of course, we need to teach these students about private conversations and appropriate responses, but they are most likely never going to understand what all the fuss is about.

We also must remember that they will find it extremely difficult to read body language and other nonverbal forms of communication. We therefore need to be careful not to condemn them for seemingly ignoring or misinterpreting our signals or misreading social situations. Our understanding of the social difficulties they experience is vital to our ability to create strategies with which they can cope.

## Teaching Social Skills

We need to be sensitive to students' levels of self-awareness when we plan to *formally* teach social skills. As the students with AS get older, the realization of their difference becomes more conscious and acute. They are aware of their social failures and their need for rules and guidance, but at the same time they don't like to be singled out and can feel very threatened or "put down" by certain forms of formal social skills training. As one young student said to a teacher, in response to a social skills lesson, "Don't give me that social skills *#*#." The best teaching opportunities come in the natural course of events—although we also need to engineer situations/ events to increase opportunities for experience and practice. We need to be alert constantly to make the most of these opportunities, as generalization of the skills is more likely to happen when the teaching is linked to a real-life experience. There are no quick fixes. From our experience in conducting an "Asperger Saturday Club," we have observed that skills and friendships develop over time, within a very supportive and nonthreatening environment. It is still questionable as to how many of these skills will be generalized. We are asked to teach students with AS the social skills that other students have acquired naturally as a result of social experience. This journey brings many challenges, and not the least of these is the necessity to teach skills that you have never even had to consider teaching to other students.

## COGNITIVE STYLE

Many teachers have found it useful to compare the cognitive style of students with AS to that of a computer. When correct data is fed into a computer, it has great capacity to produce wonderful results. It has memory files and the capacity to store amazing amounts of information. Students with AS are also great data collectors and can possess amazing "memory files." Their capacity to produce outstanding results is well evidenced by the many high achievers with AS. It is also important to understand the difficulties or differences, so that we can direct the students into areas that enhance and extend their strengths.

Here is a list of potential difficulties and stress triggers that we need to keep in mind when we do our planning:

- Too much choice
- Open-ended, vague assignments/tasks
- Activities that require sequencing and organization
- Comprehension of disguised or multiple meanings
- The need to integrate and organize information
- The need to shift to alternative solutions
- Having to imagine a scenario that they have never seen or experienced
- Determining and understanding the gist of something

## CURRICULUM

As teachers we have a set curriculum to teach, and we have prescribed accountability measures. One of the challenges, when providing support to teachers of students with AS, is to encourage them to think flexibly about curriculum. It is not only OK but also *necessary* to be lateral thinkers and planners. We need to take into consideration these students' unique learning styles and their strengths and weaknesses.

We also need to remember that their self-esteem is fragile. Many students with AS are perfectionists and are hypersensitive to criticism and failure. How can we think laterally to accommodate their needs while working within the curriculum? As teachers, we are being asked to work "outside the square." Subjects that are formula-based, factual, and involve data collection or technology are often successful endeavors for these students. The subject matter or topics for some compulsory curriculum components, however, can be extremely difficult, if not impossible, for students with AS to understand and interpret. Literature and essay or research topics, where the themes require understanding and interpretation of human relationships and interactions, are examples of problem areas. It is then necessary to adapt where we can, provide clear visual assistance in the form of step-by-step instructions or guidelines, provide time lines, limit choice (e.g., essay topics), and when possible, focus on topics that are possible for our students to understand and explore. If they can utilize their special interest areas, success and enjoyment are ensured.

These adaptations and special considerations can create difficulties within a school system where we are expected to work within prescribed requirements and curriculum. We are often faced with opposition when we attempt to stretch the boundaries to meet our students' special needs. "It is not fair to other students," "It's not equitable," "It's pandering to their idiosyncrasies" are a sample of common protestations. It makes a great difference when there is a total school commitment to accommodating individual differences. Our consultancy support to schools is an important factor here. An external consultancy expert can do much to foster understanding and bring school communities "on board." It is extremely difficult to work as an island within a school, as we all need support and encouragement. Some outstanding outcomes have resulted when schools have taken on the challenge to provide effectively for individual differences. For example, one student at a secondary school was experiencing great difficulties, and there were queries as to whether or not he should continue at the school. However, once the student's special needs and skills had been explained to the staff, they worked together to devise an alternative program. They selected some appropriate school-based subjects and put support structures in place. In addition, they organized a program with another agency for him to attend to develop his special skill area. It proved to be a turning point in this student's life.

## MOTIVATION

Motivation is an important area for teachers to consider under any circumstances, and when working with students with AS it takes on a special significance. We need to accept the fact that the student's special interest or obsession will be the most motivating factor in his or her life. It engages the student totally and provides great enjoyment and purpose. It is a means of escape when life is too hard, it provides "highs," and it can calm and soothe him or her. In the school situation we need to have limits and some control, particularly if a special interest becomes disruptive or interferes with other learning. If we can use the interest to foster focus on other studies, or as a means of reward, it becomes a powerful tool. For example, if the student successfully completes a set amount of work, then he or she can access their special interest for a prescribed amount of time. This is not "bribery," only a recognition of these students' different focus on life and their different points of motivation. We all work for our own particular rewards, and we need to appreciate that the reward for a student with AS may be quite different. If well directed, some interest areas have outstanding potential for future development and achievement (see Attwood, Chapter 6, this volume).

## SENSORY CONSIDERATIONS

We need to be aware that sensory experiences can affect the performance and behavior of students with AS. A common difficulty for our students, particularly in high schools, is coping with crowded, noisy corridors or locker areas. These situations can be absolutely overwhelming for some students, causing great stress. The resulting behaviors can be most inappropriate and unacceptable. An innocent jostle in the corridor may explode into a blatant accusation such as "That boy attacked me!" The student with AS cannot understand and will not believe that it was an unintentional jostle and not a deliberate act of aggression. If we are able to locate a locker in a quieter area, or time transition periods to avoid the "crush," we can also avoid potential difficulties. It is so easy for us to misinterpret these situations, if we don't appreciate the significant impact of these students' heightened sensibility to noise, smells, temperature, or personal space.

On the odd occasion, however, there can be another side to this issue. One very hot day, one of our teenagers turned all cooling vents toward himself. When reminded of the needs of others, he was adamant that it was justified because he had "special needs." Egocentricity abounds also!

## SENSITIVE SUBJECTS

One sensitive topic that springs to mind immediately is the study of human development and sexual issues. Considering the unique learning styles of students with AS, together with their social naiveté, some challenges become immediately apparent. In dealing with some of these issues, we need a good sense of humor, an unflappable temperament, and supremely creative diversion tactics.

Scenario one: Teenage students with AS and their teachers were on a crowded Melbourne tram passing the Royal Children's Hospital, when one student commented very loudly, "That's where I went because I have one testicle bigger than the other." In response another student began to give his family history of related problems. The teacher had to engage diversion tactics very quickly.

Scenario two: A couple of us were unashamedly eavesdropping on a discussion between two teenage students with AS. They had watched a television program on sexual issues the previous night and were wondering about the meaning of the word *orgasm*. They shared various ideas but, in the end, happily agreed that it had to be something to do with the kidneys!

Scenario three: A group of students were exploring options for work experience. The special interest of the student with AS was "love and romance" and anything related to this topic. She suggested that she would see how a business operated, and learn more about love and romance, if she did her work experience at a brothel!

When confronted with sensitive subjects, the need for understanding and sensitivity is apparent. If unsure of how to proceed, it is wise to discuss issues with a person experienced in this specialist field.

## COMMON CRIES FOR HELP

When consulting with schools, the most common cries for help concern playgrounds, physical education and sport, homework, and, of course, behavior. These arenas all contain potential stress triggers for students, parents, and teachers alike.

### Playgrounds

Whether at primary or secondary levels, one of the most difficult situations for students with AS is the playground. As teachers, the playground also presents one of the greatest challenges, because it's an area where we have least control. For the student with AS, it contains all that is most confusing and challenging. The playground is unstructured and abounds with social situations and rules that are peculiar to each school—rules that are unwritten but traditional, changeable, and "gray." The playground can be challenging for many students but is a virtual minefield for students with AS. Teachers often find the problems that arise with the students on the playground difficult to address, let alone solve. Each school has its individual logistics and issues when considering supervision and alternative solutions to playground problems. The teacher responsible for the student with AS often finds it difficult to get support within a school, unless there is a total school commitment to providing the additional effort required to overcome these special problems. When successful strategies are in place, an additional bonus is that other vulnerable students benefit from the measures taken for the student with AS. One of the most essential measures is to provide a safe place and a designated person or persons for the student to contact, if in difficulty. Schools have come up with a variety of strategies to assist these students. Some examples include reduction of the time spent in the playground, structured activities for part of the play period, availability of the library or computer room as a safe haven, buddy systems, alternative recess time activities, and designated/restricted areas in which to play. It is a very valuable exercise to share ideas and solutions with other schools.

Bullying is a common problem for all students, and much is being done to address this problem generally. Our students with AS are particularly vulnerable. They often present differently, are unable to read social situations, and are naive and easily "set up" by other students. It is up to us to provide a measure of protection and management strategies. However, the dynamics also can turn in the reverse direction. One of our teenage students becomes very upset if he believes he has been bullied, and he won't rest until the culprits have been chastised. He also reverses the dynamics and bullies his underlings. Despite all the explanations, he cannot see that the bullying rule also applies to him when he is the offender. It is not uncommon for our students to apply one rule for others but not themselves.

## Physical Education and Sports

Physical education and sports activities comprise another common area of difficulty. Many students with AS have varying degrees of fine and gross motor problems. Lack of skills in some sports can also be attributed to lack of opportunity, experience, and practice. Even if a student has the necessary skills, problems can still arise, particularly in team games. Our students are very pedantic in their interpretation of rules, and any deviation or confusion can result in disruption or outbursts of inappropriate behavior. Many students with AS find it difficult to cope if they are not best, first, and the winner. We need to start working on these issues when the students are young, cultivating the idea that it's all right to be second, or last, and to understand that they can't always win. It's a hard lesson for students to learn and for teachers to teach, and it can take considerable time and many experiences to achieve some change. We need to plan games/situations carefully, and to prepare the students by talking them through the possible scenarios, using simple language. Provide coping strategies by suggesting what they can say and do, and offer encouragement and support. Sometimes we need to think laterally if team sports continue to be problematic, to find a way of including the student with AS in these sporting activities. For example, the student might participate as a data collector or timekeeper.

## Homework

Homework is horror territory for many students with AS and their families. We need to be aware of the impact on all concerned when assigning homework for these students. There appear to be quite a few factors that contribute to the homework horror. Here are some common comments by parents:

> "He just can't organize his time or the information."
> "She doesn't know when to stop researching information."
> "He doesn't know how much to write."
> "If it's not perfect, she won't complete it."
> "He can't make a choice."
> "Without the structure, it's just too difficult for her."

One family told of working on an assignment with a student until very late in the evening. They had it almost completed when he ruled a crooked line and promptly threw the whole assignment in the trash. Many of these problems are related to difficulties experienced generally by these students—concepts of time, sequencing, organization, choice, integration and organization of information, and lack of structure. We can assist greatly by providing simple, clear, written expectations, limiting choice, and setting a timeline. We also need to ensure that these students have sufficient time available at home to debrief and relax after a hard day at school. We need to remind ourselves of the extraordinary effort it takes for these students to cope with an ordinary school day. In situations where the homework factor is creating extreme difficulties, our teachers will use any period of the day involving work that is not suitable for our students, to conduct a supervised homework session. Understanding and support make such a difference in the lives of these students and their families.

## BEHAVIOR MANAGEMENT

Our behavior management workshops are always a "sellout," because coping with the puzzling behaviors of students with AS is one of the most difficult areas. Here is where the journey toward understanding is vital. As we know, the starting point for examining problematic behaviors is to understand *why* the behavior is happening. What are the triggers? When we are able to stand in the student's shoes, even if it is in a limited way, we are often halfway to understanding the triggers and working out a management strategy.

The foundation of most school discipline/behavior policies is comprised of verbal explanation and discussion. Our natural inclination is to explain and reason with the students involved. So, once again, we need to respond in a way that is counterintuitive. The student with AS needs to hear a verbal explanation that is simple and to the point. We then need to put it in a visual form, such as making a list of rules that have clear consequences for appropriate and inappropriate behaviors. It may also be a written contract. Another useful format is a social story or a sequence of photographs or pictures. Teachers often say, "But we explained it all to him, and the behavior still occurred." The student may be able to quote the rules verbatim, but that doesn't mean that he or she really understands what underpins the explanation. Once again, it is our "gray" areas that confuse and confound these students. Remember that they are pedantic in their interpretation of rules and find it difficult to understand changes or extenuating circumstances. When struggling to find a successful management strategy, take a team approach: Talk over the problems with other staff, parents, and the consultant. No one has all the answers!

## CLASSROOM SUPPORT

Some students with AS have special funds allocated to employ a teacher assistant or aide. The assistant's role is to provide the student with additional support within the school. This situation can be both positive and negative.

On the positive side, the aide can help the student organize timetables, books, and equipment and clarify instructions or events. This assistance reduces the demands on the teacher and provides reassurance for the student. On the negative side, however, the presence of an aide can create additional difficulties. Very often it contributes to these students' feeling of being different. They hate to be singled out, and the presence of their aide exacerbates this feeling of difference. As one student repeatedly complains to us, "I hate [Mrs. Smith]! She follows me everywhere. I'm not stupid."

Some students have refused to have anything to do with the assistant, and, in some instances, the assistant has inadvertently caused further problems. A mother of a student with AS told me of an incident that occurred, resulting in her son's suspension from school for "hitting out." His aide, although well meaning, had not established an appropriate professional detachment. The unintentional social pressure placed on her son to interact with the assistant in a way that was impossible for him had resulted in his inappropriate behavior. As this mother said, "This [aide business] is just another social pressure that these students do not need." Students also may become overly dependent on this person, which has long-term negative implications.

Any situation involving the provision of classroom support needs to be planned carefully and with sensitivity. Classroom assistance can have a positive impact in some circumstances but is not beneficial for all students. *Understanding each student and his or her unique needs still remains the critical factor in all circumstances.*

## EXPLAINING ASPERGER SYNDROME

A frequently asked question is, "Will it help to explain AS to other students?" This is a sensitive issue, and there is not a clear yes or no answer. First we need to discuss the issue with parents. What are their thoughts and feelings? Do we have their permission or not? Sometimes parents want the whole school community to be educated, but for other parents it's a very private matter.

Does the student in question know that he or she has this diagnosis? We need to consider the peer group. Teachers usually have a good understanding of the group dynamics. They will have a clearer sense as to whether it would be supportive or, in fact, have the reverse effect. It therefore needs to be a joint decision with all factors taken into consideration.

## A REMINDER OF HELPFUL STRATEGIES

- Anything in written/visual form is extremely helpful (e.g., timetables, work sequences, rules, changes to routine or new situations, and instructions).
- Provide clear, written, step-by-step guidelines for assignments, homework, and any other work requirements.
- Limit choice—too much choice creates confusion and anxiety.
- Choose subjects that ensure success, based on students' idiosyncratic cognitive styles.
- Think laterally—consider the factors that are relevant, important, and motivating to the student.
- Provide stress-free activities and "safe" areas that offer respite from the constant struggle to "fit in" and succeed.
- Acknowledge and utilize their strengths and special skills to foster feelings of self-worth.
- Provide a mentor/support person so that the student knows there is someone to whom he or she can turn for guidance and comfort.

- Remember that these students may not generalize a rule, despite excellent explanations.
- Social stories can be extremely helpful in assisting these students to understand a situation.

## DEFICIT VERSUS DIFFERENCE

As our journey progresses and our understanding develops, so too does our appreciation for, and acceptance of, the person with AS. We begin to appreciate the difficulties and the supreme effort it takes just to survive a day. Hopefully we begin to look at AS not so much as representing deficits but differences. The human race is not very good at accepting and appreciating differences. Our journey helps us to make this mental shift, so that our focus turns to the strengths rather than the weaknesses. We not only accept the fact that it's OK to be different but enjoy our unique relationship with these students, in all their differences. If we are able to provide them with support strategies and channel their strong areas in directions of potential life fulfillment, our journey will be a positive and fulfilling one. As teachers, we have great opportunity and capacity to influence the lives, and affect the outcomes, of all our students. To achieve the same for our students with AS, we need to experience, and be part of, this special journey.

## A FEW SURVIVAL TIPS

- A sense of humor is vital.
- Make sure you have a support network or an understanding mentor.
- Remember the prayer of serenity.
- Be gentle on yourself—you can only do your best.
- Maintain a balance in your own life—essential, but sometimes easier said than done.

I wish you well.

## ACKNOWLEDGMENTS

I would like to acknowledge the many students, parents, and teachers who have shared their knowledge and experiences with me. Their generosity has contributed to my own personal and professional growth and enriched my continuing journey of understanding.

# 10

# School-Based Intervention for Children with Specific Learning Difficulties

RITA JORDAN

## FINDING INDIVIDUAL SOLUTIONS
## FOR INDIVIDUAL NEEDS

There is a consensus on the value of a diagnosis of an autistic spectrum disorder (ASD), whether or not specific subgroup diagnoses, such as Asperger syndrome (AS), can be justified (Autism Working Group, 2002; Howlin, 1998; Jordan & Powell, 1995a; Powell & Jordan, 1993; Seach, Lloyd, & Preston, 2002), because this diagnosis allows access to relevant literature and resources, and allows teachers and others to disengage from otherwise unhelpful labels, such as "lazy," "rude," "defiant," and so on. However, there is also a danger in such a diagnosis, in that there is a temptation to assume that there must be a specific curriculum or teaching approach to fit it, which is far from the case in autism. Even if we exclude those children who have additional general learning and structural language difficulties, the variations in abilities, disabilities, and preferred learning style within the group of children with AS and high-functioning autism (HFA) are great. Thus teaching approaches and classroom adjustments need to accommodate the autism, but also the individual.

Identifying those individual needs, however, is itself affected by the autism, because of its transactional nature; just as the child will have difficulty understanding those around him or her, so the teacher will have difficulty understanding the child. Normal intuitions may mislead, so careful observation and a willingness to consider the life of the child as a whole are crucial when interpreting behavior in particular contexts. For example, a recently diagnosed 5-year-old boy startled his teachers when he began to shout, apparently "out of the blue," "Don't spit! Don't spit!" and bang his head with his fists. No one appeared to be spitting, and the teacher's attempts to reassure him of this fact seemed to have little effect. It was only in a later conversation with his mother that the "explanation" was revealed: The little boy used to spit when anxious, was told off (in a loud voice), and then reacted by echoing the said phrase and banging his head. This reaction then generalized to any raised voice, whether or not directed at him. It is not always possible to know the natural history of all of a child's behaviors in this way, but teachers need to understand how such apparently bizarre reactions *do* have a history and may be serving a function (as in this case) of reducing the anxiety of hearing an angry voice.

In spite of the need to understand individual behavior and the tremendous individual variations in this group, however, there are also some commonalities and some principles that can guide teaching. This chapter examines the salient principles and explores what they might mean in the day-to-day life of the child with HFA/AS in school.

## SETTING EDUCATIONAL GOALS

In most developed societies, education is an entitlement and thus has a status different from any other "treatment." This status is important when considering choice of educational initiatives, especially for those with HFA/AS, where educational qualifications are one of the key factors in determining successful adult outcome (Howlin, 1998; Rutter, Greenfield, & Lockyer, 1967). Children with HFA/AS are children first and, as such, are entitled to as broad and relevant a curriculum as that available to all other children in their society. The issue then becomes one of access; what is needed in the way of support and additional resources, or additional/different teaching strategies, to enable that access? It may be the case that access is best if presented in stages, but the long-term goal of complete access remains a human right.

AS and HFA are medically defined categories and thus sometimes seen as needing remediation (if not "cure"). There are a few individuals with HFA/AS who assert their right to be different, are proud of being the way they are, and reject this notion of a "cure." For most individuals with HFA/AS and their families, however, the daily traumas of existing in a non-autism-friendly world make the disorder something whose effects they would certainly like to overcome. This potential ethical dilemma can be solved by thinking of remediation not as a cure for autism but as a way of empowering the individual him- or herself to develop the psychological strategies needed to cope with his or her own problems. These children, especially those in this higher functioning group, have a right to expect that education will do more that provide a "haven" in which they can learn; it must also equip them to cope in the wider world where such havens are harder to find.

As early as possible, the priority should be to get the child started on the learning process. During this initial period, these children need to learn how to attend to a set task, how to attend in a group, how to work independently and to finish tasks set, how to follow rules, timetables, and work schedules, and, perhaps, how to ignore certain stimuli while selectively attending to others. They also will need to learn how to modify their own behavior so that it is within acceptable norms, how to ask for help, how to calm down once upset, how to "interpret" the special language and communication style of education, how to manage motor disturbances and postured abnormalities, and so many more basic, "ready to learn" tasks. To learn all these things, they need to overcome enormous barriers and will need special support from the teacher and the environment. It is at this stage that the schools most need to adapt, when the child is developing good work habits and working so hard to overcome problems.

It is because of the need for this period of "learning to learn" that specialist input is needed in the early years (Jordan & Powell, 1995a; Rogers, 1996). Providing this input does not mean segregation; there are many examples of preschool children with ASD benefiting from integrated play with typically developing children (Roeyers, 1996; Wolfberg & Schuler, 1993). However, unsupported placement in mainstream preschools is likely to lead to a failure to learn in the most effective way and may indeed "teach" the child to fail. When there is so much to adjust to, arising directly from the autism, it is unrealistic to expect the child to make major adjustments to an unfriendly environment.

As the child develops, however, and learns to manage in the structured and adapted learning environment, it is time to help the child develop his or her own internal structures for managing the world. These internal cognitive structures should be in place *before* removing the external structure, or learning may collapse. Some children, even within this higher functioning group, are not able to develop sufficient internal structures (at least, during their time at school; some develop the capacity later, as adults, providing they have access to continuing educational opportunities), and will always require some degree of external structuring. The goal then becomes making this external support as unobtrusive as possible, to protect the child's self-image and the way he or she is treated by others.

TEACCH (Teaching and Education for Autistic and Communication Handicapped Children; Peeters, 1997; Schopler, 1997; Schopler, Mesibov, & Hearsey, 1995) provides an adaptable set of principles and techniques, for any child with an ASD in any setting, that is based on visually mediated structure and adapted to individual needs. Although exposure to only limited training can lead to less than optimal TEACCH-based environments, if done well, such an environment can offer unobtrusive and "normalized" support structures that can enable access to full curriculum opportunities (Mesibov & Howley, 2003).

An example from a mainstream setting concerns a 6-year-old boy with AS who was causing mayhem in morning school assemblies. The decision was about to be made to exclude him from these formal gatherings. In some instances exclusion might be the correct decision, given that assemblies are not part of the academic curriculum and some children may find the sheer numbers and crowding unable to bear. Yet assemblies are part of the social and moral ethos of the school (and, in some schools affiliated with a religion, may also provide spiritual experience), deemed of benefit for all children and, it might be argued, even more so for the child with an ASD. Furthermore, this boy was not overly disturbed by noise and had overcome his fear of others; what disturbed him about assemblies was his perception of a lack of structure, because there were different topics and a different class presenting each time. Yet there *was* a structure; it was just not apparent to him. The boy was provided with a little clipboard to take into assembly, on which the elements of the structure (file in to music, Head of School talks, one teacher reads from a book, one class presents work, music, Head makes announcements, file out to music) were pictured and attached by paper clips, which could be turned over when that part had passed. In this way, the boy was able to sit content, without drawing undue attention to himself, while the structure unfolded in a predictable way.

An older child who has relied on TEACCH-based support over the years might be helped to face a similar situation in a different way. He might have the structure pointed out first visually, but then be encouraged to develop his own strategies for marking the passing of the elements. For example, he might note that there were seven elements to the structure, and that he could learn to "tick them off" mentally. Once this method was mastered, he would be given practice at analyzing similar situations (e.g., a meeting or a church service) for him to determine the structural elements and then mentally mark their passing. The idea is to prevent the panic response to seeing the world as chaotic and unstructured, by helping the person perceive existing structures or impose them, if they do not exist. For many of us, when faced with a tedious amount of work to get through, compiling a list in which the work is broken down into elements, to be ticked off as accomplished, provides a degree of meaning and satisfaction where otherwise none might exist. People with an ASD have the same needs; it is just harder for them to see meaning or structure unaided.

## INCLUSION

To oppose inclusion is like opposing peace and love; it depends on what is meant. Some apparent examples (Jordan & Powell, 1994) are travesties of inclusion, where a child with an ASD in a mainstream school remains totally isolated, or where the experience is traumatic for the individual concerned (Exley, 2001; Gerland, 1997; Joliffe, Lansdown, & Robinson, 1992). Others are well planned and supported, with every child's education benefiting from the experience (Hesmondhalgh & Breakey, 2001; Seach et al., 2002). It is important to recognize that inclusion is not about location but about how the child is educated and the attitudes, understanding, and experiences of those involved. As I have said, "There is a need to research how children with an ASD are benefiting from their mainstream 'experience' rather than assuming it is an outcome measure of success" (Jordan, 2001, p. 137). It is this more able group of children with HFA/AS who are most at risk of our misunderstanding and neglect of their needs, as a recent parental survey has indicated (Hart & Geldhart, 2001).

The long-term goal is social inclusion in the wider society. Generally, this societal level is best achieved through inclusive schooling, but that may not be best in every case. Some children with HFA/AS are very sensitive to all forms of stimulation and find the physical conditions in most mainstream schools impossible to tolerate. Proximal supports (head phones, colored lenses, tactile buffers) may reduce the distress, and some physical adaptations can be made to the school (reduced lighting, screening of fluorescent lighting to reduce the flicker effect, changing school uniforms to loose tracksuits, and so on), but there are practical limits to these accommodations as well as instances when other children's needs are in conflict. In such instances it may be best to limit integration to times and activities when the child can be supported, while working on programs to increase the child's tolerance levels.

In some cases, behavior has been "managed" inappropriately so that the child now manifests significant problems with challenging behavior that puts others at risk. This is a common cause of exclusion in the United Kingdom (National Autistic Society, 2000), and although it is an unacceptable one in a system committed to inclusion, it may be best for a particular child and his or her family until the behavior can be brought under control and a more supportive environment engineered. It is a mistake to think that one mainstream school is much like another (many parents have found that a child whom one school has found impossible to include is happily included in another). Jordan and Powell (1995b) discuss the elements and qualities parents can use when trying to select an "autism-friendly" school for their child; others (Cumine, Leach, & Stevenson, 1997; Hesmondhalgh & Breakey, 2001; Seach et al., 2002) suggest ways mainstream schools can adapt to become "autism friendly."

## CURRICULUM ISSUES

Many countries have national curricula, although the extent to which they are centrally determined varies. In the United Kingdom, educational entitlement is taken to mean entitlement to the National Curriculum for all children, although adaptations and exemptions may be applied. Although it is a debatable point whether this National Curriculum is the most appropriate course of study for children with an ASD, the arguments against its use are no more telling for children with HFA/AS than for other children. Certainly, there are no good grounds for excluding any particular subject or curriculum area in any blanket way for children with HFA/AS, although particular cases may be made for particular children. Even special schools normally follow the National Curriculum in the United Kingdom, although independent schools are not obliged to do so. However, to introduce a radically different form of curriculum is to erect barriers to future inclusion opportunities—which is a significant reason for the emphasis on adaptation and inclusion rather than difference and exclusion. Although there are no subject areas which should automatically be excluded, there are particular problems that may be anticipated.

### English

When students with HFA/AS study English, problems are liable to arise in regard to understanding the motivation of characters in stories or dramas, especially if the motivations are implicit. In addition, problems in perceiving narrative structure are common (Bruner & Feldman, 1993). At a young age, children with HFA/AS need to be taught to actively listen to stories by using puppets or dolls to enact the action being described. In this way these young students come to understand that stories are "about" certain characters, who may be represented by proper nouns (names) but also by pronouns such as "you," "me," "I," "she," "he," "they," or "it." Later they can apply this knowledge to written scripts, using highlighter pens to show all the references (by noun or action) to the main character, then the subplot (in another color), and so on. They thereby learn to listen to and appreciate the narrative structure of storytelling. Sherratt and Peter (2002) suggest that children with ASD can be taught to role play parts in learned scenarios, and the learning may even generalize to new symbolic play acts. The children who participated in Sherratt's (2002) study and were able to learn to pretend play were children with additional learning difficulties. So using the same techniques of structured (but not rigid) role play with children with HFA/AS should yield even better results. Sherratt also evoked high emotional engagement, which may help to explain the better results obtained in this study than in others using more laboratory-based teaching techniques (Libby, Messer, Jordan, & Powell, 1998).

Although structural language problems are not a distinguishing feature of HFA/AS, there is a genetic link between autism and dyslexia, and many children with an ASD have additional specific problems in learning to read and write (Martin, 2002). When the autism is mild, the associated specific learning difficulties may constitute the bigger problem in education, at least at certain stages. However, both disabilities and their interaction must be recognized and addressed. Children with an ASD and dyslexic difficulties share common problems in organizing material for learning, sequencing activities, and perceiving underlying meaningful structures. Many of the techniques and strategies that are effective for children with dyslexia are also helpful for children with an ASD (see Preston, 1996, for practical strategies for children with dyslexia). Certainly, there is a shared need for explicit structures in teaching.

Tjus, Heimann, and Nelson (1998) showed how computer-generated study material for teaching literacy skills can help children with an ASD, and earlier work (Green, 1985) showed how computer keyboard skills, found essential in the teaching of children with dyslexia, also serve the same function of physically representing material to children with an ASD (in whom tactile and procedural memory may well be better than visual, and certainly than verbal, memory). Using a computer, therefore, should involve the teaching of typing skills to establish these motor memory patterns. Using computers also may help students with HFA/AS who have motor coordination problems and whose handwriting is illegible, even to themselves. They also may need to learn to write by hand as a life skill (and some techniques used for children with cerebral palsy can help here, such as the use of pencil grips to control grip tension and posture supports). The ease of production on a computer, however, can free them to be more expressive and can greatly enhance their self-esteem and willingness to work. Using computer word processing also makes revisions and corrections part of the process of producing a final copy, rather than being seen as making a mistake or getting it wrong. This helps students with HFA/AS reduce their anxiety and the consequent difficult reaction. Including the notion of multiple versions from the beginning also encourages critical reflection on their own work, and culminating in a final "perfect" copy to keep. (Ideally, the teacher records the process as well as the product, to monitor how the child is learning.)

Just as many children with dyslexia overcome their initial difficulties with decoding words but go on to develop "reading without understanding," children with HFA/AS have difficulty analyzing all texts (including spoken ones) to abstract meaning and develop a similar ability to understand individual spoken words or phrases but not to see how the meaning changes with the textual context (as well as the social one). This problem with abstracting meaning from experience (often incorrectly assumed to be a problem with the abstract nature of the concepts themselves) is a well recognized feature of "autistic" thinking (Blackburn, 2000; Grandin, 1992; Powell & Jordan, 1997) and presents a significant barrier to learning incidentally or in unstructured settings. Children with these problems need to have their attention drawn to overall meaning in clear, structured ways.

Teaching meaning from text at the simplest level is best tackled through written instructions to actions. This can be done for academic tasks but also for practical or even "fun" activities, in the form of written rules for social games with others. More advanced understanding may come from drama and play teaching, where improvised scenarios (e.g., ordering food in a café, cheering up a friend who is sad) are recorded and transcribed, becoming scripts for more formal enactment of the scene in a drama.

## Mathematics

Mathematics, in contrast to English, is often seen as a strength in ASD, but this is not always the case. Aspects of mathematics can present a challenge. There has been no systematic review of the existence of dyscalculia in people with HFA/AS, but anecdotal evidence from teaching experience suggests it is not uncommon. The feats of calculation that feature so often in accounts of autistic savants might indeed be viewed as more akin to "hyperlexia" than true understanding of mathematics. As with other areas of learning, what appears to be relatively easy are rote skills that do not require an analysis of meaning and are not necessarily tied into a body of knowledge. Even the actual processes by which these feats are achieved are not conscious and so cannot be used or adapted. A young man with AS, known to me, had a remarkable calculating ability. He was as accurate as an electronic calculator and a great deal faster (given the human user). The staff in a secure unit (for habitual arson) where he resided were trying to teach him a job in the hospital, to occupy his time and give him a possible vocational skill. They attempted, at various times, to get him to use a calculator for bookkeeping, to enter data on computer spreadsheets, and to manage the cash register at the hospital canteen. These "low-level" skills would appear to be far below his calculating ability, and yet he could not master them. He had no insight into his own capacity to calculate, and slowing it down and making it explicit and transparent seemed to destroy the ability. At a practical level, then, his remarkable ability reduced to a "party piece," and training him to do a job required starting from "scratch."

For those with HFA/AS, most problems with mathematics do not involve calculation but generalizing procedures to other contexts, including real-life ones, and understanding processes such as estimation where there is no exact correct answer. Many children with HFA/AS enjoy doing pages of "sums" at school but have little idea of what they mean or how to use them as problem-solving tools. Thus the practice of doing sums using duplicate examples should be limited and perhaps reserved for homework, when at least it can serve the function of keeping the child happily occupied. Some children with HFA/AS resist even this task, seeing no point in doing something they can already do, over and over again. Rather than viewing this resistance as a challenge to their authority, teachers need to see it as an opportunity to justify their practice and make the reasons explicit.

In school, the repetition may be part of a TEACCH-based program of training the child in independent work skills. Or it may be that the child is working too slowly and needs practice at speeding up and working against the clock, which is a helpful skill in examinations and makes the skills more automatic and fluent—and thus easier to generalize. Another way of getting a reluctant child to practice the same skill (which the teacher may feel is necessary to consolidate it) is to ask the child to "help" another student tackle the task. This tutoring fosters cooperative skills, raises the child's esteem in the peer group, and helps the child develop some reflective awareness of his or her own capacity.

The child with HFA/AS needs explicit teaching to learn how to apply these basic skills to real-life scenarios. Shopping, for example, involves more that the ability to add up costs and calculate change. First there are perceptual and social challenges in even determining the price. I learned a valuable mathematics exercise for all children from Mary Harris, a talented mathematics educator. The teacher supplies an array of wrappers from candy bars (or supply an array of the candy bars and the children are allowed to empty them—so much the better). The task for the children is to examine the wrappers and note all the information on them that might relate to the cost of the item. The children then report back, whereupon amazing sources of confusion are revealed (especially for children with HFA/AS, but also for others). Some wrappers have the word "free" across them, but it turns out not to refer to the cost but to some special offer if wrappers are saved; some prices are crossed through and a new one added; sometimes it is hard to distinguish weight information from price, and so on. This task often leads (or can be guided to lead) to a discussion about the information the students need to know to understand the price. They need to know that shopkeepers are most unlikely to be giving candy away free; and they need to have a rough idea of the cost of items before setting out to purchase them. Without that, they do not know whether they will need $50 or 50¢ to buy a loaf of bread, nor will they know if they have been grossly cheated or a big mistake has been made. Setting homework tasks (in cooperation with parents) in which the child conducts neighborhood surveys of prices, and helping him or her understand that prices vary, but only within limits, can be a really useful way of improving life skills as well as practical mathematics.

It is unusual to have problems with basic mathematical processes in this higher functioning group, but even these may occur sometimes. Young children, including those with HFA/AS, often have their first experience of counting as an ordinal task: using 1 to trigger 2 to trigger 3, and so on. This learning often occurs in the context of counting the stairs as the toddler climbs them or through simple action songs and rhymes. At this stage, the young child has no knowledge of the number system and does not integrate counting into a knowledge base; it is an isolated skill. The child may be able to count to 10 or even 20, but cannot start at 6, because each step (number) needs the trigger of the preceding one to prompt it. To manipulate numbers effectively and deal with mathematical operations beyond mere counting, this limited skill needs to transfer to an integrated knowledge system about numbers. Part of that knowledge system must include the fact that numbers are both ordinal and cardinal (although, of course, that knowledge may never be explicit). Thus each number has a place in a numbered system but it also "stands for" a set number of items in the real world; "7" is the number after "6" and before "8," but it also means a category of seven items (i.e., its cardinal meaning), and these items may include anything. There are two reasons why children with HFA/AS may get stuck at this stage: (1) They may have problems abstracting the "sevenness" from their experience of groups of seven items, and (2) they may have difficulty accepting the dual meaning of "7," which requires switching from the ordinal meaning they first learned.

Teaching mathematics to children with HFA/AS needs to be explicit and support them in developing an understanding of the dual meaning of numbers and applying that knowledge. However, teachers of young children are often themselves unaware of these properties of numbers, at an explicit level, and their teaching may then further confuse the child. For example, presenting the child with a set of items and asking "How many?" is fine, as long as the number group can be ascertained without counting (i.e., it is small—perhaps three or four items, or items arranged in an easily distinguishable pattern, as on a die). If the child is presented with seven items, however, and asked the same question before he or she has had the relevant experience with smaller numbers to appreciate the switch in meaning to a cardinal grouping, then the teacher's attempt to "help" the child by getting the child to count the items will only reaffirm the ordinal meaning. What usually happens in these circumstances is that the child happily counts on, and it is the teacher who has to get the child to stop at seven, without the child understanding why. In most cases, the teacher is encouraging one-to-one counting at this stage (getting the child to move blocks or put his or her finger on the items, in turn), and some children do then learn to stop counting when they "run out of" items. However, this is still far from understanding the switch between cardinal and ordinal numbers; it is just another "trick" to get by in a puzzling world, but it does not equip the child to deal with situations where the trick cannot be used.

## The Humanities

History is one of those subjects where certain aspects may be readily grasped by children with HFA/AS, but other aspects may cause real difficulties. Most children with HFA/AS will take great delight in learning lists of battles, dates of sovereigns or treaties, and so on, and in the past, when this kind of memorization formed a significant part of the curriculum for this subject, these children were able to excel. There comes a time, however, when children are asked to analyze the reasons behind events and discuss contemporary politics and human motivation. For children with HFA/AS, such tasks constitute severe stumbling blocks to further progress. Increasingly, understanding the processes by which history is constructed and appreciating that different explanations and even descriptions of events may arise from alternative viewpoints, both at the time and in hindsight, have come to take an even more dominant role in the history syllabus. Even young children are encouraged to imagine and feel empathy for other lives and times (Jordan & Guldberg, 2002). These more complex and nuanced learning objectives may readily become impediments to progress and understanding for children with HFA/AS.

One "solution" has been to exempt children with an ASD from history after a certain level, because of these difficulties, and to devote more time to what are seen as more essential aspects of the curriculum, such as personal and social skills. This shift may constitute a valid choice in any particular case. However, we also need to remember that where there is a challenge, there is also an opportunity. The very tasks that children with HFA/AS find difficult about history involve areas with which they need to become familiar in order to develop life skills and a greater understanding of the world. In a crowded mainstream curriculum, here is a time-tabled opportunity to teach these important skills and concepts, which will have a much wider benefit than the sole context of a particular history class. Furthermore, it is often difficult to obtain extra resources to teach something different in a mainstream setting; it is assumed that if something different is required, the child is not really "mainstream." Obtaining extra resources and support to provide "access" to part of the mainstream curriculum, however, is easier to accomplish under existing legislation that encourages inclusion.

The study of geography also has undergone changing conceptualizations over time. When there is an emphasis on physical geography, the child with HFA/AS can usually excel, although sometimes an obsessional interest with one aspect can dominate the child's attention and interfere with the learning of other aspects. Increasingly, however, geography studies have focused more on human geography, where social knowledge and application become important. The same problems can arise as in history, as noted, where children are encouraged to use empathy to explore the lives of people beyond their experience, or to consider the human implications of physical resources and their exploitation. Just as with history, the imaginative teacher can use these "difficulties" as opportunities to teach children with HFA/AS about these important aspects of knowledge.

Adopting the principle of using the child's interests and developing them (Grandin, 1995) has its place but needs to be applied with caution. The task of "reinterpretating" the subject matter in terms of this one particular aspect can place a tremendous burden on already overstretched mainstream teachers. Furthermore, there is always the possibility that the child will change obsessions partway through a project. Having said that, the humanities curriculum often lends itself to project work, which does allow children to use their own interests for broadening knowledge across other subject areas and exploring their real-life applications. In cases of a fixed and dominating interest, the TEACCH principle of "work then play" requires the child to tackle less favored aspects of the subject before being allowed time to research his or her favorite topic.

## Languages

The "dead" languages of ancient Greek and Latin are often attractive to this group of children, when they are sufficiently able, and have the opportunity, to study them. These languages are attractive because they have a clear and mostly logical structure, much of which can be learned in a rote way. Meanings are also ossified, not subject to the ever-changing variations of a living language, and although students might have to learn how meanings changed over the time span of certain ancient writers, the entire time period remains a fixed event, without the possibility of current change. Sadly, the career opportunities for students of these languages are increasingly limited, although there are a few in teaching and academia. The idea of studying the classics to "improve the mind" is no longer widely supported, and people with HFA/AS are unlikely to compensate for their condition-related difficulties in managing work situations by increasing their logical and analytical abilities in relation to esoteric areas of knowledge. However, fostering quality of life is currently an important goal in education; quality-of-life issues have a real impact on children's overall satisfaction with school and their ability to cope and feel good about themselves, so this area should not always be sacrificed to what is regarded as more relevant to some future quality of life. The capacity to enjoy learning opportunities is worthwhile in itself and something that most children with HFA/AS need to be taught.

When it comes to modern foreign languages, the story is very different. The temptation to exclude children with HFA/AS from these learning opportunities on the grounds of further possible confusion, however, is also questionable. Many, though by no means all, children with HFA/AS excel at these subjects, sometimes taking them through to degree level. Given that many of these students struggle with some aspects of language (the semantic, pragmatic aspects) even in their native tongue, there is no clear explanation for achievement in this area. It may be that learning a foreign language makes forms of knowledge and language use explicit, whereas these forms remain implicit when learning one's mother tongue. Thus, often for the first time, children are taught explicit rules for speaker addressee forms, for polite forms, conversational exchanges, cultural influences on pragmatic forms, and so on. They are also taught about idioms and that nonliteral forms of English cannot be translated literally; they are thereby alerted to the problem and also may receive specific instruction in how to "translate" the idiom (in their own understanding, as well as in the foreign language). Understanding that a single item or event can be described with equal accuracy using totally different language forms can transform these children's understanding of the arbitrary language and its nature and teach them to pay attention to the speaker's intentions as well as the actual language forms used.

Even those students for whom foreign language is not an area of strength usually benefit from this (perhaps sole) opportunity in a mainstream curriculum to learn about how to behave in cafes, restaurants, shops, public places, and so forth. Thus, while learning how to order food in a French restaurant or read a train timetable in German, children with HFA/AS will also be learning how to act appropriately in any restaurant or how to make sense of any train timetable, in addition to learning the French or German vocabulary, syntax, and appropriate idiomatic phrases.

The fact that the information is in a foreign language is less important for them than the clarity and progression with which its structure is explained.

## Science and Technology

The area of science and technology is often assumed to be a strength for students with HFA/AS, and indeed that is usually the case, although some aspects may become problematic. Some authors are happy to acknowledge this expertise in science that often characterizes this group of learners, while still maintaining that they have problems with "abstract" concepts. This is an anomaly that has not gone unnoticed by those with autism who are also scientists (Grandin, 1992, 1995). It is hard to think of a subject area that constitutes more abstract concepts than science and technology, but as Grandin notes, it is this very abstractness that helps her acquire the concepts. Her difficulty, as with others with an ASD, is experienced when attempting to "abstract" from human experience; it is everyday ("fuzzy") concepts, acquired from this distillation of experience, that are affected in individuals with HFA/AS, not the abstract scientific concepts that are typically defined in unambiguous mathematical language, chemical formulas, or by criterial features (e.g., a biological system of classification).

Researchers such as Baron-Cohen (1995) have suggested that being good at science is typical of a cognitive style exhibited by people with HFA/AS, by which "folk physics" (understanding how things work) is a natural strength and "folk psychology" (understanding how people work) is a natural weakness. Earlier work by Carey (1985) on the development of conceptual knowledge in childhood had suggested that young children typically interpret the world through folk psychology and that they have to be taught formally to replace this intuitive understanding with more scientific concepts and theories of how the world works. Carey claimed that confusions often lasted through to university level. If Baron-Cohen is correct, then people with HFA/AS would not have to struggle to replace their intuitive folk psychology with these more scientific concepts, and this should be an advantage in this subject.

Some aspects of science do present problems for children with HFA/AS. Science involves a view of "the truth" that is dependent on evidence and peer support and is open to continual revision, as new evidence emerges. Most science curricula at school do not contain much philosophy of science, of course, but nevertheless, the child is confronted with the inherent uncertainty and the necessity of hypothesizing, almost from the start. Most children with HFA/AS are not comfortable with uncertainty. They want to know if it is "this" or "that," not that we will "see what happens," and even after the results, still be faced with a 95% chance of it being "this" and only a 5% chance of it being "that." However, taking the opportunity to teach about statistics and probability can assist with this problem (and lead, on occasions, to a life-long fascination with statistics).

The particular learning style shared by many individuals with HFA/AS, whereby painstaking attention is given to detail and a dogged persistence applied to following topics to their conclusion, can be very conducive to the study of one of the sciences. Many can do well in the biological sciences, at the theoretical level, but may be impeded by their motor clumsiness in dissection and the preparation of samples for the microscope. Theoretical physics and mathematics may be an attraction, in the more able, because they do not require consensus skills; the language for understanding them is the language of mathematics or the visual language of modeling, and these can be tackled logically and systematically. Applied sciences and technology (especially computer technology) are almost always attractive to this group of children for many of the same reasons, although some technological subjects require a degree of manual dexterity and control that is beyond those with additional dyspraxic difficulties.

Learning via a computer seems to provide an ideal learning environment for many subject areas (Murray, 1997), although there are obvious dangers in the child becoming obsessed with this way of learning and not increasing his or her ability to learn in other ways. It can be a way of ensuring that a child's academic learning is not held back because of a difficulty in learning in the social way of the other children. By helping the child acquire the basic knowledge and understanding of a topic in this way, he or she may then be able to join others in a social learning context for the same topic area; the other children may be learning about the topic for the first time, whereas the child with HFA/AS is learning how to learn about that topic in a social context.

## The Arts

People with HFA/AS may excel at any area of the arts, although many will not, and artistic savant skills are still uncommon in this group (although they are more common in the ASD population than in the population as a whole). When a particular talent is present, it needs to be fostered, partly because of the vocational opportunities that it may afford, but mostly because of the social and personal value of having a particular skill. Even with talent, the way in which the art is learned and practiced is very different from the norm, so teachers need to be sensitive to how the child is best able to work. There is always the danger of forcing a child to do things in the accepted way, without allowing the child to demonstrate what works for him or her. It may be that the talent can only flourish in certain conditions, as in the case with children who sing beautifully, in tune, but not in the company of others, or play a solo instrument but are not able to follow ensemble playing or the timing of the conductor.

Apart from the rare, particular talents that need to be fostered, the arts are a valuable part of a full education for children with HFA/AS, and can be a vehicle for engaging the emotions in learning in a way that may benefit the development of a sense of self and further cognitive development (Damasio, 2000; Hobson, 2002; Jordan, 2002). The once pessimistic view of the limited participation possible by people with an ASD has been challenged by many arts initiatives (Beyer & Gammeltoft, 2000; Lord, 1997; Sherratt & Peter, 2002), and further opportunities await. Contrary to what was once believed, some greatly enjoy, and do quite well with, drama.

Music has a role not just as a skill at which children with HFA/AS may excel, or as a future vocational choice, but as a medium to influence mood and assist in the learning process. Music has been used extensively in the United Kingdom to structure (and thus foster) social interaction skills and emotional bonding (Christie, Newson, Newson, & Prevezer, 1992), enabling a relationship between the child and a key worker (i.e., the teacher, parent, or preschool worker) rather than a therapist, where the benefits tend to be limited to that context. Music through headphones is also being used as a way of encouraging listening, blocking out distracting and disturbing noise, and encouraging a focus on tasks such as painting, crafts, and even mathematics. Children, with and without an ASD, are being encouraged to relax and calm down, or to become energized and focused, with the help of music. None of these methods has been properly evaluated, but there are anecdotal reports of success.

## Physical Education

Physical activities and games have always had an important role in the full curriculum in the United Kingdom. In Japan, the emphasis on daily aerobic exercise, which is a characteristic of all schools, has gained special significance with its use in Daily Life Therapy (Quill, Gurry, & Larkin, 1989) in relation to Higashi schools for children with autism. It has long been reported that aerobic exercise has a beneficial effect on reducing challenging behavior and increasing task-related skills in people with an ASD (Elliott, Dobbin, Rose, & Soper, 1994; Rimland, 1988; Rosenthall-Malek & Mitchell, 1997), although only recently has this finding influenced the curriculum (mainly in specialist schools) for children with an ASD. Swimming, jogging, and trampolining are common features of the physical education programs in specialist schools for children with an ASD, where they enable exercise in an enjoyable way and are often used to foster additional skills of turn taking, and engaging in group activities. In some schools more adventurous programs such as canoeing, rock climbing, cycling, and sailing provide ways of extending leisure opportunities, increasing motor coordination skills, permitting opportunities for risk analysis, experiencing the thrill of danger in controlled conditions, and relying on the group and self (Evans, 1997).

In terms of the physical education program in mainstream schools, however, the opportunities are often more limited, and children with HFA/AS may have problems in gaining full access even to these. Some of these individuals have additional postural or motor coordination problems, which make them fearful of some apparatus work, for example. They may find it difficult to be even a short distance off the ground or to walk (or keep their balance at all) on uneven surfaces such as sand or grass. Children's reluctance or refusal to engage in such activities may be dismissed as behavioral problems, when what is needed is the help of an occupational therapist or physiotherapist to improve balance and posture and reduce fear.

The actual space in which physical education takes place also may present a problem for children with HFA/AS, who often have difficulty in marking the boundaries of their own body space (Williams, 1996) and may need to wear clothing that provides them with a clear signal of where their body ends and the environment begins. Faced with a large "empty" space, they may become very fearful and seek the security of the periphery, making contact with the outside walls. The fear may be increased if the other children are running around in a disorderly and unpredictable way. When children with HFA/AS are required to take up a position in a relatively large, unstructured space, it often helps to give them a mat to stand on or a hoop to stand within, thereby marking out that space and making the instruction clear. When there are different sets of apparatus to be negotiated in a particular order, and when that order may change from lesson to lesson, problems may be avoided if the child can see the layout on a plan before each lesson, to prepare him- or herself for the change.

The other part of physical education classes in many mainstream schools is taking part in team games. Added to the problems that may arise through physical incoordination are the problems of adjusting to a social context, understanding complex rules, and reacting to ever-changing situations at speed. Motivation is also a problem, as many will not see the point of the game or be motivated by competition, especially when it is for the glory of the team, rather than for themselves as individuals. Their lack of skill and enthusiasm make them, at best, indifferent players of team games and, more usually, a distinct disadvantage to any team. Forcing the issue adds to their unpopularity in the class, increases the stress and distress of the child in question, and usually does little to improve matters, since team members are most reluctant to include this player, and the resulting lack of practice means that skills never get better. The most helpful strategy is to organize extra "training" in the appropriate skills and then to conduct short, "friendly" games, in which the class teams take their turn in having the child on their team. By encouraging other children to support the child (e.g., setting buddy scheme targets, perhaps) and the child to engage more purposefully with the activity, some improvement can be made. However, most children with HFA/AS are unlikely to participate in team games in the long term, so it may be better to concentrate on physical activities that they do enjoy and where they have a reasonable chance of success.

## COMMUNICATION PROBLEMS

The effects of the communication difficulties experienced by children with an ASD, regardless of structural language ability, are pervasive throughout the curriculum and the general duration of school life. These children often talk "well," in the sense that they have a mature (even pedantic) grammatical structure and a vocabulary that is at least age-appropriate and may even be precocious. These abilities can seem like an advantage and, indeed, having language does make it easier for these children to learn some things and for teachers to teach in the ways to which they are accustomed. However, the level of language acquisition also can be a disadvantage in that it may mislead others regarding the true degree of understanding, and it may result in children being denied the very support they most need. If a child is not speaking, there is the immediate realization that something is wrong and a natural intuitive adjustment in the level of language we use and the time given to the child to respond. This need for shorter utterances and more time is unlikely to be recognized when the child has HFA/AS. When the teacher is confronted by an apparently high level of language ability, instead of adjusting his or her speech to accommodate the child's special needs, the teacher is more likely to attribute any failure in response to willfulness rather than disability and act accordingly, putting more pressure on the child to respond in the expected way. As Blackburn (2000) notes, the child's apparent ability then becomes his or her biggest "disability," in that it leads to false expectations and a lack of appropriate support.

All nonautistic children learn to communicate before they learn to speak, and the interaction and routine formats of early childhood are designed to foster that basic communicative understanding and competence. When they come to school, such children may need to adjust to the different forms of communication used there, but their basic understanding is not affected, because that has been well established at home; they simply learn a new set of rules for school. Children with HFA/AS, in contrast, often learn to speak without that underpinning of communicative understanding and skill and may only just have reached the stage of learning about communication when they enter school. The communication environment in a school is a special one, adapted to the special purposes of education, and the "crowd control" measures adopted in most schools are not designed to foster basic communicative understanding and skill. Thus children who are basing their understanding of communication on school experience are liable to be misled about the rules of that communication. It is not just that raising a hand to signal that the child wants a turn to speak is going to look odd at home, or on the playground. Getting the impression that hand raising is the signal for wanting a turn means the child is failing to pay attention to the actual cues that denote this communicative intent (e.g., making eye contact, leaning toward the current speaker, making preparatory hand gestures) and so is even less likely to learn when and how to relinquish the floor as a speaker.

Similar problems arise in the area of understanding how to join in conversations, maintain the topics under discussion, and end conversations. Contrary to "normal" situations, wherein having something to contribute to a topic is a common (if not exclusive) reason for joining a discussion, classroom rules often preclude this reason. The teacher may be faced with a sea of eager children with hands raised, ready and eager to contribute to the topic, and yet the child who is at the back, trying to be ignored (perhaps suspected by the teacher of not doing the set homework reading) is the one chosen to contribute; it must make little sense to someone trying to work out the basic rules and not realizing that this set of circumstances is a particular variant.

And what if the teacher is the model for topic introduction and maintenance? What evidence does the child see that the teacher selects a topic to interest the others in the discourse, gives way to topics introduced by others, or lets a topic die when others have ceased to show any interest? The teacher is more likely to provide a model that children with HFA/AS have already mastered: They introduce a topic of their own choosing, irrespective of the negotiated interests of the listeners, they continue talking, ignoring all signs of inattention, irritation, or boredom (and even berating any listener who displays such signs openly); they resist any attempt by the listeners to modify or change the topic; and they end the topic in an arbitrary way (e.g., the bell signaling the end of the lesson rings) or when they decide it is at an end, regardless of the reaction of their listeners. It is optimistic to expect a once-a-week session on conversation skills to compete with this daily example of the contrary.

Further sources of confusion arise with the use of questions in schools. Many children with HFA/AS have a particular problem with the use of questions, especially repetitive questions (which are extremely taxing for parents and teachers alike), and questions to which it is apparent the child already knows the answer. Yet if the teacher refuses to answer a child's question on the grounds that "You already know the answer to that," what is the child to understand when the teacher spends a large part of the day asking questions to which (one hopes) he or she certainly knows the answer? The fact is that teachers rarely ask questions that conform to what linguists call "sincere" questions—ones where the questioner is genuinely seeking an answer that is not known. Most classroom questions fall into one of the following categories: They are rhetorical, in order to make a point; they are display questions designed to test knowledge; they are ways of encouraging children to think more deeply or differently; or they are sarcastic, having the opposite meaning to the apparent one. It is not surprising that children with HFA/AS are unable to detect the sincere purpose of questions from these examples. Nor are these children likely to be using a sincere form themselves. They are not usually aware of their own lack of knowledge (at least, when young), nor do they realize that the teacher could know something that they do not, so it is most unlikely that they would be asking for information they did not already have. Thus the teacher's response will be simply bewildering.

Children with HFA/AS are also likely to be bewildered, and often distressed, by the usual conduct of a question-and-answer session between the teacher and the class, often used to introduce the topic of the lesson. In a typical example of this method, some stimulus object will be held up to the class or pointed at while on display. The teacher will then ask a question about the stimulus, to elicit what has been remembered from previous sessions and to set the scene for the current topic of this lesson. The most common question format is "What is this?" The teacher also might use an implied question through an instruction such as "Tell me about this." A child in the class volunteers an answer that is correct but clearly does not match the teacher's intention, so it is greeted by a "Yes" from the teacher, but the response is delivered with an intonation that indicates to the initiated (in this educational "game") that the teacher cannot say it is incorrect but it will not do as the required answer. Several more volunteered responses may get the same response from the teacher (and there may be an incorrect response that gets a clear "No"), but the questioning goes on until someone gives the desired answer (probably by remembering the context of what was done last session and the likely content of today's session), to which the teacher says another "Yes," with a different intonation pattern, and the questioning ceases. What is the child with HFA/AS to make of this exchange? Intonation patterns can be perceived (and sometimes echoed exactly) but the meaning inherent in the different patterns is not understood. As far as this child is concerned, there are one or more "yeses" and the questioning continues, and then another "yes" and it comes to an end. The child is unlikely to understand the educational game of guessing what is in the teacher's mind, and so he or she will often search in desperation for the rule governing this behavior. Perhaps one has to say "yes" three times before it is correct—but then that does not work the next time!

The good news is that the teaching solutions to all these difficulties are fairly straightforward. The first principle remains one of trying to understand the reason for the child's responses and confusion and, wherever possible, to preempt that confusion by making intentions explicit. The conversational rules for classroom discourse need to be spelled out clearly and distinguished from the conversational rules that apply when in less formal (and less peopled) situations. In other words, the child needs to learn two sets of "how to communicate" rules—but that is a better alternative than getting conflicting messages about the rules and never developing any consistent way to sort them. In introducing topics, teachers could use techniques that would benefit other children, as well as those with HFA/AS: First remind the class of the general topic area (e.g., "Remember, we have been studying light") and then be far more explicit with the questioning probe (e.g., "I want you to tell me something about this object that describes it in relation to light").

Repetitive questions from the child require more detective work to understand what particular function they are serving in a particular instance and thereby respond appropriately. As with other people, those with an ASD often ask repetitive questions when they are anxious about something and want to feel the reassurance of hearing the same answer repeated. Just as the anxious lover will not be reassured to have a "Do you love me?" question answered with a "I refuse to answer that because you already know the answer" or "I'm going to answer that twice and then no more," so too the child with HFA/AS looks for added doses of reassurance and is unlikely to rest until they are obtained. The more the reassurance is withheld, the more frantic the child's questions become. What is needed is another way of offering reassurance that does not involve getting locked into this question-and-answer routine. How to answer the repeated question of what is happening next or when some particular event is going to happen (whether its occurrence is looked upon with eager anticipation or dread) can be "solved" by having a visual timetable at hand to which the child can be redirected (preferably by a gesture, without any verbal response). In this way the child learns to seek out his or her own means of reassurance (e.g., checking the timetable and learning when the event is going to happen).

However, repetitive questions also may have other underlying causes. Sometimes the questioning is a way of following the teacher-inspired model and is the child's only known way of introducing a favorite topic. In that case, the child needs to be taught explicitly how to introduce topics in other ways. In addition, the child may need guidance in limiting his or her time to talk on that topic by making agreed-upon rules and a timetable of occasions when he or she is free to do so, as well as specified occasions when the topic must not be broached. It is unreasonable (and unrealistic) to expect a child never to talk about an obsessional interest at school, but it is equally unreasonable, and not in the child's long-term best interests, to allow unrestricted talk about the single topic.

Lastly, the child may use repetitive questions much more knowingly— that is, wanting to hear the same answer, not due to anxiety but because he or she likes the sound of the answer (or even the shape of someone's mouth as he or she is saying it). All we can do about the latter is to have a sense of humor and let the child know we will indulge it once but not repetitively.

## PROBLEMS WITH SOCIALIZATION AND THE SOCIAL CONTEXT

Given the social complexity of most schools and the inherent problems in understanding and coping with social demands, it is not surprising that many of school-related problems stem from this area of difficulty. The social context makes all learning more problematic, since children with HFA/ AS (especially when young) are unable to learn new information while processing social information at the same time. Once the social information is familiar (i.e., they know the members and understand the group rules) or the task is familiar, then it is possible for them to manage to complete that task in the social group. Even a teacher's attentions may interfere with the child's efforts to understand the task, particularly if the teacher is too intrusive or confusing. A child with HFA/AS may learn new tasks best through asocial means, such as via a computer, or by working independently with a clear visual template, and only later come to learn how to perform tasks in the presence of others.

Teachers need to exercise a sensitive discernment to judge when it is appropriate to support the child in joining in a group activity and when the child would do better sitting alone (but perhaps near the group) or even protected by screens. Children with HFA/AS are particularly apprehensive about invasions of body space that arise from behind them, so it is important to consider that vulnerability when determining seating arrangements for the class. Forcing a child to occupy a particular seat even though that position induces fear in the child all the time he or she is in it, will only result in ongoing distraction and anxiety, an inability to concentrate on the task at hand (even when the "task" is eating lunch), and possibly even a violent eruption. There are times when the child should be helped to tolerate some conditions to which he or she will be regularly exposed, but a gradual approach is nearly always preferable to force.

Problems in the social domain are not all about learning to tolerate others. Many difficulties arise because the child has not understood the social rule or does not accept that it applies in this case. Being unable to predict others' behavior and having limited means (through communication or social manipulation) of exerting control over others makes children with HFA/AS extremely anxious to resist attempts to control them, while they desperately seek to control others. This dynamic is a serious challenge to teachers and to school authority. Working around the problem, rather than trying to confront it directly, is likely to lead to the best results, since confrontation usually leads to increased resistance. Making clear rules, preferably displayed in written form, enables the teacher to insist on adherence to the *rules*, which is far more easily accepted than insistence on obeying the *teacher*. Putting the child in charge of "policing" the rule is a step further in getting the child not just to obey a rule but to monitor his or her own behavior in relation to that rule—a useful step toward self-control. Teachers need to monitor the situation, however, ensuring that the child with HFA/AS does not become bossy and objectionable to others, and that others also take this "policing" role in turn.

This principle of putting the child in charge of his or her own learning, whenever possible, was followed by Barber (1996) in helping a 14-year-old boy with AS integrate into a mainstream school. An initial step was to allow him to study subjects in which he excelled at an accelerated pace. He was put in several classes whose students were 2 years older than he, and who were seriously engaged in preparing for exams. He flourished in this hardworking atmosphere, where he was not teased for working and where he did not have time to "waste" (he had no idea how to use free time). However, although this placement solved his academic problems, he was still in trouble repeatedly, with staff or students, because of his unusual and often difficult and disruptive social behavior. One approach might have been to identify his "problem" behavioral areas, select targets, and then try to motivate him to work on these specific behaviors. However, given the difficulties discussed above concerning control and a lack of understanding, such a program is unlikely to be successful, at least in a way that would enable the boy to retain his dignity and develop insight into, and control over, his own behavior. Instead, Barber developed an ingenious way of getting *him* to identify his own problem behaviors, set the targets to be worked on, negotiate the recording of progress with staff, and monitor and display his results.

Problems with peers also need careful analysis, since they are rarely simple matters of bullying on the part of peers, or inappropriate behaviors on the part of the child with HFA/AS. The transactional nature of the problem means that intervention needs to involve both peers and the target child as having roles in both the problem and its solution. One incident with a 12-year-old boy with HFA was reported by his carer as one of systematic and significant bullying, including abuse about autism. The view of the school, however, was that the boy himself was provocative and would react violently to behavior that was, at most, teasing and no different from that shown to all the boys. From observing the situation, it became clear that the conflict did start, as the school claimed, with the other boys teasing him in just the way they teased one another. They were making fun of his diagnostic label, but there was little sign of malevolent intent—just a funny name they did not understand—and they also picked on "unfavorable" characteristics of one another, such as calling one boy "fatty" and another "spotty." None of this was pleasant or desirable, and school staff were trying to reduce such name calling, but there was no evidence that the boy with HFA was singled out for abuse in any way.

Yet the incidents involving this boy were more serious than the others, because of the boy's reactions. He did not understand the difference between teasing and bullying, nor did he recognize the overall friendly tone in which such comments were made. Even more importantly, he did not recognize the attempts other boys made to pacify and mollify him, when they saw that he was upset and that they had "gone too far." He took their clumsy attempts to give him a friendly and gentle punch on the arm and to place an arm around his shoulders as further examples of bullying, and he reacted with his own anger and violence. It was necessary to work with his peers to help them understand the nature of autism and how that boy was feeling, and to help them develop other ways of interacting with him that would be mutually enjoyable. At the same time, the boy with HFA needed help to understand the behavior of the other boys and to appreciate the difference between being unkind to cause harm and being insensitive because one does not understand. This explanation made sense to him because he had taken time to understand and accept his own diagnosis, and he could readily appreciate that it might be a problem for others. He also could accept that he was insensitive to others sometimes, and useful and supportive plans of action were agreed within the group. It would be naive to think that all examples of bullying are as innocent and equitably solved as this case, but the principle of working with all parties on an agenda for change, rather than dispensing recrimination, does seem to be the best approach in almost all cases.

Some schools have approached the problem of relationships with peers and vulnerability to bullying much more systematically by setting up "buddy" schemes or "Circles of Friends." As the name implies, buddy schemes are interventions whereby a peer (or sometimes an older child) is assigned as a buddy to the child with HFA/AS, usually during informal times such as playtimes and lunch breaks, although possibly during other lessons, such as physical education. In a survey of educational provision for children with autism in Scotland, Jordan and Jones (1997) found many different kinds of buddy systems, with the most successful being ones where working with the children with autism was seen as a privilege to be earned rather than a social duty. Most buddy systems have something to offer, and Seach and colleagues (2002) recommend their use in mainstream schools. However, problems may easily arise if the buddies are not well supported; they may even be victimized and bullied themselves, or may feel too embarrassed to continue the work at the secondary level. Buddy schemes seem to work well in primary schools and where there are two buddies to share the support for each child with HFA/AS.

"Circles of Friends," whereby peer volunteers are paired with a target child to work out problems and find solutions together, have become a widespread source of support for children with HFA/AS in mainstream schools in the United Kingdom. Bozic, Croft, and Mason-Williams (2002) provide a recent example of how this method can work well. An interesting problem, noted by the parent in this report, was that the increased confidence her son with AS gained by his participation in the Circle of Friends encouraged him to attempt more overtures to noncircle children, but, sadly, these noncircle children were not knowledgeable or confident enough to respond appropriately. Generalizing results outside of the trained peer groups, so that the child is not rebuffed, remains a challenge that needs to be resolved. There also is a need to help children with HFA/AS do more of the "work" in the circles and rely less on the support and understanding of the Circle peers. Hesmondhalgh and Breakey (2001) teach about friendship as part of a program on relationships and sexuality and have adapted the very useful "friendship guide" (pp. 128–129) that was developed by a young man with AS (Segar, 1997). This guide explains about "false friends" as well as true ones and how to distinguish between them and avoid the problem of vulnerability and being "set up" by others. This set of guidelines offers one way of dealing with a problem that is seldom addressed in the literature but is evident in practice; many young people with HFA/AS become very suspicious of the intent of others, even paranoid, because they do not know how to distinguish the sincere from the insincere. Learning how to make this distinction is not an easy matter, but it is an important life skill that needs to be tackled, for its absence leads only to further social withdrawal.

## SPECIFIC LEARNING PROBLEMS

Specific problems in learning arise from HFA/AS and yet do not constitute general learning difficulties. These include lack of motivation, overreliance on rote memory, and the limited expressions of self-control and responsibility.

## Motivation

A significant problem when addressing socially based challenges is the apparent lack of motivation (at least, toward teacher-directed activities) that appears to characterize many children with HFA/AS. The lack of enthusiasm for curriculum tasks is often in direct contrast to the obsessional interest in certain activities, often to the exclusion of all else. The problem with motivation is threefold: (1) the direct competition with the preferred activity; (2) impaired ability to "pick up on" intent and consequent unawareness of what is expected; and (3) a difficulty in establishing relationships with others, so that the normal motivations to please others simply do not apply.

All three sources of the motivational difficulty need to be tackled. Firstly, patterns of activity and good work habits need to be established, so that preferred activities come at the end of a chain of progressively more favored activities; as in the TEACCH framework, visual schedules showing what has been done and what is left to do, before the favored activity can be followed, are recommended. Second, an ongoing cognitive program can be enacted, in which teachers make their intentions explicit and teach children to understand what instructions are, in effect, commands, even when formulated as queries (e.g., "Would you like to get on with your work now?") or even statements (e.g., "All I want to see are children busy working at their desks"). Finally, children with HFA/AS may still need help establishing relationships with adults as well as peers and may need ongoing work by staff to engage in mutually reinforcing exchanges to compensate for missed experiences of early development, but in more age-appropriate ways. For example, teachers should take the opportunity to join the child in favored activities, thereby establishing a relationship that may transfer to teacher-selected tasks.

## Memory

Overreliance on good rote memory ability leads to ineffective learning; children with HFA/AS generally do not grasp the meaning of the task, nor can they recall spontaneously, without cues. These children need explicit instruction regarding the key elements of meaning in any task, how the task relates to what is already known, and how the knowledge might be used in future contexts. The dependence on cued memory needs to be recognized and accommodated in teaching, so that cues are identified and rehearsed at the time of learning, and then rehearsed again in a reflective process after the event. This process of teaching children with HFA/AS how to initiate a "plan, do, reflect" sequence in relation to their learning has been advocated in the preschool area (Jordan & Powell, 1990) and is part of a broader cognitive curriculum, for which principles have been developed (Jordan & Powell, 1991; Powell & Jordan, 1991).

Keeping a homework diary not only acts as a key reminder for the child but also requires him or her to identify the key aspects of the assignment to be recorded, which later serve as efficient cues for recall of the homework task. Furthermore, diary keeping enables the child to think about the pragmatic aspects of communication by becoming aware of what is shared knowledge (i.e., between the child and the teacher, who were both present at the lesson to which the homework relates) and what is not (i.e., parents were not present in class, so they will have to be told things explicitly if they are to help with the homework). It is important to set parameters around the time spent on homework, because the child may be very anxious about it and spend hours (as may his or her parents) trying to ensure that it is done absolutely correctly. Reinforcing the notion of drafts that can be corrected in a word-processing context is helpful here to reduce the obsession about "perfect" work. Myles and Southwick (1999) suggest other ways parents can help the child with HFA/AS deal with homework problems.

## Developing Self-Control and Responsibility

Aside from our need to manage children's behavior, there are also educational issues that relate to fostering a sense of responsibility and self-control in the children in our care. It is a common experience that children with HFA/AS focus on the consequences of their actions only to the extent that there are sanctions. In spite of an apparent understanding of the reason why the sanction has been employed, these children do not relate it to the point at which they had a choice to behave differently. All their energies are focused on getting the sanctions removed or on blaming the person responsible for applying the sanctions as being the one who needs to alter his or her behavior. Without a way of understanding their choice in the situation, and thus their responsibility for the consequences of their own actions, it is unlikely that they will be able to behave more appropriately in the future, at least not without others exerting external controls.

Visually representing a particular type of situation on a flow chart (see Figure 10.1) can make the choice point explicit and help the child make an informed choice and exhibit self-control. Illustrate the triggering event in a picture, with a question mark above it to indicate this scenario is the point of choice. The child is then given an alternative (acceptable) reaction (ideally, this alternative is a negotiated choice) to the one that is being "punished." The agreed-upon alternative is illustrated in another picture on the same piece of paper and linked to the choice point by a railway track (such tracks are one-way and their characteristics are usually well under-

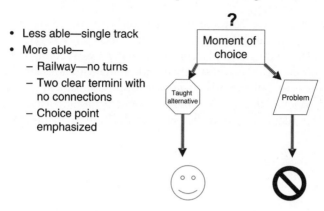

- Less able—single track
- More able—
  – Railway—no turns
  – Two clear termini with no connections
  – Choice point emphasized

**FIGURE 10.1.** Teaching consequences.

stood by children with HFA/AS) with an arrow going from the choice point toward it (i.e., the alternative). The railway track then extends beyond this second picture to a third depiction, this one of a happy child enjoying the item whose removal is going to be the sanction (e.g., using a computer). At this stage the procedure is an illustrated form of behavior therapy; the cognitive element comes from adding a second track that emanates from the choice point and leads first to a picture of the unwanted response. From there the track continues to the terminus, which is an illustration of the sanction (e.g., a computer with a big cross through it). The child's attention is drawn to the fact that once on a particular track, there is no turning back until the terminus to that track is reached (i.e., either the happy outcome or the sanction). It is further pointed out (and clearly indicated by the visual representation) that there is no connection between the unwanted reaction and the "happy" terminus. The only way of reaching that terminus is to take that track from the choice point. The child may still need support in choosing the "right" track at the choice point, but the process takes a step toward putting children in control of the consequences they experience in a way that helps them make more sense of their environment and their own role within it.

## CONCLUSION

Although the needs of children with HFA/AS are complex, they can be accommodated within mainstream contexts in most cases, providing that the school administration and staff understand these needs and are willing to adapt teaching and structures to accommodate those needs. There may be a need to prepare these children for entry and to make available additional resources to help the children, teachers, and peers work together to achieve mutual understanding. No placement can work by expecting the child with HFA/AS to make all the adjustments, and no mainstream school can be expected to execute all the adaptations. Mutual adjustment is required, the benefit of which is the creation and experience of an inclusive environment that is better adapted to meet the needs of all children, including those with an ASD.

## REFERENCES

Autism Working Group. (2002). *Autistic spectrum disorders: Good practice guidance*. London: DfES/DH.

Barber, C. (1996). The integration of a very able pupil with Asperger Syndrome into a mainstream school *British Journal of Special Education, 23,* 19–24.

Baron-Cohen, S. (1995). *Mindblindness: An essay on autism and theory of mind.* Cambridge, MA: MIT Press.

Beyer, J., & Gammeltoft, L. (2000). *Autism and play.* London: Jessica Kingsley.

Blackburn, B. (2000). Logically illogical: A view from within and without autism. *Good Autism Practice, 1*(1), 1–3.

Bozic, N., Croft, A., & Mason-Williams, T. (2002). A peer-support project for an eight-year-old boy with an autistic spectrum disorder: An adaption and extension of the Circle of Friends approach. *Good Autism Practice, 3*(1), 22–30.

Bruner, J., & Feldman, C. (1993). Theories of mind and the problem of autism. In S. Baron-Cohen, H. Tager-Flusberg, & D. J. Cohen (Eds.), *Understanding other minds: Perspectives from autism* (pp. 267–291). Oxford, UK: Oxford University Press.

Carey, S. (1985). *The construction of mind.* Cambridge, MA: MIT Press.

Christie, P., Newson, E., Newson, J., & Prevezer, W. (1992). An interactive approach to language and communication for non-speaking children. In D. Lane & A. Miller (Eds.), *Child and adolescent therapy.* Milton Keynes, UK: Open University Press.

Cumine, V., Leach, J., & Stevenson, G. (1997). *Asperger syndrome: A practical guide for teachers.* London: Fulton.

Damasio, A. (2000). *The feeling of what happens: Body and emotion in the making of consciousness.* London: Harcourt Brace.

Elliott, R. O., Dobbin, A. R., Rose, G. D., & Soper, H. V. (1994). Vigorous aerobic exercise versus general motor training: Effects on maladaptive and stereotypic behavior of adults with autism and mental retardation. *Journal of Autism and Developmental Disorders, 25,* 565–576.

Evans, G. (1997). Outdoor pursuits. In S. Powell & R. Jordan (Eds.), *Autism and learning: A guide to good practice* (pp. 152–170). London: Fulton.

Exley, R. (2001). Foreword. In M. Hesmondhalgh & C. Breakey, *Access and inclu-*

sion for children with autistic spectrum disorders: Let me in (p. 1). London: Jessica Kingsley.

Gerland, G. (1997). *A real person.* London: Souvenir Press.

Grandin, T. (1992). An inside view of autism. In E. Schopler & G. B. Mesibov (Eds.), *High functioning individuals with autism* (pp. 105–125). New York: Plenum Press.

Grandin, T. (1995). How people with autism think. In E. Schopler & G. B. Mesibov (Eds.), *Learning and cognition in autism* (pp. 137–158). New York: Plenum Press.

Green, I. (1985, Spring). Training autistic children in keyboard skills. *Communication,* pp. 10–12.

Hart, A., & Geldhart, H. (2001). Inclusion: The parent's view. In G. Linfoot (Ed.), *2001: An autism odyssey* (pp. 141–150). Sunderland, UK: Autism Research Unit, Autism North.

Hesmondhalgh, M., & Breakey, C. (2001). *Access and inclusion for children with autistic spectrum disorders: Let me in.* London: Jessica Kingsley.

Hobson, P. (2002). *The cradle of thought: Exploring the origins of thinking.* Oxford, UK: Macmillan.

Howlin, P. (1998). *Children with autism and Asperger syndrome: A guide for practitioners and carers.* Chichester, UK: Wiley.

Jolliffe, T., Lansdown, R., & Robinson, T. (1992). *Autism: A personal account.* London: National Autistic Society.

Jordan, R. (2001). Research into policy in autistic spectrum disorders: The development of evidence-based practice in the British Isles. In G. Linfoot (Ed.), *2001: An autism odyssey* (pp. 129–139). Sunderland, UK: Autism Research Unit, Autism North.

Jordan, R. (2002). What's love got to do with it? Making sense of emotions in autism: Biology, cognition and treatment. In G. Linfoot (Ed.), *Building bridges: Proceedings of Durham Conference, 2002* (pp. 15–24). Sunderland, UK: Autism Research Unit, Autism North.

Jordan, R., & Guldberg, K. (2002). Web wise: New training opportunities in autistic spectrum disorders. *Special Children, 11,* 24–26.

Jordan, R., & Jones, G. (1997). *Educational provision for children with autism in Scotland: Final report of a research project for the SOEID.* University of Birmingham, School of Education, United Kingdom.

Jordan, R., & Powell, S. (1990). High Scope: A cautionary view. *Early Years, 11*(1), 29–34.

Jordan, R., & Powell, S. (1991). Teaching thinking: The case for principles. *European Journal of Special Needs Education, 6,* 112–123.

Jordan, R., & Powell, S. (1994). Whose curriculum? Critical notes on integration and entitlement. *European Journal of Special Needs Education, 9,* 27–39.

Jordan, R., & Powell, S. (1995a). Autism: The case for early specialist intervention. *Early Years, 16,* 46–51.

Jordan, R., & Powell, S. (1995b, Winter). Factors affecting school choice for parents of a child with autism. *Communication,* pp. 5–9.

Jordan, R., & Powell, S. (1995c). *Understanding and teaching children with autism.* Chichester, UK: Wiley.

Libby, S., Messer, D., Jordan, R., & Powell, S. (1998). Spontaneous play in children with autism: A reappraisal. *Journal of Autism and Developmental Disorders, 28,* 487–497.

Lord, S. (1997). Movement in the arts curriculum. In S. Powell & R. Jordan (Eds.), *Autism and learning: A guide to good practice* (pp. 79–99). London: Fulton.

Martin, N. (2002). A study of the possible indicators for specific learning difficulties in children with Asperger's syndrome. *Good Autism Practice, 3*(1), 58–62.

Mesibov, G., & Howey, M. (2003). *Accessing the curriculum for pupils with ASD.* London: Fulton.

Murray, D. (1997). Autism and information technology: Therapy with computers. In S. Powell & R. Jordan (Eds.), *Autism and learning: A guide to good practice* (pp. 100–117). London: Fulton.

Myles, B. S., & Southwick, J. (1999). *Asperger syndrome and rage: Practical solutions for a difficult moment.* Shawnee Mission, KS: Autism Asperger Publishing.

National Autistic Society. (2000). *Inclusion and autism: Is it working?* London: Author.

Peeters, T. (1997). *Autism: From theoretical understanding to educational intervention.* London: Whurr.

Powell, S., & Jordan, R. (1991). A psychological perspective on identifying and meeting exceptional needs. *School Psychology International, 12,* 315–327.

Powell, S., & Jordan, R. (1993). Diagnosis, intuition and autism. *British Journal of Special Education, 20,* 26–29.

Powell, S., & Jordan, R. (1997). Rationale for the approach. In S. Powell & R. Jordan (Eds.), *Autism and learning: A guide to good practice* (pp. 1–14). London: Fulton.

Preston, M. (1996). *Four times harder.* Birmingham, UK: Questions Publishing.

Quill, K. A., Gurry, S., & Larkin, A. (1989). Daily life therapy: A Japanese model for educating children with autism. *Journal of Autism and Developmental Disorders, 19,* 637–640.

Rimland, B. (1988). Physical exercise and autism. *Autism Research Review International, 2,* 3.

Roeyers, H. (1996). The influence of nonhandicapped peers on the social interaction of children with a pervasive developmental disorder. *Journal of Autism and Developmental Disorders, 26,* 303–320.

Rogers, S. J. (1996). Brief report: Early intervention in autism. *Journal of Autism and Developmental Disorders, 26,* 243–246.

Rosenthal-Malek, A., & Mitchell, S. (1997). Brief report: The effects of exercise on the self-stimulatory behaviors and positive responding of adolescents with autism. *Journal of Autism and Developmental Disorders, 27,* 203–202.

Rutter, M., Greenfeld, D., & Lockyer, L. (1967). A five to fifteen year old follow-up study of infantile psychosis. II. Social and behavioural outcome. *British Journal of Psychiatry, 113,* 1183–1199.

Schopler, E. (1997). Implementation of TEACCH philosophy. In D. J. Cohen & F. R. Volkmar (Eds.), *Handbook of autism and pervasive developmental disorders* (2nd ed., pp. 767–798). New York: Wiley.

Schopler, E., Mesibov, G. B., & Hearsey, K. (1995). Structured teaching in the TEACCH system. In E. Schopler & G. B. Mesibov (Eds.), *Learning and cognition in autism* (pp. 243–268). New York: Plenum Press.

Seach, D., Lloyd, M., & Preston, M. (2002). *Supporting children with autism in mainstream schools.* Birmingham, UK: Questions Publishing.

Segar, M. (1997). *Coping: A survival guide for people with Asperger's syndrome.* London: Kith and Kids.

Sherratt, D. (2002). Developing pretend play in children with autism. *Autism: The International Journal of Research and Practice, 6,* 154–160.

Sherratt, D., & Peter, M. (2002). *Developing play and drama in children with autistic spectrum disorders.* London: Fulton.

Tjus, T., Heimann, M., & Nelson, K. E. (1998). Gains in literacy through the use of a specially designed multimedia computer strategy: Positive findings from thirteen children with autism. *Autism: The International Journal of Research and Practice 2,* 139–154.

Williams, D. (1996). *Autism: An inside-out approach.* London: Jessica Kinglsey.

Wolfberg, P. J., & Schuler, A. L. (1993). Integrated play groups: A model for promoting the social and cognitive dimensions of play. *Journal of Autism and Developmental Disorders, 23,* 1–23.

# 11

# The Ideal Classroom

## LINDA KUNCE

Structured educational intervention targeting multiple domains of functioning is the mainstay of treatment for individuals with pervasive developmental disorders (National Research Council, 2001; Volkmar, Cook, & Pomeroy, 1999). Often, younger and more severely impaired children with autism are educated according to the relatively well-defined principles and methods of comprehensive treatment programs (Harris & Handleman, 1994; Olley & Reeve, 1997). In contrast, children with high-functioning autism (HFA) or Asperger syndrome (AS) are more likely to be educated in regular classroom settings by teachers who have little or no prior knowledge of autism and recommended interventions (Helps, Newson-Davis, & Callias, 1999). Although many children with AS or HFA "survive" or even prosper at school, disheartening proportions either experience significant distress or fail to reach their long-term potential (Attwood, 2000).

Desires to minimize student distress and optimize student learning naturally lead to the question, *What is the ideal classroom for individuals with AS?* Reflection upon this question, however, triggers a cascade of queries:

What type of teacher is best?
How big should the classroom be?
What learning goals should receive the most attention?
Who should make curricula decisions—parents, teachers, or students?
Does diagnosis matter?

Compared to a decade ago, professionals and parents have a wealth of relevant resources to help them answer such questions. These resources include (1) an ever-richer clinical literature (e.g., Mercier, Mottron, & Belleville, 2000), (2) an expanding body of descriptive research (e.g., Miller & Ozonoff, 2000), (3) empirically based theoretical explanations that have opened up new avenues of treatment (e.g., Hadwin, Baron-Cohen, Howlin, & Hill, 1997), (4) a small but influential body of research on the effectiveness of social interventions (e.g., Bauminger, 2002), (5) substantial reviews of the research on educational interventions for classic autism (e.g., National Research Council, 2001), (6) published practice parameters (e.g., Volkmar et al., 1999), and (7) specific discussions of intervention strategies for students with AS or HFA. The explosion of resources in this last category has been phenomenal. Early works (e.g., Mesibov, 1992) have been followed by edited volumes for professional and parent audiences (Klin, Volkmar, & Sparrow, 2000; Quill, 1995; Schopler, Mesibov, & Kunce, 1998), general parent and professional guides (e.g., Mesibov, Shea, & Adams, 2001; Myles & Simpson, 1998; Ozonoff, Dawson, & McPartland, 2002), numerous "tips" and "strategies" articles in the education literature (e.g., Myles & Simpson, 2001), as well as a profusion of Internet-based resources.

Although I draw heavily on the resources identified above, my goal in this chapter is not to conduct a critical review of these literatures. Neither do I intend to present a "how-to" set of strategies. Instead, my goal is to provide an integrated model of effective education for high-functioning individuals who have an autism spectrum disorder (ASD). To create a background context for the proposed model, I first discuss four major challenges in the field and their implications for educational intervention.

## MAJOR CHALLENGES

Professionals and parents designing educational programs for individuals with AS or HFA confront four substantive difficulties, each of which has implications for intervention planning. First, there is a paucity of empirically sound research on the efficacy of educational interventions for AS and HFA. Therefore, intervention recommendations and models, *including those presented in this chapter*, must be considered open to revision and disconfirmation based on future research.

Second, educational intervention is complicated by the characteristics associated with AS and HFA. The list of affected domains is daunting: social functioning, communication, interests, play, sensory responses, motor coordination, adaptive behavior, self-organization, and abstract thinking (American Psychiatric Association, 2000; Ozonoff, 1998; World Health Organization, 1993). As illustrated in Table 11.1, these characteristics often clash with the physical, social, and instructional characteristics of regu-

**TABLE 11.1. Selected Examples of the Potential Mismatch between Student and Classroom Characteristics**

| Characteristics of students with AS or HFA | Characteristics of traditional classroom environments |
| --- | --- |
| Cognitive–organizational | |
| Difficulty organizing time, tasks, materials. | Students expected to start, complete, and turn in work with appropriate independence. |
| Absorption in own unique interests. | Teachers use age-typical interests to motivate students. |
| Facility with facts and details versus abstract reasoning. | Emphasis on conceptual themes; facts used in service of more complex understanding. |
| Social communication | |
| Less engagement in group activities (e.g., on periphery at recess, "lost" in class). | Group learning activities; formation of group identity; emphasis on group rules. |
| Impaired understanding of others' nonverbal communication. | Teacher intentions communicated through emotional expression, voice tone, gestures. |
| Impairments in complex auditory comprehension. | Emphasis on teaching through talk (i.e., lectures, verbal instructions, etc.). |
| Behavioral–emotional | |
| Desire for sameness and repetition. | Changes in school routines (e.g., assembly) expected to delight students. |
| Reduced control over outbursts, especially in response to sensory stimuli. | Student outbursts interpreted (and punished) as intentionally disruptive. |
| Limited understanding of own and others' emotional responses. | Teacher use of social–emotional reasoning (e.g., "How would you feel if . . . ?") |
| Other | |
| Impaired application of concepts and skills in real-life contexts. | Limited inclusion of real-life skills in academic curriculum. |
| Atypical sensory reactions and related problematic behaviors. | Teacher use of contingency management to address problematic behavior rather than modifying antecedent stimuli. |
| Impaired gross and fine motor skills. | Value group sports and athletic prowess; emphasis on written work. |

*Note.* Selected research and clinical references for student characteristics include American Psychiatric Association (2000); Attwood (2000); Dunn et al. (2002); Ghaziuddin et al. (1998); Konig et al. (2001); Landa (2000); Mercier et al. (2000); Minshew et al. (1997); and Ozonoff (1998).

lar classroom environments, further impairing the individual's ability to learn. Two major implications emerge from this complex and perplexing situation: (1) Intervention needs to target multiple domains of student functioning, and (2) the natural focus on changing *student* behavior must be balanced by an emphasis on changing the *classroom* environment, in order to make it more meaningful for students with AS or HFA (cf. Mesibov et al., 2001).

Third, debate over the empirical validity of AS has caused confusion for professionals and parents alike (Klin, Volkmar, & Sparrow, 2000; Schopler, Mesibov, & Kunce, 1998). The position in this chapter is that, at the current time, subgroup diagnosis (i.e., AS vs. HFA) does not provide a meaningful basis for intervention planning. This conclusion is based on the lack of data demonstrating subgroup differences in response to treatment, on evidence that clinicians and researchers do not diagnose AS in a consistent and thus reliable manner (Szatmari, 2000), and on recent research findings revealing markedly similar neuropsychological profiles associated with AS and HFA (e.g., Manjiviona, & Prior, 1999; Miller & Ozonoff, 2000).

Finally, the uncertainty associated with working toward unpredictable long-term goals presents a fourth major challenge. Follow-up studies suggest that individuals with AS or HFA do make significant progress over time. Yet, too often these adults function at a level below what is expected, given their age and IQ (Howlin, 2000). For example, social difficulties, underemployment, and ongoing reliance on parents all occur frequently. Given the nature of these difficulties, educational intervention must explicitly address long-term goals that range far beyond traditional markers of academic success.

Considered together, these major challenges reveal that the question posed at the beginning of this chapter—*What is the ideal classroom for individuals with AS?*—is far too specific. Instead, we need to ask: *What are the essential elements of effective educational intervention for high-functioning individuals with an ASD? And: How are these elements related to one another and to student outcome?*

## AN INTEGRATIVE MODEL OF EFFECTIVE EDUCATIONAL INTERVENTION

In the remainder of the chapter I present an integrative model to organize and explore what is recommended with regard to educational intervention for school-age students with AS or HFA. The model draws heavily upon existing clinical, theoretical, and research literature as well as my own training and work with North Carolina's comprehensive network of autism services known as Division TEACCH (Treatment and Education of Autistic and related Communication handicapped CHildren; Schopler, 1997). Following an overview of the proposed model, I explain the elements in greater detail by providing a rationale and illustrative strategies for each.

## Overview

The proposed model, depicted in Figure 11.1, includes multiple elements hypothesized to be vital to educational intervention for students with AS or HFA. The arrows in the model illustrate pathways along which the elements are thought to influence one another and, ultimately, student outcome. The *foundational elements* (first column) provide essential groundwork and ongoing support for the development of a *meaningful educational plan* (second column) and, by extension, for the student's entire educational program. The *structural elements* (third column) provide the infrastructure for the educational program by ensuring that necessary supports are offered across the curriculum, which is defined in relation to seven content or *curricular elements* (fourth column). The quality of programming in the curricular elements is hypothesized to be (1) dependent on the foundational and structural elements, and (2) predictive of student outcome. *Student outcome* is defined in a multifaceted manner, encompassing both short- and long-term functioning across multiple domains. These do-

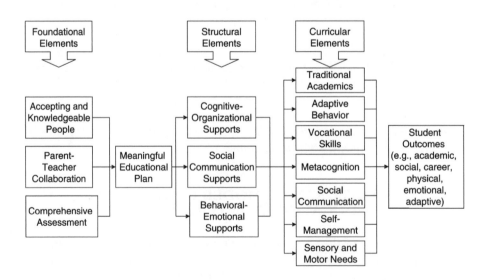

**FIGURE 11.1.** Proposed integrative model of effective educational intervention for students with AS or HFA.

mains are listed in the fifth column of Figure 11.1 and explained through illustrative examples in Table 11.2.

## Foundational Elements

According to the proposed model, effective educational intervention, at its most basic level, requires (1) an accepting and knowledgeable school community, (2) ongoing parent–teacher collaboration, and (3) comprehensive assessment of the student's unique learning profile.

### Accepting and Knowledgeable People in the School Community

The social communication difficulties, cognitive characteristics, and restricted interests of students with AS or HFA result in classroom behaviors that may be misinterpreted by others in the school community, particularly in the absence of accurate information about ASD. Helps and colleagues (1999), for example, found that only 5% of mainstream teachers and 50%

**TABLE 11.2. Short- and Long-Term Outcome Variables across Six Domains for Students with AS or HFA**

| Domain | Sample outcome variables | |
| | Short term | Long term |
| --- | --- | --- |
| Academic | Content mastery | Continued/more complex learning |
| | Personal enrichment | Scientific/professional advancement |
| Social | Connects with others | Forms and maintains relationships |
| | Follows important school rules | Follows social rules at work |
| Career | Exploration of own interests | Personal satisfaction in work |
| | Develops effective work habits | Financial security |
| Physical | Regular exercise | Healthy habits (e.g., nutritional diet) |
| | Remediation of motor impairments | Physical well-being |
| Emotional | Fewer behavioral outbursts | Less anxiety/depression, greater joy |
| | Learns coping strategies | Self-initiated use of coping strategies |
| Adaptive functioning | Reduced prompt dependence | Makes decisions about own life |
| | Basic self-care skills | Independent living (as per own potential) |

of specialist teachers had received extra training specific to autism. Without appropriate information, teachers and peers alike may be hurt or frustrated by the child's perplexing behaviors, and the risks to the classroom community multiply. For example, teachers may view the students' behaviors as manipulative and themselves as incompetent. Peers may feel rejected or threatened and, in turn, neglect, reject, or even victimize students with AS or HFA (Tantam, 2000).

Accepting and understanding teachers can have a major impact on students with HFA or AS, in part, because of the direct support they offer and, in part, because of the role they play in helping others accept the student. For example, Odom and Watts (1991) illustrated the importance of teacher prompting in promoting interactions between typical peers and students with autism. Clinical wisdom suggests that "ideal" teachers for students with AS or HFA are (1) caring, trustworthy, respectful of the student, and predictable with regard to these qualities, as well as (2) knowledgeable about ASD (e.g., Asperger, 1944/1991; Ozonoff et al., 2002). In addition, teachers who are flexible and open to diversity may be more adept at putting themselves in the student's shoes and more open to making needed accommodations.

Five illustrative strategies for creating an accepting and knowledgeable school community are listed below.

1. Given the centrality of the classroom teacher to creating a safe and effective learning environment, teachers are selected *thoughtfully*, with attention given to characteristics such as those described above, and *early*, at least by the end of the prior academic year.
2. Classroom teachers and individual aides are provided with ongoing education about autism through print and electronic resources, workshops and conferences on autism, interactions with children and adults with an ASD, access to a knowledgeable consultant, and other methods (see Ozonoff et al., 2002, for a resource list).
3. Teachers are educated about the individual needs and strengths of specific students (e.g., through discussions with parent, reading reports, talking with prior teachers).
4. Additional school staff are educated about autism and, as needed, the specific student's needs. This staff education effort includes (a) administrators, who require a working knowledge of autism, training resources, intervention methods, and available local services (cf. Klin & Volkmar, 2000), as well as (b) specialist teachers (e.g., music) and school support staff (e.g., secretaries), who require an understanding of the specific student's "visible" problems and need for environmental supports.
5. Peers are (a) educated about ASD, (b) given suggestions for interacting with students with ASD, and (c) supported in their own con-

cerns. Resources include: parent guest speakers, supportive class meetings, adults who model acceptance, children's books about ASD, and programs such as the Circle of Friends (Whitaker, Barratt, Joy, Potter, & Thomas, 1998).

## Ongoing Parent–Teacher Collaboration and Communication

In collaborative approaches to parent–teacher relationships, parents are viewed as active and integral partners in their child's education (Gareau & Sawatzky, 1995). By identifying parent–teacher collaboration as a foundational element, I propose that these working relationships are fundamental to effective educational intervention. This view has a long history in the autism field (Schopler, 1997), and current consensus among autism professionals is that parents need to be involved in the assessment, treatment planning, and treatment implementation processes (e.g., Marcus, Kunce, & Schopler, 1997; Volkmar et al., 1999).

The rationale for parent collaboration is multifaceted, reflecting teacher, child, and parent variables. First, as noted earlier, many teachers of students with AS or HFA lack sufficient formal training and experience. Second, the very nature of the child's characteristics—such as social communication difficulties, idiosyncratic responses, and problems applying academic knowledge in real-life—requires direct parent–teacher communication. Third, parents are the best experts on their children (Schopler, 1997). Parents observe and guide their child over the greatest variety of settings and over the longest span of time. In addition, parents often assume an explicit treatment provider role by teaching their child, coordinating services, and remaining a substantial source of support far into adulthood (Howlin, 2000; Marcus et al., 1997). Parent–teacher collaboration, therefore, has multiple advantages. By taking advantage of parental expertise, teachers can avoid past mistakes, make the school environment more appealing to the student, and help ensure continuity of goals and strategies over settings and time.

Strategies to promote collaborative relationships include, but go beyond, any parent participation mandated by law (e.g., in the United States, Public Law 94-142, Individuals with Disabilities Education Act, Public Law 105-17; Simpson, 1995). Five qualities illustrative of "ideal" parent–teacher collaboration are described below.

1. Information, support, and provision of resources flow from teacher to parent *and* from parent to teacher.
2. Educators make a commitment to engage in intensive and ongoing communication with parents—*and they receive the administrative recognition and resources needed to honor this commitment.*
3. Parent–teacher communication is comprehensive enough to address

the complex needs and strengths of students with AS or HFA. Parents and teachers discuss (a) learning goals and objectives, (b) environmental supports, (c) child's application of knowledge across settings, (d) child's work habits, especially with regard to homework, and (e) the full range of the child's characteristics, as well as effective and ineffective adult responses to those characteristics.

4. Parents and teachers have access to autism-relevant parent–teacher support groups and behavior management groups, either within the school system or through outside agencies (e.g., Sofronoff & Farbotko, 2002).

5. Because parent involvement changes in frequency and intensity over time (Marcus et al., 1997), the degree of parent–teacher collaboration should be matched to parents' current preferences and capabilities as well as the child's needs.

### Comprehensive Assessment

No one neuropsychological or symptom profile typifies all individuals with AS or HFA. Furthermore, highly uneven patterns of skills and abilities may occur within individuals (Klin, Sparrow, Marans, Carter, & Volkmar, 2000). Assessment of individual strengths, weaknesses, and interests across multiple domains, therefore, is fundamental to successful educational intervention for students with AS or HFA. Not surprisingly, comprehensive assessment is included as the third and final foundational element in the proposed model (Figure 11.1).

No single evaluation protocol exists for AS and HFA, and many recommended tests are the same as those that would be used with other populations (see Mesibov et al., 2001, for specific measures). Because formal tests appear to overestimate the real-world competence of students with AS or HFA (Landa, 2000), however, informal measures are often needed (e.g., unstandardized rating scales, observations). Fortunately, more sensitive standardized measures are becoming available for purposes of screening, diagnosis, and functional assessment (e.g., Ehlers, Gillberg, & Wing, 1999).

The five illustrative examples provided below were drawn from the general autism and AS/HFA-specific assessment literatures (e.g., Klin, Sparrow, et al., 2000; Mesibov et al., 2001; National Research Council, 2001).

1. Evaluation extends beyond a focus on clinical diagnosis to include assessment of intellectual and neuropsychological functioning, academic abilities, social and communication skills, adaptive behavior, vocational skills, sensory responses, fine and gross motor skills, in-

terest and behavior patterns, medical concerns, and family and community resources.

2. Evaluators have expertise in (a) the tests they administer, (b) ASD, and (c) the current best assessment procedures available for AS and HFA.

3. Teachers conduct *ongoing* informal assessment of student behaviors and learning across settings, academic subjects, tasks, and intervention strategies.

4. Evaluators write reports that are understandable and include pragmatic recommendations. Teachers review these reports and implement recommendations in light of the student's educational plan and classroom-based assessments of student progress and needs.

5. Parent input is valued and encouraged at all levels of the assessment process.

## Meaningful Educational Plan

The student's educational plan (second column in Figure 11.1) is the overall "road map" that identifies student learning goals and objectives, the strategies used to help the student attain those goals and objectives, and the individuals responsible for implementing the various strategies. In the United States, the written document that captures this plan and is mandated by law is referred to as the Individualized Education Plan (Simpson, 1995). Too often, however, written educational plans for students with AS or HFA meet the "letter of the law" but are not truly meaningful for the child.

Five illustrative strategies for creating a *meaningful* educational plan for students with AS or HFA are outlined below (for practical assistance, see Fouse, 1999).

1. The educational plan builds on the three foundational elements, in that it is (a) grounded in an understanding of AS and HFA and respect for the student, (b) developed in collaboration with the student's parents, and (c) individualized, based on an assessment of the student's unique strengths, weaknesses, and interests.

2. In the language of the proposed model, the educational plan addresses both structural elements (i.e., the environmental supports to be provided) and curricular elements (i.e., learning goals and objectives for content domains in which student needs have been identified).

3. Identified learning objectives and goals are optimistic, attainable, and address meaningful short- and long-term outcomes.

4. Because students with AS or HFA often receive services from multiple professionals, the educational plan clearly identifies all involved indi-

viduals, their responsibilities, and their place in the overall plan. In addition, a primary coordinator or case manager is identified.

5. The educational plan includes content and strategies that are appealing and meaningful to the *student* (e.g., by incorporating special interests, allowing the student to take advanced courses in areas of strength, including the student in plan development).

## Structural Elements

The *structural elements* involve the provision of environmental modifications and supports to compensate for the learning and behavioral differences that typically characterize students with AS or HFA. Because these supports generally are needed across the student's curriculum, they are placed prior to the curricular elements in Figure 11.1. In other words, the support provided by the structural elements is assumed to enable student learning in traditional academics as well as other content domains. Based on intervention recommendations for AS and HFA (e.g., Klin & Volkmar, 2000; Myles & Simpson, 2001; Ozonoff et al., 2002) as well as autism intervention program descriptions (e.g., Harris & Handleman, 1994; Olley & Reeve, 1997), three overlapping areas of need were identified: cognitive-organizational supports, social communication supports, and behavioral–emotional supports.

### Cognitive-Organizational Supports

Researchers have used constructs such as executive functioning (Ozonoff, 1998), central coherence (Frith & Happé, 1994), and complex information processing (Minshew, Goldstein, & Siegel, 1997) to describe the cognitive impairments exhibited by individuals with AS or HFA. Cognitive impairments are thought to be evident in students' real-world difficulties with organizing their responses, identifying relevant information in assignments, managing time, and understanding complex language. In contrast, strengths generally are demonstrated in students' relative facility with rote learning, rule learning, factual or detailed information, maintaining a passion for special interests, verbal expression and, for some, visual spatial ability (e.g., Mesibov et al., 2001; Miller & Ozonoff, 2000; Minshew et al., 1997; Ozonoff, 1998).

As described earlier, this general pattern of strengths and weaknesses matches poorly with characteristics of traditional learning environments. Therefore, environmental modifications and supports are often needed to ensure that students with AS or HFA are not punished inadvertently for their different learning and thinking styles. Descriptions of cognitive-organizational supports can be found in the literatures on AS and HFA (cited previously), classic autism (e.g., Olley & Reeve, 1997), structured teaching (e.g., Kunce & Mesibov, 1998; Schopler, Mesibov, & Hearsey, 1995), and executive dysfunction (e.g., Denckla & Reader, 1993; Ozonoff, 1998). Five major groups of strategies are listed below.

1. Across the curriculum, teachers implement cognitive-organizational strategies in order to compensate for the individual's relative weaknesses, to build on the individual's strengths, and to utilize the individual's special interests.

2. Educators use a broad range of structured teaching approaches to increase the predictability and meaningfulness of the school environment for the student. Specific strategies include (a) *using routines* to capitalize on student preference for, and ability to learn in the context of, familiar activity sequences; (b) creating an *organized and visually clear classroom environment* (e.g., preferential seating and a semiprivate work area); (c) providing students with *strategies for organizing materials* (e.g., labeling, checklists); (d) using *individual written or picture schedules* to smooth transitions; and (e) *communicating work expectations* in a way that the student readily understands, remembers, and is motivated to follow (e.g., work systems, checklists, use of timers and time lines). (See Mesibov et al., 2001, for a pragmatic and extended discussion.)

3. Tasks are presented in ways that increase the likelihood of understanding, such as by (a) presenting information visually (e.g., in writing); (b) providing explicit, step-by-step instructions; (c) introducing topics and materials prior to class lessons (i.e., priming); and (d) providing "graphic organizers" that help students figure out what is relevant in a reading or lecture (e.g., outlines, flow charts).

4. When needed, tasks are simplified by (a) reducing work load (e.g., shorter assignments), (b) breaking work into smaller units (e.g., giving instructions one at a time), (c) providing hands-on activities, and (d) using other creative ways to simplify input (e.g., larger print).

5. Teachers are actively engaged in (a) monitoring student understanding and progress; (b) identifying adults responsible for developing, implementing, and evaluating supports; and (c) ensuring that effective cognitive-organizational supports are shared across settings and years of schooling.

### Social Communication Supports

By definition, "social impairments" are universal to ASDs (American Psychiatric Association, 2000; World Health Organization, 1993). Many authors therefore consider enhancement of social competence and communication to be a central aspect, if not "the most important component[,] of the intervention program for individuals with AS" and related disorders (Klin & Volkmar, 2000, p. 350). Despite relatively intact formal language, students with AS or HFA may have difficulty attending to others' speech, understanding and using nonverbal communication, forming peer relationships, and sharing emotions and interests in a mutual manner (American Psychiatric Association, 2000). Researchers have attempted to identify core deficits underlying observed impairments and have variously emphasized constructs such as theory of mind, affective reciprocity, and joint attention (Hadwin et al., 1997; Mundy, 1995; Robertson, Tanguay, & L'Ecuyer, 1999). However, there is no one agreed-upon scheme for understanding or remediating social communication problems in individuals with AS or HFA (Attwood, 2000; Waterhouse & Fein, 1997).

According to the proposed model, educators address social and communication impairments in two ways: first, by changing aspects of the school social environment (as discussed here) and, second, by targeting student skills for development (discussed later under curricula elements; refer to Figure 11.1). Five illustrative social communication supports are listed below. (For additional information, see Attwood, 2000; Gray, 1998; Landa, 2000; Myles & Simpson, 1998; Quill, 1995.)

1. Educators learn to enhance student understanding by adjusting their *own* communication (e.g., use shorter statements, less figurative language, positive yet matter-of-fact tone).

2. Teachers make the social environment more meaningful and less overwhelming by providing appropriate structure. Depending on student needs, teachers might provide (a) unobtrusive supports (e.g., verbal script), (b) assistance during unstructured activities (e.g., recess), (c) alternate activities (e.g., student watches a school assembly on video rather than attending), or (d) a less demanding classroom environment (e.g., fewer students, more structured routines).

3. Teachers provide student with *explicit* explanations of social situations and expectations through any one of a variety of techniques (e.g., social stories, cartooning, social scripts, individualized social rules).

4. Educators understand and respect the student's social interests and preferences (e.g., building social activities around the student's interests, allowing some "alone" time).

5. Educators promote social interaction on at least three levels by (a) providing opportunities for structured social interactions, (b) encouraging more informal connections with typically developing peers (e.g., identifying peer activity partners), and (c) identifying social activities that genuinely engage and delight the student.

## Behavioral–Emotional Supports

Several research groups have reported that individuals with AS or HFA are at risk for clinically significant symptoms reflecting both internalizing and externalizing patterns (e.g., Kim, Szatmari, Bryson, Streiner, & Wilson, 2000; Tantam, 2000). Hyperactivity symptoms appear to dominate in childhood, whereas depressive symptoms are reported most frequently in adolescents and adults (Ghaziuddin, Weidmer-Mikhail, & Ghaziuddin, 1998). Additionally, rates of repetitive behavior, circumscribed interests, and insistence on sameness are elevated and can interfere with learning and social relationships (e.g., Mercier et al., 2000). Preliminary reports indicate that psychotropic medications are used frequently to treat symptoms such as hyperactivity, depression, anxiety, and aggression in this population (Martin, Scahill, & Klin, 1999).

Stresses in the school environment may increase the risk of internalizing and disruptive behaviors in students with AS or HFA—especially if educators fail to recognize the student's special needs (Tantam, 2000) or if the student is overwhelmed by social and organizational demands (Klin & Volkmar, 2000). Tantam (2000) has argued that the management of psychological problems "almost always involves consideration of the environment, particularly the social environment, and the reaction to it by the person with Asperger syndrome" (p. 59).

Similarly, the integrative model proposed here places the use of behavioral–emotional supports in a broad context. First, as illustrated in Figure 11.1, effective design of behavioral–emotional supports is hypothesized to depend on knowledgeable professionals, parental input, and individualized assessment. Second, the use of behavioral–emotional supports is hypothesized to influence student learning across the curriculum and, eventually, long-term outcome. The following five illustrative support strategies were drawn from the general intervention literature and the literature on emotional and behavioral issues (e.g., Ghaziuddin, Ghaziuddin, & Greden, 2002; Mesibov, 1992; Quill, 1995; Tantam, 2000).

1. Teachers minimize emotional and behavioral problems by proactively using cognitive-organizational and social communication supports (described earlier) in order to make the classroom environment more meaningful and welcoming for students with AS or HFA.

2. Key support people are identified (e.g., "safe" person at school; therapist to provide problem-solving support), and coordination is ensured with regard to medication management and strategy implementation.

3. Crisis plans and coping strategies (e.g., safe place, take-a-break routines) are established in advance, practiced with the student, and followed by adults.

4. Teachers help students develop self-esteem and confidence by providing daily opportunities for student success, pleasure, and interest. Because students with AS or HFA often have atypical interests and motivations, these activities are built around the *student's* patterns of interest and strength.

5. Adults "choose their battles wisely"; asking themselves questions such as, What do I know about AS and HFA that can help me understand this behavior? Is the behavior interfering with the student's learning?

## Curricular Elements

The *curricular (or content) elements* comprise the third major set of elements in the proposed model (Figure 11.1, fourth column). Olley and Reeve (1997) noted that although autism professionals have focused heavily on intervention strategies, "curriculum is an essential component of any effective education or treatment plan" (p. 484). The majority of children with AS or HFA will probably receive most of their education in regular classrooms governed by standard curricula; academic curricula alone, however, appear insufficient for ensuring successful long-term functioning (e.g., Howlin, 2000). Therefore, the curriculum for students with AS or HFA must be broad enough to target the multiple associated impairments.

Based on a review of the relevant literature, seven content areas or "curriculum elements" were selected for inclusion in the proposed model. The first area, traditional academics, parallels standard academic curricula. The second two areas, adaptive behavior and vocational/career preparation, are familiar to special education professionals. The last four areas, however, reflect the more unique needs associated with ASD. These areas include metacognition, social communication, self-management, and sensory and motor needs.

### Traditional Academics

Intervention in this domain typically involves modification of standard academic curricula to compensate for relative academic weaknesses (e.g., listening and reading comprehension, completing open-ended assignments) and to build on relative academic strengths (e.g., reading decoding, spelling; Griswold, Barnhill, Myles, Hagiwara, & Simpson, 2002; Siegel, Goldstein, & Minshew, 1996). Teachers use cognitive-organizational and social communication supports to modify instructional methods (e.g., supplementing lectures with written outlines) and assignment expectations (e.g., breaking assignments into chunks). Teachers enhance student motivation by incorporating student interests into lessons and by providing advanced education in areas of special aptitude. Further, even for college-bound individuals, an emphasis on functional academics may be needed to ensure that students can apply academic concepts in real-life situations (e.g., use of math skills to manage money). Often, modifications such as these fit within the bounds of the standard curriculum. At other times, however, individualized plans will conflict with educational requirements (e.g., course credit expectations). In such instances, flexible adaptation of requirements is recommended in order to help the students reach long-term goals.

## Adaptive Behavior

Klin and Volkmar (2000), among others, have argued that "adaptive skills should be one of the central points of any program for a child with AS" (p. 346). Individuals with AS or HFA not only exhibit significant deficits in adaptive behavior (e.g., Liss et al., 2001), but these deficits are significantly correlated with functioning in adulthood (e.g., Carter et al., 1998). Assessment of adaptive deficits for students with AS or HFA is typically based on teacher observations, parental input, and structured data gathered using the Vineland Adaptive Behavior Scales. Learning goals and objectives in this domain address a student's ability to perform daily life skills such as personal care, domestic maintenance, community functioning, basic safety measures, and leisure skills. Needed skills are taught explicitly, and the student is given multiple opportunities for practice across settings (Klin & Volkmar, 2000; Myles & Simpson, 1998).

## Vocational Skills and Career Preparation

The relatively high rates of under- and unemployment of people with AS or HFA (Howlin, 2000) have been linked to the individuals' cognitive and social impairments as well as to failures in the educational and vocational support systems (Gerhardt & Holmes, 1997). Vocational and career preparation needs to start early: Effective work routines can be taught from the earliest school years, explorations of job skills should start by adolescence, and work on an explicit school-to-work (or college) transition plan should begin, at least, by age 16. Content to be covered in this domain includes (a) job-relevant social skills (e.g., interview skills, appropriate use of free time), (b) use of external supports to improve work performance (e.g., written directions, written schedules), (c) effective work habits and problem-solving strategies, and (d) applying skills in real-life work practice ranging from in-class to in-school to community jobs. (See Smith, Belcher, & Johrs, 1997, for detailed information.)

## Metacognition

Learning goals and objectives in this domain explicitly target students' thinking and learning strategies. In the autism literature, these sorts of strategies have been referred to as metacognitive strategies, flexibility training, cognitive-behavioral strategies, and other terms (e.g., Jordan & Powell, 1995; Klin & Volkmar, 2000; Koegel & Koegel, 1995; Ozonoff, 1998; Quinn, Swaggart, & Myles, 1994). These somewhat disparate methods all share an emphasis on teaching the student to exert control over his or her own thinking, learning, and problem-solving processes—hence the selection of the term *metacognition* for this domain. Specific curricular content in this domain might include helping students learn (1) when and how to use environmental supports, (2) how to select an appropriate problem-solving strategy, and (3) abstract thinking skills, such as identifying the main point, drawing inferences, understanding figurative language, and flexible problem solving (e.g., McAfee, 2002; Ozonoff, 1998; Siegel et al., 1996).

## Social Communication

The domain of social communication focuses directly on enhancing the social communication skills and knowledge of students with AS or HFA. Published social curricula are now available to guide educators (e.g., McAfee, 2002); however, there is no "gold standard" social curriculum. Important content is assumed to include friendship skills, conversational skills, social problem-solving strategies, and understanding of emotions and mental states (e.g., Attwood, 2000; Landa, 2000; Ozonoff et al., 2002). Therapy or consultation with a speech–language pathologist, trained in pragmatic language impairments, is often essential to appropriately identify and address student needs.

Board games, academic-type projects, computer programs, and virtual reality environments all have been proposed as strategies for teaching social–emotional concepts (e.g., Attwood, 2000; Beardon, Parsons, & Neale, 2001). Teaching specific social skills individually, using an explicit step-by-step strategy in combination with modeling, role plays, feedback, and real-life practice, also has been emphasized (e.g., Bock, 2001; Myles & Simpson, 2001). In addition, group social skills training is frequently recommended. Several researchers have reported that group-based social intervention leads to improvement in targeted skills, but that generalization of gains to more global measures is relatively disappointing (e.g., Hadwin et al., 1997; Ozonoff & Miller, 1995). Bauminger (2002) reported preliminary positive results with a program that may be appealing to educators due to its broad focus (i.e., targeting social cognition, emotional understanding, and social interaction), its high level of structure (i.e., curriculum available), and its relevance to typical school settings (i.e., intervention implemented in classroom setting).

## Self-Management

Self-management approaches increase the ability of students with AS or HFA to regulate their own behavior, typically without requiring insight or deep self-awareness (Olley & Reeve, 1997). Instead, these approaches promote self-regulation by emphasizing skills such as self-observation, self-description, and self-monitoring. For example, a student might observe and then record instances of his or her on-task behavior. Among these approaches, self-management training (Koegel & Koegel, 1995) has received notable empirical support. This approach, as well as formal cognitive-behavioral therapy (e.g., Ghaziuddin et al., 2002; Hare, 1997), may be best implemented by experienced clinicians. Other techniques can be implemented in the classroom environment fairly easily. These strategies include helping students (1) label or describe their feelings, behaviors, and interests, (2) make connections between environmental stimuli and emotional reactions, (3) develop and use coping strategies, (4) explore what it means to have AS or HFA, and (5) self-monitor on-task behavior (e.g., Quinn et al., 1994). Self-determination, defined as active participation in making decisions that affect one's life, is a related long-term goal (Ward & Meyer, 1999). Teachers can promote healthy self-determination by offering choices, respecting student choices, and including the student in the development of educational and behavioral management plans (Myles & Simpson, 2001).

## Sensory and Motor Needs

Although not included in official diagnostic criteria (American Psychiatric Association, 2000; World Health Organization, 1993), sensory abnormalities and motor impairments are common in students with AS or HFA. Hypo- and hypersensitivities can occur across the full range of sensory stimuli (e.g., touch, smell, hearing) and are frequently associated with problematic behaviors (e.g., Dunn, Myles, & Orr, 2002). Classroom intervention typically involves identifying problematic sensory responses and avoiding or minimizing "trigger" stimuli. In addition, sensory issues may be directly addressed, most often with the assistance of an occupational therapist who may or may not use sensory integration therapy. Despite enthusiastic anecdotal accounts, well-designed efficacy studies of traditional occupational therapy and sensory integration therapy are lacking for this population (Dawson & Watling, 2000).

Gross and fine motor impairments have been documented in individuals with AS or HFA (Dawson & Watling, 2000; Miller & Ozonoff, 2000). In the classroom, motor impairments often translate into difficulties with handwriting, physical education activities, adaptive behaviors (e.g., tying shoes), and social skills (e.g., coordinating movements in the presence of others). Effective assessments are needed to help identify appropriate learning goals, needed modifications, and required special services (e.g., occupational therapy, physical therapy, adaptive physical education).

## CONCLUSION

Earlier in this chapter two pivotal questions were posed: *What are the essential elements of effective educational intervention for high-functioning individuals with an ASD?* And: *How are these elements related to one another and to student outcome?* In the body of the chapter, an integrative model was presented in order to explore answers to these questions and, perhaps, to provide a guide for professionals and parents designing or studying educational interventions for school-age individuals with AS or HFA.

Because of the complexity of AS and HFA, it is all too tempting to selectively emphasize specific deficits. For example, one professional may emphasize problems in nonverbal communication, another abnormal sensory responses, and still another executive dysfunction. As a result, each professional may concentrate exclusively on a single intervention approach, such as social skills training, sensory integration therapy, or the use of organizational supports. Although such heightened focus can be beneficial when professionals coordinate their efforts, it also can cause conflict and a lack of balance in the student's education.

The integrative model proposed in this chapter can be used to promote a more holistic approach to educational intervention for school-age individuals with AS or HFA. First, the *foundational elements* place the student's needs in a broad ecological context (i.e., school community, family variables, and person variables). Second, use of the *structural elements* ensures that a broad range of instructional and support strategies are implemented to compensate for the poor match between student learning characteristics and the school environment. Third, identification of learning goals and objectives across seven *curricular elements* targets a broad range of student needs and thus multiple aspects of student outcome.

By taking an integrative and holistic approach, such as the one presented here, parents and professionals may be better able to design educational intervention programs with the qualities identified by Volkmar and colleagues (1999) as desirable in autism intervention. That is, the educational intervention is more apt to (1) provide individualized support broad enough to target the full range of impairments; (2) be grounded in reality yet include a long-term vision for the individual; (3) address the individual's unique strengths and deficits; and (4) promote parent involvement and interdisciplinary coordination of services.

On the other hand, there are several limitations or qualifications that must be kept in mind when considering the proposed model. First, it is important to remember that the model is just that, a model. Because any model involves simplification of complex real-world processes, some distortion is inevitable. For example, the divisions between the three major groups of elements and those between specific elements are not as distinct in real life as illustrated in the model. Further, the arrows in the model suggest only a limited number of unidirectional paths of influence, and other directional and bidirectional paths are probable.

Second, the model does not prescribe any one educational setting. Although it would be reassuring to be able to identify one "ideal" setting for students with AS or HFA, given the wide range of individual characteristics, a continuum of services is far more appropriate. In general, however, given the nature and complexity of student needs, smaller settings may be more effective. Furthermore, to reduce the likelihood that these students will be victimized or mimic potentially dangerous behavior, placement with peers who have conduct disorder should be avoided (cf. Klin & Volkmar, 2000).

Third, with only a few exceptions, resource needs are not explicitly addressed in the model. Most of the recommended educational strategies can be implemented in regular classroom settings with, for the most part, inexpensive technology. Nevertheless, a *genuinely* individualized, coordinated, and comprehensive intervention plan designed to maximize meaningful long-term goals requires substantial human resources (Mesibov et al., 2001).

Fourth, caution is warranted when setting expectations for student outcome. AS and HFA are considered challenging neurodevelopmental disorders with life-long impact. Outcome cannot yet be predicted reliably for individuals or with regard to specific intervention strategies (Howlin, 2000). In addition, long-term outcome is apt to be influenced by many factors outside of educator control, such as availability of community resources, individual temperament, severity of cognitive deficits, and degree of autistic symptoms.

Fifth, if used to guide educational intervention planning for specific students, this model must be applied in a truly individualized manner. As a result, the relative emphasis placed on elements in the model will vary across students, and no two educational plans will be identical. For example, one student may require supports in all three structural domains and have learning goals in all seven curricular areas. In contrast, another student may need supports in only one structural domain and individualized learning goals in only three curricular domains.

Finally, the history of autism intervention is replete with examples of treatments and "cures" that generated substantial enthusiasm but, once subjected to well-designed empirical testing, were not shown to have significant effects (e.g., facilitated communication, steroid treatment, auditory integration training; Volkmar et al., 1999). Until additional efficacy research is available on educational interventions for students with AS or HFA, careful evaluation of individual student progress will continue to be crucial in monitoring intervention effectiveness. From an empirical standpoint, researchers need to conduct studies on distinct elements of educational programs as well as on combinations of those elements. From a clinical standpoint, it is important to remember that everyday, despite numerous challenges, parents and professionals *can and do* design educational plans that help individuals with AS or HFA learn, adapt, connect with others, and expand their personal boundaries.

## REFERENCES

American Psychiatric Association. (2000). *Diagnostic and statistical manual of mental disorders* (4th ed., text rev.). Washington, DC: Author.

Asperger, H. (1991). Autistic psychopathy in childhood. In U. Frith (Ed.), *Autism and Asperger syndrome* (pp. 37–92). Cambridge, UK: Cambridge University Press. (Original work published in German 1944)

Attwood, T. (2000). Strategies for improving the social integration of children with Asperger syndrome. *Autism, 4*, 85–100.

Bauminger, N. (2002). The facilitation of social–emotional understanding and social interaction in high-functioning children with autism: Intervention outcomes. *Journal of Autism and Developmental Disorders, 32*, 283–298.

Beardon, L., Parsons, S., & Neale, H. (2001). An interdisciplinary approach to investigating the use of virtual reality environments for people with Asperger syndrome. *Educational and Child Psychology, 18*, 53–62.

Bock, M. A. (2001). SODA strategy: Enhancing the social interaction skills of youngsters with Asperger syndrome. *Intervention in School and Clinic, 36*, 272–278.

Carter, A. S., Volkmar, F. R., Sparrow, S. S., Wang, J. J., Lord, C., Dawson, G., Fombonne, E., Loveland, K., Mesibov, G., & Schopler, E. (1998). The Vineland Adaptive Behavior Scales: Supplementary norms for individuals with autism. *Journal of Autism and Developmental Disorders, 28*, 287–302.

Dawson, G., & Watling, R. (2000). Interventions to facilitate auditory, visual, and motor integration in autism: A review of the evidence. *Journal of Autism and Developmental Disorders, 30*, 415–421.

Denckla, M. B., & Reader, M. J. (1993). Education and psychosocial interventions:

Executive dysfunction and its consequences. In R. Kurlan (Ed.), *Handbook of Tourette's syndrome and related tic and behavioral disorders* (pp. 431–451). New York: Marcel Dekker.

Dunn, W., Myles, B. S., & Orr, S. (2002). Sensory processing issues associated with Asperger syndrome: A preliminary investigation. *American Journal of Occupational Therapy, 56*, 97–102.

Ehlers, S., Gillberg, C., & Wing, L. (1999). A screening questionnaire for Asperger syndrome and other high-functioning autism spectrum disorders in school age children. *Journal of Autism and Developmental Disorders, 29*, 129–142.

Fouse, B. (1999). *Creating a win–win IEP for students with autism: A how-to manual for parents and educators.* Arlington, TX: Future Horizons.

Frith, U., & Happé, F. (1994). Autism: Beyond "theory of mind." *Cognition, 50*, 115–132.

Gareau, D. E., & Sawatzky, D. (1995). Parents and schools working together: A qualitative study of parent–school collaboration. *Alberta Journal of Educational Research, 41*, 462–473.

Gerhardt, P. F., & Holmes, D. L. (1997). Employment: Options and issues for adolescents and adults with autism. In D. J. Cohen & F. R. Volkmar (Eds.), *Handbook of autism and pervasive developmental disorders* (2nd ed., pp. 650–664). New York: Wiley.

Ghaziuddin, M., Ghaziuddin, N., & Greden, J. (2002). Depression in persons with autism: Implications for research and clinical care. *Journal of Autism and Developmental Disorders, 32*, 299–306.

Ghaziuddin, M., Weidmer-Mikhail, E., & Ghaziuddin, N. (1998). Comorbidity of Asperger syndrome: A preliminary report. *Journal of Intellectual Disability Research, 42*, 279–283.

Gray, C. A. (1998). Social stories and comic strip conversations with students with Asperger syndrome and high-functioning autism. In E. Schopler, G. B. Mesibov, & L. J. Kunce (Eds.), *Asperger syndrome or high-functioning autism?* (pp. 167–198). New York: Plenum Press.

Griswold, D. E., Barnhill, G. P., Myles, B. S., Hagiwara, T., & Simpson, R. L. (2002). Asperger syndrome and academic achievement. *Focus on Autism and Other Developmental Disorders, 17*, 94–102.

Hadwin, J., Baron-Cohen, S., Howlin, P., & Hill, K. (1997). Does teaching theory of mind have an effect on the ability to develop conversation in children with autism? *Journal of Autism and Developmental Disorders, 27*, 519–537.

Hare, D. J. (1997). The use of cognitive-behavioural therapy with people with Asperger syndrome: A case study. *Autism, 1*, 215–225.

Harris, S. L., & Handleman, J. S. (Eds.). (1994). Preschool education programs for children with autism. Austin, TX: Pro-Ed.

Helps, S., Newsom-Davis, I. C., & Callias, M. (1999). Autism: The teacher's view. *Autism, 3*, 287–298.

Howlin, P. (2000). Outcome in adult life for more able individuals with autism or Asperger syndrome. *Autism, 4*, 63–83.

Jordan, R., & Powell, S. (1995). *Understanding and teaching children with autism.* Chichester, UK: Wiley.

Kim, J. A., Szatmari, P., Bryson, S. E., Streiner, D. L., & Wilson, F. J. (2000). The prevalence of anxiety and mood problems among children with autism and Asperger syndrome. *Autism, 4,* 117–132.

Klin, A., Sparrow, S. S., Marans, W. D., Carter, A., & Volkmar, F. R. (2000). Assessment issues in children and adolescents with Asperger syndrome. In A. Klin, F. R. Volkmar, & S. S. Sparrow (Eds.), *Asperger syndrome* (pp. 309–339). New York: Guilford Press.

Klin, A., & Volkmar, F. R. (2000). Treatment and intervention guidelines for individuals with Asperger syndrome. In A. Klin, F. R. Volkmar, & S. S. Sparrow (Eds.), *Asperger syndrome* (pp. 340–366). New York: Guilford Press.

Klin, A., Volkmar, F. R., & Sparrow, S. S. (Eds.). (2000). *Asperger syndrome.* New York: Guilford Press.

Koegel, R. L., & Koegel, L. K. (Eds.). (1995). *Teaching children with autism: Strategies for initiating positive interactions and improving learning opportunities.* Baltimore: Brookes.

Konig, C., & Magill-Evans, J. (2001). Social and language skills in adolescent boys with Asperger syndrome. *Autism, 5,* 23–36.

Kunce, L. J., & Mesibov, G. B. (1998). Educational approaches to high-functioning autism and Asperger syndrome. In E. Schopler, G. B. Mesibov, & L. J. Kunce (Eds.), *Asperger syndrome or high-functioning autism?* (pp. 227–261). New York: Plenum Press.

Landa, R. (2000). Social language use in Asperger syndrome and high-functioning autism. In A. Klin, F. R. Volkmar, & S. S. Sparrow (Eds.), *Asperger syndrome* (pp. 125–155). New York: Guilford Press.

Liss, M., Harel, B., Fein, D., Allen, D., Dunn, M., Feinstein, C., Morris, R., Waterhouse, L., & Rapin, I. (2001). Predictors and correlates of adaptive functioning in children with developmental disorders. *Journal of Autism and Developmental Disorders, 31,* 219–230.

Manjiviona, J., & Prior, M. (1999). Neuropsychological profiles of children with Asperger syndrome and autism. *Autism, 3,* 327–356.

Marcus, L., Kunce, L. J., & Schopler, E. (1997). Working with families. In D. J. Cohen & F. R. Volkmar (Eds.), *Handbook of autism and pervasive developmental disorders* (2nd ed., pp. 631–649). New York: Wiley.

Martin, A., Scahill, L., & Klin, A. (1999). Higher-functioning pervasive developmental disorders: Rates and patterns of psychotropic drug use. *Journal of the American Academy of Child and Adolescent Psychiatry, 38,* 923–931.

McAfee, J. L. (2002). *Navigating the social world: A curriculum for individuals with Asperger's syndrome, high functioning autism, and related disorders.* Arlington, TX: Future Horizons.

Mercier, C., Mottron, L., & Belleville, S. (2000). A psychosocial study on restricted interests in high-functioning persons with pervasive developmental disorders. *Autism, 4,* 406–425.

Mesibov, G. B. (1992). Treatment issues with high-functioning adolescents and adults with autism. In E. Schopler & G. B. Mesibov (Eds.), *High-functioning individuals with autism* (pp. 143–155). New York: Plenum Press.

Mesibov, G. B., Shea, V., & Adams, L. W. (2001). *Understanding Asperger syndrome and high-functioning autism.* New York: Kluwer Academic/Plenum Press.

Miller, J. N., & Ozonoff, S. (2000). The external validity of Asperger disorder: Lack of evidence from the domain of neuropsychology. *Journal of Abnormal Psychology, 109,* 227–238.

Minshew, N. J., Goldstein, G. G., & Siegel, D. J. (1997). Neuropsychologic functioning in autism: Profile of a complex information processing disorder. *Journal of the International Neuropsychological Society, 3,* 303–316.

Mundy, P. (1995). Joint attention and social–emotional approach behavior in children with autism. *Development and Psychopathology, 7,* 63–82.

Myles, B. S., & Simpson, R. L. (1998). *Asperger syndrome: A guide for educators and parents.* Austin, TX: Pro-Ed.

Myles, B. S., & Simpson, R. L. (2001). Effective practices for students with Asperger syndrome. *Focus on Exceptional Children, 34,* 1–14.

National Research Council. (2001). *Educating children with autism.* Washington, DC: National Academy Press.

Odom, S. L., & Watts, E. (1991). Reducing teacher prompts in peer-mediated interventions for young children with autism. *Journal of Special Education, 25,* 26–43.

Olley, J. G., & Reeve, C. E. (1997). *Issues of curriculum and structure.* In D. J. Cohen & F. R. Volkmar (Eds.), *Handbook of autism and pervasive developmental disorders* (2nd ed., pp. 484–508). New York: Wiley.

Ozonoff, S. (1998). Assessment and remediation of executive dysfunction in autism and Asperger syndrome. In E. Schopler, G. B. Mesibov, & L. J. Kunce (Eds.), *Asperger syndrome or high-functioning autism?* (pp. 263–289). New York: Plenum Press.

Ozonoff, S., Dawson, G., & McPartland, J. (2002). *A parent's guide to Asperger syndrome and high-functioning autism: How to meet the challenges and help your child thrive.* New York: Guilford Press.

Ozonoff, S., & Miller, J. N. (1995). Teaching theory of mind: A new approach to social skills training for individuals with autism. *Journal of Autism and Developmental Disorders, 25,* 415–433.

Quill, K. A. (Ed.). (1995). *Teaching children with autism.* New York: Delmar.

Quinn, C., Swaggart, B. L., & Myles, B. S. (1994). Implementing cognitive behavior management programs for persons with autism: Guidelines for practitioners. *Focus on Autistic Behavior, 9,* 1–13.

Robertson, J. M., Tanguay, P. E., & L'Ecuyer, S. (1999). Domains of social communication handicap in autism spectrum disorder. *Journal of the American Academy of Child and Adolescent Psychiatry, 38,* 738–745.

Schopler, E. (1997). Implementation of TEACCH philosophy. In D. J. Cohen & F. R. Volkmar (Eds.), *Handbook of autism and pervasive developmental disorders* (2nd ed., pp. 767–795). New York: Wiley.

Schopler, E., Mesibov, G. B., & Hearsey, K. (1995). Structured teaching in the TEACCH system. In E. Schopler & G. G. Mesibov (Eds.), *Learning and cognition in autism* (pp. 243–268). New York: Plenum Press.

Schopler, E., Mesibov, G. B., & Kunce, L. J. (Eds.). (1998). *Asperger syndrome or high-functioning autism?* New York: Plenum Press.

Siegel, D. J., Goldstein, G., & Minshew, N. J. (1996). Designing instruction for the high-functioning autistic individual. *Journal of Developmental and Physical Disabilities, 8,* 1–19.

Simpson, R. L. (1995). Individualized education programs for students with autism: Including parents in the process. *Focus on Autistic Behavior, 10,* 11–16.

Smith, M., Belcher, R., & Johrs, P. (1997). *A guide to successful employment for individuals with autism.* Baltimore: Brookes.

Sofronoff, K., & Farbotko, M. (2002). The effectiveness of parent management training to increase self-efficacy in parents of children with Asperger syndrome. *Autism, 6,* 271286.

Szatmari, P. (2000). The classification of autism, Asperger syndrome, and pervasive developmental disorder. *Canadian Journal of Psychiatry, 45,* 731–738.

Tantam, D. (2000). Psychological disorder in adolescents and adults with Asperger syndrome. *Autism, 4,* 47–62.

Volkmar, F., Cook, E. H., & Pomeroy, J. (1999). Practice parameters for the assessment and treatment of children, adolescents, and adults with autism and other pervasive developmental disorders. *Journal of the American Academy of Child and Adolescent Psychiatry, 38,* 32S–54S.

Ward, M. J., & Meyer, R. N. (1999). Self-determination for people with developmental disabilities and autism: Two self-advocates' perspectives. *Focus on Autism and Other Developmental Disabilities, 14,* 133–139.

Waterhouse, L., & Fein, D. (1997). Perspectives on social impairment. In D. J. Cohen & F. R. Volkmar (Eds.), *Handbook of autism and pervasive developmental disorders* (2nd ed., pp. 901–919). New York: Wiley.

Whitaker, P., Barratt, P., Joy, H., Potter, M., & Thomas, G. (1998). Children with autism and peer group support: Using "Circle of Friends." *British Journal of Special Education, 25,* 60–64.

World Health Organization. (1993). *International classification of diseases: Tenth revision.* Geneva: Author.

# 12

## Longer-Term Educational and Employment Outcomes

PATRICIA HOWLIN

## SECONDARY SCHOOLING

Difficulties in meeting the educational, social, and emotional needs of individuals with an autistic spectrum disorder (ASD) often become more pronounced as the children age. In contrast to the vast literature on teaching methods and educational programs for pre- and primary school children, there are few systematic studies of interventions for secondary school-age pupils with autism or Asperger syndrome (AS). Moreover, research on children with mixed intellectual disabilities indicates that although inclusion may succeed in the early years, relatively few studies have reported on successful integration of these students within secondary school. Acceptance by normally developing peers and mainstream teachers tends to decrease with age (Beveridge, 1996) and studies over the last two decades have consistently reported that children whose problems are more pervasive, such as those with autism, may experience increasing difficulties in mainstream placements as they grow older (Carlberg & Kavale, 1980; Deno, Maruyama, Espin, & Cohen, 1990; Rich & Ross 1989). Indeed, unless appropriate support is available, these children may receive less attention and less individualized instruction in normal classes than in segregated classes. All too often, within mainstream settings, lack of adequate training or of systematic, ongoing support for teachers and classroom assistants leads to a focus on minimizing behavioral difficulties rather than enhancing skills. Thus, although children with special needs may be tolerated, they are not necessarily assimilated or accepted (Farrell, 1997; Howlin, 2002). Furthermore, social interactions with typically developing peers do not tend to occur unless the environment, teaching materials, and children's activities are appropriately structured (Lord, 1995; Wolfberg & Schuler, 1993), and even then, close, reciprocal friendships are unlikely to develop (Burack, Root, & Zigler, 1997; Gottlieb, 1990; Saintano, Goldstein, & Strain, 1992).

Arguments for and against inclusive education are as rife in the field of autism as for any other disability (see Burack et al., 1997; Farrell, 1997; Mesibov, 1990; Simpson & Myles, 1993). Although some studies (mostly conducted with very young children in experimental settings) conclude that academic and social attainments are enhanced by inclusion (Harris et al., 1991; Hoyson, Jamieson, & Strain, 1984), others report few positive effects on social, cognitive, or communication skills (Burack et al., 1997; Harris, Handleman, Kristoff, Bass, & Gordon, 1990; Sigafoos, Roberts, Kerr, Couzens, & Baglioni, 1994). Moreover, the highly structured, individualized, adult-directed, and predominantly visually based learning environments that seem most likely to facilitate learning in children with an ASD may be very difficult to achieve within the mainstream classroom (Rouse & Florian, 1996).

Although full inclusion should certainly be the *goal* for higher-functioning children with autism or AS, alternatives also should be available. Properly planned and adequately financed resource bases, or units, within mainstream settings may provide one solution. Such facilities offer the opportunity for children to be integrated gradually into mainstream classes, allowing full-time inclusion (with support, as necessary) for those children who can cope with this option, while providing others with the daily opportunity to mix with their mainstream peers. Another solution is to provide specialist peripatetic services that can offer advice and practical support to mainstream school staffs on ways of dealing with specific problems and, more generally, ensure that the teaching environment is "autism friendly " (Cumine, Leach, & Stevenson, 1998; see Gill, Chapter 9, this volume). This approach is often more appropriate for academically able children who would not wish to be singled out from their peers by attending, even part time, a special unit. However, success depends on close liaison and good working relationships between classroom teachers and support staff, and such coordination can sometimes be difficult to achieve when many different teachers are involved, as is the case in most secondary schools

Despite the problems faced in providing appropriate education for children with autism and AS, it is apparent that schooling has improved over recent decades. In the early follow-up studies (e.g., DeMyer et al.,

1973; Lockyer & Rutter, 1970; Lotter, 1974a, 1974b; Rutter, Greenfield, & Lockyer, 1967; Rutter & Lockyer, 1967), the majority of children, even those with higher IQs, had received less than 5 years schooling in all. One-third of children in the Lockyer and Rutter studies, for example, had never attended school. In more recent outcome studies, almost all the children, whatever their intellectual level, had remained in school of some sort for at least 10 years. Inclusion, however, still appears to be the exception rather than the rule. In the United Kingdom, studies (Howlin, Goode, Hutton, & Rutter, in press; Mawhood, Howlin, & Rutter, 2000) that focused on higher functioning individuals with autism found that between 80 and 90% had spent most of their school years in segregated, mostly autism-specific, classrooms. Even in countries such as the United States and Canada, where historically there has been a greater emphasis on inclusion, the proportion of high-functioning individuals in mainstream schools has tended to hover around 50% (Rumsey, Rapoport, & Sceery, 1985; Szatmari, Bartolucci, Bremner, Bond, & Rich, 1989; Venter, Lord, & Schopler, 1992; see Table 12.1).

It is also clear that, despite the many arguments in favor of inclusion, mainstreaming does not necessarily meet children's academic, social, or emotional needs. In their outcome study of a group of boys with autism and a group with receptive language disorder, matched for early IQ and language development, Mawhood and colleagues (2000) reported that the children with autism had spent significantly more time in specialist provision. However, their educational history was much more stable; schooling generally seemed more appropriate to their needs, and they actually obtained higher levels of formal qualifications than did the language-disordered group. Nevertheless, in both groups academic and occupational attainments were well below the levels that would be expected of typically developing peers of similar age and IQ.

Access to the normal school curriculum is crucial for the future academic and employment prospects of higher-functioning children with autism, but unless their very specific needs and difficulties are adequately understood, they are likely to become extremely isolated, lonely, and dejected. Bullying by peers is another major potential problem. Therese Jolliffe, a woman with autism who has a PhD in psychology, writes:

> I hated school. . . . Although ordinary schooling enabled me to leave school with . . . a few A levels and then to obtain a degree, it was not worth all the misery I suffered. . . . The teachers pretended to be understanding but they were not. I was frightened of the girls and boys and everything there. . . . I was kicked, hit, pushed over and made fun of by the other children. When I attended a place for autistic people life was a little more bearable and there was certainly less despair. . . . Parents of autistic children should never think of

**TABLE 12.1. Reported Educational Histories in Follow-Up Studies of Adults with Autism**

| Study (1st author) (n) | Year | Age (yr) | IQ | Years in school | % mainstream school | % attending college/ university | % with degree or diploma |
|---|---|---|---|---|---|---|---|
| Mittler (26) | 1966 | 7–27 | 24–111 | | 22 | | |
| Lockyer (38) | 1970 | 16+ | $\bar{X} = 62$ | 33% no school | 2 | | |
| Kanner (96) | 1973 | 22–29 | | | 3 | 9 | 7 |
| DeMyer (120) | 1973 | $\bar{X} = 12$ | | 68% < 5 yr | 8 | | |
| Lotter (29) | 1978 | 16–18 | 55–90 | 55% < 5 yr | 0 | | |
| Rumsey (14) | 1985 | 18–39 | 55–129 | | 57 | 14 | 14 |
| Szatmari (16) | 1989 | 17–34 | 68–110 | All > 5 yr | 50 | 50 | 43 |
| Chung (66) | 1990 | > 12 yr | 24% > 70 | 12% no school | 21 | | |
| Kobayashi (201) | 1992 | 18–33 | 23% > 70 | | 27 | 2 | |
| Venter (22) | 1992 | 18+ | $\bar{X} = 90$ | | 52 | 7 | 4 |
| Ballaban-Gil (45) | 1996 | 18+ | 31% > 70 | | 1 | | |
| Tuffreau (49) | 1995 | 12+ | 89% > 50 | | 0 | 0 | 0 |
| Larsen (18) | 1997 | 32–43 | 78% > 50 | | 44 | 0 | 0 |
| Mawhood (19) | 2000 | 21–26 | 70–117 | All > 10 yr | 10 | 22 | 11 |
| Howlin (68) | 2002 | 21+ | 51–137 | All 10 yr | 15 | 7 | 4 |

*Note.* Includes only follow-up studies in which there are specific data on schooling and/or further education.

sending their children to ordinary schools because the suffering will far outweigh any of the benefits achieved. (in Jolliffe, Landsown, & Robinson, 1992, p. 13)

Many more reports of the difficulties experienced by high-functioning individuals with autism are contained in Clare Sainsbury's book *Martian in the Playground* (2000). The very title conveys the isolation these children experience. On the other hand, if they do not have access to the normal curriculum, their chances of making progress in later life will be severely limited. Mainstream education, particularly for more able children, can and should work, but it will not do so without adequate support and training for teachers and appropriate modifications of the school environment (Jordan & Jones, 1999). Unless these resources are made available, the social exclusion experienced by the children in school may well extend into adult life.

## LEAVING SCHOOL

Access to tertiary education should be possible for all high-functioning individuals with an ASD, and indeed the situation seems to have improved somewhat over the years, with more individuals in the follow-up studies conducted post 1980 continuing their education beyond secondary school age. Nevertheless, it is clear that we are still a long way from meeting the goal of full inclusion. In the majority of the outcome studies listed in Table 12.1, few individuals had gone on to further education, attended college or university, or obtained a degree or similar qualification. Among the remainder, the average proportion attending college was around 16% (range 2–50%). Fourteen percent (range 4–43%) had obtained university degrees, with the numbers higher in groups of higher ability (e.g., Mawhood et al., 2000; Rumsey et al., 1985; Szatmari et al., 1989).

It appears from these studies that, once schooling comes to an end, integration becomes progressively more difficult to achieve. Moreover, the failure to provide continuing education for pupils with autism and AS beyond their midteens ignores research indicating that many of these individuals show considerable improvements with age (Gilchrist, Green, Cox, Rutter, & Le Couteur, 2001; Howlin et al., 2000; Mawhood et al., 2000; Mesibov, Schopler, Schaffer, & Michal, 1990; Piven, Harper, Palmer, & Arndt, 1996). Indeed for some (particularly those who become more aware of their difficulties), midadolescence often can be a period of remarkable improvement and change (Kanner, 1973).

Moving from the relatively supportive environments of home and school into the adult world of college or university is a time of potential upheaval and stress for many "normal" young people. However, for most students the social environment coupled with the removal of parental restraints actively foster personal development and maturity. For someone with autism, however, successful transition will require much greater help and support.

In the wake of the movement toward inclusion, there have been some improvements in facilities to help people with special needs participate in higher education. Transitional support services have been well established in the United States for some time. For example, over 15 years ago, Wehman and his colleagues (Wehman, Moon, Everson, Wood, & Barcus, 1988) described, in detail, the facilities and programs used to help individuals with disabilities make the transition from school. In particular, they stressed the importance of long-term planning and the roles that both teachers and parents can play in preparing students for this significant stage of their lives.

In Britain, the situation was improved by the 1992 Further and Higher Education Act, which placed an obligation on colleges in England and

Wales to "have regard for students with learning difficulties or disabilities." Subsequently there has been a steady increase in college placements for people with learning disabilities, together with the establishment of "Learning Support Units" or other support services for individuals attending college. The development of courses leading to a wider range of vocational qualifications has also helped to ensure that a higher proportion of students with special needs has access to courses that suit both their interests and their ability.

Unfortunately, however, staff in further education facilities frequently receive little or no training in how to work with students who have special needs, and the uneven profile of students with autism presents a considerable dilemma for many lecturers. It can be especially difficult for college or university staff to understand a student with autism or AS whose academic knowledge in a certain area may be second to none, but whose behavior in other domains is, at best, unusual and, at worst, totally unacceptable. Progress is also frequently hampered by these students' very poor organizational skills, low standards of written work, failure to understand the importance of meeting deadlines, and inability to convey the knowledge that they do possess in an acceptable way. Whereas factual information may be learned and memorized without difficulty, more abstract issues (such as considering different sides of an argument) can present enormous problems. Exams are often a major source of difficulty, not only because of slowness, but also because of problems in understanding the intent that underlies many questions.

Meeting the challenge of autism is not an easy task for staff in tertiary education, but many potential problems can be avoided if there is close liaison, not only between college and school, but also with families. Teachers from the parent school are likely to be familiar with the difficulties that can interfere with an individual student's learning, and they are likely to have developed strategies for dealing with these that can then be passed on to college staff. The importance of collaboration between school and parents is now widely recognized. Unfortunately, since one of the major goals of most tertiary education centers is to foster students' independence, it is often more difficult for staff in these settings to accept that parents' knowledge of their sons or daughters may be vital for educational outcome. Few students with autism, no matter how high their intellectual ability, will have acquired the social competence or level of independence required to survive when they first enter college. To expect them to be able to cope without support from their families is to deprive them of a vital backup system and to deprive college staff of a valuable source of information.

Achieving liaison with families or the parent school can obviously present difficulties when mainstreamed pupils move to universities or colleges that are far away from home. One solution has been the development of specialist autism advice services, which offer support for both students and staff in universities or colleges. Another recent initiative has been the development of programs to help students with autism acquire the skills necessary to enter college. In the United States, the support offered by the TEACCH organization in North Carolina has enabled many students with autism to benefit from further education. In Britain, there are organizations such as INTERACT (Graham, 1999), which teach social, communication, and problem-solving skills and provide on-site support for students and advice and assistance to college staff, as necessary. Other schemes may provide students with a key worker at college and offer training for college staff to help them improve their knowledge of, and ability to deal with, the problems associated with autism (Morgan, 1996). In addition, for staff working in further education settings there is an increasing number of postgraduate and distance learning courses that are designed to improve understanding and management skills. On occasion, placement in a college for people with special needs also may prove to be a useful steppingstone for some individuals with autism or AS, who initially find the social and academic demands of a regular course overwhelming. Unfortunately, it not always possible to arrange provision of this kind and for many students the support systems on which they had depended at secondary school disappear entirely once they reach the age of 18. Moreover, in Britain, at least, there are no statutory obligations on further education colleges to accept, or offer specialist help to, students with autism, and hence access to appropriate support to enter college, or maintain a place, once accepted, varies considerably across the country.

## PRACTICAL PROBLEMS AND WAYS OF COPING

Although access to further education is becoming more widely available, it is evident that many barriers to inclusion persist even for high-functioning students with autism. Difficulties occur because of lack of understanding, misinterpretation of behavior, and inflexibility, either on the part of staff, other students, or within the organizational structure. Moreover, even the best intentioned of staff may have difficulties coping with the communication and social impairments that are characteristic of autism. As noted above, they may find the characteristically uneven pattern of skills and deficits particularly difficult to understand. They are also likely to find the very direct comments made by someone with autism (e.g., questioning even the most trivial of facts, correcting them in lectures, complaining about the quality of teaching, or personal comments about appearance or style of dress) very unnerving. Many students with autism show no reticence in giving voice to their complaints, nor do they learn to express these in a more diplomatic or effective way. Understandably, such behaviors can result in students being viewed as rude or as "trouble makers." Rather than recognizing their need for more help, lecturers whose competence is called into question in this way are likely to become markedly less sympathetic and may even call for the student's exclusion. As in school, the risk of teasing, bullying, provocation, or rejection by other students can continue unless staff are alert to this possibility and take steps to prevent it. Students with autism may be taunted for their "stupidity" if they are unable to cope with more complex or academic components of the course, and their social vulnerability makes them prey to abuse of many other kinds. For example, other students may take a delight in "setting them up" to attempt things they cannot possibly manage or achieve (e.g., drinking 30 pints of beer, dating the most popular woman student, or running for president of the Student Union). Worse, these students may be duped into acting as an unwitting stooge for illegal activities, such as collecting drug supplies. Individuals with an ASD also can be the source of considerable irritation and disruption to other students because of their constant requests for help, explanation, or reassurance.

Despite such problems, success at this level is crucial if the individual with autism is to have any real chance of living and working independently. As with school-based programs, there are some general procedures that can help to circumvent or minimize difficulties. People with autism function at their best in settings that are stable and under their control. If they are unsure what should be done—if the situation is unpredictable or if rules vary from time to time, place to place, or individual to individual—then progress will be slow and inappropriate behaviors difficult to change. Many problems can be overcome, or avoided entirely, if there are clear and explicit rules concerning the standard of work required and if appropriate guidance is provided. Thus, a clear supervisory and monitoring system is needed to help students manage their interactions with the various faculty members with whom they will come into contact. A key worker should be assigned to ensure that the needs of the student with autism are adequately recognized and supported. The value of the TEACCH approach (Kunce & Mesibov, 1998) for school-age children and the need for a high level of cues and checks have already been noted in Chapter 11, and these strategies also need to be incorporated into adult education programs.

At whatever level the student with AS is enrolled, whether for a PhD or a precollege preparatory course, the task structures and requirements must be clearly specified. Self-motivation and self-direction are frequently lacking, and even the most able students may need to be told explicitly where they should go, what they should be doing at all times, and to whom they should turn if problems occur. Additional help is likely to be needed when they are required to complete longer work assignments. The timing of these assignments needs to be precisely specified, otherwise the work probably will never be finished. Complex tasks should be broken down as far as possible, so that individual components are each completed by a fixed date. Help in understanding the importance of exams and developing effective strategies for revision and "exam technique" generally is also vital.

The relative freedom of college can lead to considerable problems for individuals with autism, who may have little understanding of the many unwritten rules governing social interactions. Their attempts to socialize may appear naive, inappropriate, or even offensive to other students, and difficulties in relating to members of the opposite sex are particularly common. The rejection and isolation that can follow can be deeply distressing and, for many, can result in their leaving (or being asked to leave) the college. Some colleges provide a "buddy" system, whereby the person with autism is offered support from another student acting as a mentor or guide. However, difficulties can and do occur if the person with autism misunderstands the nature of this supportive relationship and expects the buddy to fulfill the role of an intimate friend or even potential partner. Such systems tend to work most effectively if the limitations of the buddy's role are made clear from the outset and if the mentors themselves have support from a designated staff member, should problems arise. Staff must also be prepared to give explicit guidance to individuals with autism, if their social interactions with other students are viewed as inappropriate for any reason.

In addition, firm rules about regular attendance at college are crucial. By the time most students enter higher education, it is generally considered that they should be responsible for their own behavior, so that failure to attend lectures is their own concern. However, for people with autism, this freedom may be entirely inappropriate and counterproductive. They may begin to attend very erratically, or even, over time, cease to go altogether, drifting gradually back into a life of ritual and isolation. Self-regulation is unlikely to occur, so if the student is to profit from the educational opportunities, the requirement of punctual and daily attendance must be imposed from the outset.

Finally, providing clear and explicit feedback about the acceptability of the student's work and social behavior is essential at all times. If the standard of work is poor or if behaviors are socially unacceptable, the person with autism has no way of knowing unless he or she is told so directly. If mistakes go uncorrected they will persist, often leading to more and more difficulties as time goes on.

In planning entry to college, at whatever level, specific agreements are needed concerning who will be responsible for monitoring progress, what strategies will be implemented if problems occur, and to whom the student should turn for support. A well-established structure that is acceptable to everyone concerned, and which is agreed upon before the student enters the college, is almost always the most effective way of avoiding or minimizing subsequent problems and ensuring academic success.

## FLEXIBILITY OF APPROACH

Although these guidelines might seem relatively straightforward, in practice, they may prove difficult to implement, given the many other demands faced by teachers in further and higher education. Students with autism may find the move from the relatively protected environment of school to the college or university particularly difficult. Thus, in some cases, *gradual* introduction into college life may be necessary, if the transition is to be accomplished without undue difficulty on both sides. For example, some students find it easier to cope if they can begin by completing only certain modules of a course, rather than attempting to gain a full degree or diploma. If successful, they may later transfer to a full-time program. Similarly, in the first year or two of a course it may be better for them to live at home, rather than attempting to cope with the additional demands of living with other students or independently.

Greater flexibility is also required with respect to funding. Whereas students with physical or sensory difficulties may have relatively little difficulty in accessing financial support to help them overcome barriers to learning, obtaining such funding can be much more difficult for students with AS. However, providing initial support (to get around college, to ensure work assignments are completed satisfactorily, to provide feedback on social behavior, etc.) can avoid major problems, and even failure, later on in the course.

In conclusion, further educational opportunities for individuals with autism AS have improved greatly over recent years. Eventually, tertiary education should become the norm rather than an exception. A wide range of *potential* provision is available, but in order to gain access to, and profit from this provision, the special needs of students with AS will require greater recognition, as will the necessity of covering the costs, in terms of time and extra staffing, that may be essential to meet these needs.

## EMPLOYMENT

For individuals with any form of disability, the chances of finding or keeping employment in the open work market are limited. It is estimated, for example, that even among individuals with mild intellectual disabilities, have unemployment rates are as high as 60–70%. Although specialist vocational training programs do exist (Kunce & Mesibov, 1998), these tend to be geared to a very low level, so that many potential trainees fail to gain access to courses that adequately meet their needs (Harrison, 1996). Moreover, even for those who manage to find work, job status and stability are typically low (Zetlin & Murtaugh, 1990), and work experience is frequently very negative (Szivos, 1990).

The situation is little different for individuals with an ASD, even those who are intellectually very able. Problems begin, as the previous section indicates, well before the time comes for seeking work. Many people leave school without the formal qualifications needed for further education or vocational training schemes, and very few go on to college or university, so that they fall progressively further and further behind their peer group. Even for those few who successfully complete mainstream education and go on to obtain college or university qualifications, follow-up studies indicate that employment levels in adulthood are disappointing. Even if individuals are successful in getting through the interview process (a major stumbling block for many), jobs tend to be of low status and/or to end prematurely—often because of difficulties related to social competence.

Table 12.2 summarizes the frequency of employment in follow-up studies into adult life. Although, over the years, there appears to have been some increase in the proportion of individuals with autism who do find work, the numbers are still relatively low, with an average of around 24% employed, according to post-1980 studies. Szatmari and colleagues (1989) reported the highest proportion in work (around 47%), but theirs was a particularly able group, both in terms of cognitive ability and general levels of independence. In other studies with a focus on high-functioning individuals, such as that by Mawhood and colleagues (2000), only 16% of adults were was employed. It is not clear whether these differences in outcome are related to the cognitive and social abilities of the individuals concerned or to the accessibility of support networks that could help individuals with special needs find employment. Moreover, although in most studies several individuals were described as obtaining high-level, well-paid, responsible jobs, the majority had rather menial positions, such as kitchen labor, unskilled factory work, or back-room supermarket duties. In addition, jobs had often been procured through the efforts or personal contacts of families rather than through the normal channels (Howlin & Goode, 1998). Employment stability, too, was poor, with many individuals experiencing lengthy periods without paid work, even among those who had obtained tertiary qualifications.

There are significant financial and social implications related to such low-employment rates. The costs of adequately educating individuals with special needs, whether in integrated or special schooling, are substantial. Failure to transfer the skills acquired through education to the workplace is a clear waste of resources. Continuing and unnecessary reliance on state benefits is also extremely expensive, as are the indirect costs of treating emotional and psychiatric disorders related to long-term unemployment (Howlin, 1997).

**TABLE 12.2. Reported Employment Outcomes in Follow-Up Studies of Adults with Autism**

| Study (1st author) (n) | Year | Age (yr) | IQ | % in work | Type of jobs | |
|---|---|---|---|---|---|---|
| | | | | | Highest level | Lowest level |
| Mittler (26) | 1966 | 7–27 | 24–111 | None | | |
| Lockyer (38) | 1970 | 16+ | $\overline{X} = 62$ | 11 | No information | Factory work |
| Kanner (96) | 1973 | 22–29 | | 9 | Military, bank, clerk, chemist, accountant | Store hand; kitchen work |
| Lotter (29) | 1978 | 16–18 | 55–90 | 4 | No information | |
| Rumsey (14) | 1985 | 18–39 | 55–129 | 29 | Librarian, cab driver, data input | Janitor; most sheltered workshops |
| Szatmari (16) | 1989 | 17–34 | 68–110 | 47 | Librarian, teacher, salesman | Factory; workshop |
| Kobayashi (201) | 1992 | 18–33 | 23% > 70 | 22 | Bus conductor, mechanic, cook | Industrial work |
| Venter (22) | 1992 | 18+ | $\overline{X} = 90$ | 27 | Bartender | All but one low level |
| Von Knorring (38) | 1993 | 10–29 | | 5 | No information | |
| Ballaban-Gil (45) | 1996 | 18+ | 31% > 70 | 11 | | All "menial" |
| Tuffreau (49) | 1995 | 12+ | 89% > 50 | None | | |
| Larsen (18) | 1997 | 32–43 | 78% > 50 | 22 | Driver, office boy, gardener | Sheltered factory work |
| Mawhood (19) | 2000 | 21–26 | 70–117 | 16 | Lab technician | Voluntary, sheltered work |
| Stein (28) | 2001 | 21–36 | 30–94 | None | | |
| Howlin (68) | 2002 | 21+ | 51–137 | 34 | Scientific officer, computing, accounts, cartographer, office and electronic work | Washing up, supermarket, grave digger, charcoal burner, factory jobs |

*Note.* Includes only follow-up studies in which specific data on adult employment are reported.

## SUPPORTED EMPLOYMENT SCHEMES

Over the last two decades a variety of specialist employment schemes has emerged, with the aim of finding jobs for individuals with sensory or physical disabilities, general psychiatric problems, or global learning difficulties (Wehman et al., 1988; Williams, 1995; Pozner & Hammond, 1993). The supported employment model, which originated in the United States in the early 1980s, has enabled many people, particularly those with learning disabilities, to enter competitive paid employment. Supported Employment is defined as "the process of enabling a person with a disability to secure and maintain a paid job in a regular work environment, by supplying all appropriate training support to them in the workplace where they will be doing the job" (Pozner & Hammond, 1993). In the United States these schemes have attracted significant financial support from state and federal support agencies. Outcome appears to be superior to sheltered workshop and day-service options, achieving greater financial gain for workers, wider social integration, increased worker satisfaction, higher self-esteem, and savings-on-service costs (Bass & Drewett, 1998; Kilsby & Beyer, 1996; McCaughrin, Ellis, Rusch, & Heal, 1993). The key elements associated with successful programs include careful job placement, prior job training, advocacy, follow-up monitoring, and long-term support to ensure job retention (Keel, Mesibov, & Woods, 1997).

Evaluative studies in the United States suggest that, although the initial cost of such schemes is considerable, the financial burden decreases steadily over time. For example, analysis of the costs and benefits of 30 supported employment programs in Illinois, from 1986 to 1990, indicated that by the fourth year financial returns to the taxpayer (in the form of benefit reductions, etc.) exceeded program costs (McCaughrin et al., 1993; Rusch, Conley, & McCaughrin, 1993). In a Virginia-based program, all participants increased their income, and it was estimated that, on average, the return to the taxpayer was $1.87 for every $1.00 invested. After 8 years, the return had increased to $2.93 per dollar invested (Hill et al., 1987).

Although the financial "payoff" may not always be so large (Beyer & Kilsby, 1997; Noble, Conley, Banerjee, & Goodman, 1991), the supported employment model has been widely adopted in the United Kingdom. Between 1986 and 1995 the number of these programs increased from five to 210 (Beyer, Goodere, & Kilsby, 1996). However, Beyer and Kilsby (1997) cautioned against the temporary nature of many of these schemes and noted that almost 60% of the funding came from local authority social services departments, whereas only 3% came from central government employment services. Moreover, the main focus of such programs has been clients with learning disabilities, and most supported jobs have been unskilled, with low hourly rates of pay. Beyer and colleagues (1996) reported that 17% of individuals in supported employment experienced no change in income at all—they merely substituted earned income for welfare benefits; only 2% earned substantially more than they had received from benefits. Indeed, Bass and Drewett (1998) warn that it is essential to provide skilled advice to prevent employees from *losing* income if they move from long-term disability benefits to earned income.

Although the effectiveness of supported employment schemes for people with intellectual disabilities is now well established, it is only relatively recently that schemes have been developed specifically for individuals with autism. Smith, Belcher, and Juhrs (1995) describe a wide variety of successful job placements for clients in their Maryland service. These included manufacturing jobs, such as simple assembly-type work (25 clients); backroom retail work (44 clients); printing and mailing jobs (31); food services (23); warehouse work (20); recycling and delivery (12); and jobs with government organizations, mainly as janitors or office clerks (15). The program is remarkable not only for the large number of clients finding work, but also because of its success in placing individuals with very limited language, low intellectual ability, and challenging behavior, as well as those who were more able.

In another U.S.-based support program, Keel and colleagues (1997), evaluating job outcomes for 100 TEACCH clients, found that almost all were employed in work of some kind. Sixty-nine were in individual placements, 20 worked in "enclaves" (i.e., small groups with a job coach in one setting); and seven of the least able clients worked in "mobile crews" providing housecleaning services. Jobs were mostly in the food service field (38%), but 24% of individuals worked in clerical or technical services.

The results of schemes such as these clearly demonstrate how much the employment situation for individuals with autism could be improved by means of specialist help. Nevertheless, the levels of occupation attained remained relatively low, and they were not specifically geared to meet the needs of more intellectually able adults with autism or AS. Despite the fact that individuals with HFA/AS have a high potential for success, given their generally high level of cognitive ability and often exceptional expertise or knowledge in certain areas, they can find it much more difficult to access help in the workplace than individuals who are more globally impaired. It was for this reason that Mawhood and Howlin (1999) focused on the outcome of a specialist employment scheme designed especially for high-functioning individuals with autism. In association with the National Autistic Society in the United Kingdom, they evaluated outcome in a group of 30 young adults (27 males and 3 females) living in the Greater London area, who were supported by the scheme. All had a formal diagnosis of autism or AS, a WAIS IQ score of 70 or above, and had been actively seeking work for some time. Their work outcomes, over a 2-year pilot period, were compared to those of a matched comparison group of 20 individuals living in other metropolitan regions. Twenty percent of the supported group and 25% of the controls had obtained a university degree; over two-thirds of both groups had other academic or vocational qualifications.

Once individuals were registered with the scheme, detailed information was obtained on their level of functioning and on their past educational and job histories. When a suitable job was identified and the client began work, guidance from the support worker was provided on a full-time basis for the first 2–4 weeks of employment. The support workers were responsible for job finding, work preparation, and ensuring that clients could cope with all the social and occupational requirements of the job. They also spent much of their time educating and informing potential employers and advising work colleagues or supervisors about how to deal with or avoid problems. (For full details of the job-finding process, the nature of support offered, and the types of problems addressed, see Mawhood & Howlin, 1999.) The overall costs of the scheme declined steadily over time, in line with previous research. In the first month job coaches provided an average of around 10 hours support per week, but by the fourth month this time expenditure had declined to around 1¼ hours per week. Eventually, most clients required only occasional (but planned) meetings between employee, line manager, and support worker. However, a support worker could always be contacted at any time in an emergency.

In the course of the 2-year evaluation period, over two-thirds of the supported group had obtained paid employment. Four other clients were supported in work-experience placements. In contrast, only one-quarter of the control group found paid work. Moreover, in the supported group the majority of jobs was clerical or administrative in nature whereas only one individual among the controls obtained a job at this level. Earnings were significantly higher for the individuals in the supported group, and there was a high level of satisfaction with the scheme, both among employers and the people with autism themselves.

Financial support for the continuation of this scheme, which is now based at the National Autistic Society, has been provided via government funds normally available to support individuals with sensory or physical disabilities within the workplace. The money is used to provide job coaches rather than wheelchair ramps or interpreters, etc. Over the first 7 years of the scheme, 177 jobs were found in all, with around 63% in computing, accounting, or administration fields. The range of jobs found is considerable and includes secretarial, nursery, film processing, and consultancy work; jobs in science and government departments; and positions in housekeeping, sales, warehouses, and telephone and postal services. It is also important to note that when one placement has been successful, several companies have been only too willing to take on another employee with autism.

Employers have included major retail companies, local and national government departments, health services, the police, British Broadcasting Corporation, banks, charities, museums, transport, and British Telecom. Also encouraging is the fact that, at a time when temporary work contracts are becoming the norm, over 50% of the placements are permanent. Furthermore, to date, only two individuals have been dismissed or have had their contract terminated prematurely.

## MAKING SUPPORTED EMPLOYMENT WORK

### Job Finding

Matching the job to the client is probably the most crucial ingredient for success in any supported employment scheme. Achieving this match requires detailed information about the client's particular skills and difficulties, his or her ambitions, likes and dislikes, and a thorough task analysis. In the National Autistic Society program, careful details are kept on each potential client, and when jobs become available these are then matched to the client's characteristics as closely as possible. Jobs themselves have come from a variety of different sources. Links with the Employers Forum on Disability and specialist employment services and agencies have helped to identify companies that specifically aim to offer employment opportunities to people with disabilities. Once a potential employer has been identified, direct contact is made with personnel managers to discuss the benefits that can accrue from employing someone with autism. Punctilliousness, loyalty, honesty, excellent memory, no time wasted in social gossip, and willingness to perform repetitive and sometimes mundane tasks are just some of their positive attributes. The academic attainments of many are also substantial. Employers are advised on the types of jobs and working environments that are most likely to suit people with autism generally, and individual clients in particular. They are also assured of the continuing support of the job coach to whom they can turn at any time for advice.

If a vacancy exists, appropriate means of assessing a particular client's suitability are then addressed. Interviews are not usually considered to offer "equal opportunities of access" for people with autism. The hidden agenda behind many questions, the highly sophisticated social requirements, and the need for rapid responses to abstract issues are all loaded against them. However, if the employer is willing and flexible, there are various alternatives to the traditional job interview. Instead of answering unpredictable questions from an unknown panel, the client with autism may be asked to make a prepared presentation, indicating how his or her particular skills fit the requirements of the job and/or company. Alternatively, questions may be provided in advance, so that the job support coach can help the client "interpret" the meaning behind questions and prepare suitable responses. In some situations the job coach may accompany the client to the interview, "interpreting" on the spot if necessary. In other cases, the interview has been waived in favor of a short-term job trial, which gives a much more accurate indication of the client's capabilities.

## Ensuring an "Autism-Friendly" Working Environment

When a client has been accepted for work, the job coach spends time with immediate managers, and work colleagues if appropriate, in order fully to inform them of the nature of the "triad" of impairments that is typically associated with autism. Potential problems related to difficulties in reciprocal conversation, understanding, social unawareness, ritualistic tendencies, and coping with change are discussed and ways of dealing with them are recommended. Among the principal recommendations are the need for consistency; clear and explicit (usually written) guidelines; direct and immediate feedback; a designated line manager with whom to discuss problems; and an environment that, initially at least, is as free from unnecessary noise or distraction as possible. The job coach usually remains on site during the first few weeks, so employers are given the opportunity to observe how these issues can best be managed in practice, rather than having to cope by themselves.

## Problems and Problem Solving

Despite their age and intelligence, the clients involved in the supported employment scheme described above all shared similar problems. Many difficulties arose from their failure to understand or respond to social cues, resulting in their unwittingly offending people in a variety of ways, such as by inappropriate dress, undesirable personal habits, failure to respect others' "personal space," talking too much or too little or about inappropriate topics (e.g., one person talked at great length about the birthing problems of Arabian mares; another about chasing hares with dogs). Other problems were associated with their previous lack of work experience and included poor time keeping, slowness, failure to meet deadlines, overreliance on supervisors, and poor organization of assigned tasks. High anxiety levels, lack of self-drive and/or motivation, and rigid patterns of behavior also gave rise to difficulties. In almost every case the problems that gave rise to most complaints by other staff were related to these areas rather than to inability to cope with the demands of the job itself.

Difficulties of these sorts had frequently prevented individuals in the past from finding work or, if they did manage to do so, would lead to fairly rapid termination of contracts. Nevertheless, it became evident that such problems generally could be dealt with relatively easily, if clients and their employers were given appropriate support and advice.

### Socially Inappropriate Behaviors

In many cases, the most effective solution was simply to provide immediate feedback on what aspects of behavior were unacceptable and what should be done to modify them. Without clear and direct information of this kind, there is no way someone with autism can know whether his or her behavior is offensive. Sidelong glances, deep groans among colleagues, or other signs of annoyance or irritation are unlikely to be noticed, and even if they are, will probably not result in behavior change. Instead, the person needs to be informed directly that his or her dress or personal hygiene is unacceptable; that colleagues do not wish to hear, endlessly, about his or her particular topics of interest; or that he or she is behaving in an inappropriate way (e.g., standing too close, intruding into others' work space, upsetting female members of staff, etc.).

However, reporting the complaint is not enough; advice also must be given on how to change the behavior in question. Such advice might include identifying concrete cues, such as marking out desk areas with tape or indicating how close to colleagues it is acceptable to stand. If topics of conversation are offensive (or just downright boring) the individual should be informed of this problem, told to stop, and if possible provided with suggestions about alternative topics for discussion. More intimate issues such as hygiene or appearance also need to be addressed directly. Although colleagues may find such frankness very difficult, most people with autism are neither embarrassed about, nor resentful of being given, personal advice of this nature. On the contrary, it is *not* being able to understand what to do, *not* being informed if their actions are unacceptable that causes them most concern. Temple Grandin, in a lecture to the Autism Society of America in 1991, recalled being given a can of deodorant by her boss and told to use it; his secretary was also instructed to take her to buy more suitable clothes. She added, "This is part of the learning process. I was lucky enough to have people who helped me."

Social difficulties are often more likely to arise during unstructured periods, such as break or mealtimes, when individuals with autism may have no clear idea what is expected—where they should go; where they should sit; whether access to certain areas of the canteen, or even to certain lavatories, is restricted to particular staff groups; whether and where it is admissible to eat their own food from home, and so forth. There can be a myriad of unwritten rules of this kind, which individuals with autism only become aware of (if then) when they are inadvertently infringed. Appropriate support in the workplace involves not only ensuring that they are familiar with the demands of the *job*, but also that they are given adequate information on how to behave during leisure times.

## Work-Related Problems

For anyone who has been out of work for many years, learning to adjust to the regime of the workplace can be very difficult. The situation is likely to be even more problematic for someone with autism or AS, who may never have had an outside placement. Understanding what is required and recognizing the need to meet deadlines and produce work of an acceptable level within a specified period will not come automatically. Instead, work standards should be made absolutely explicit, with goals stated in writing. It is also usually much more effective to break down tasks into a series of small, short-term goals initially (i.e., specified jobs to be completed by the end of the morning) and only gradually to extend deadlines and task complexity. At all times it is preferable to have aims or instructions clearly written down. Reliance on verbal instruction is unlikely to be successful. Checklists and "Post-its" have the advantage of being used by other staff, as well, and allow each step to be systematically cued. Further advice on variety of other practical strategies for improving work performance (as well as finding work) is provided by Meyer (2001), who has AS.

Honest, direct, and immediate feedback is needed at all times. Few people with autism are driven by the competitive spirit and will rarely strive to outperform, or even keep up with, colleagues. Hence, unless work quality is closely monitored, standards are very likely to fall. Moreover, because of the rigidity that tends to be associated with autism, unacceptable practices that pass uncorrected can be very difficult to change in the future. The burden of monitoring work output, however, should not fall entirely on the supervisor or manager. With guidance, individuals can learn to monitor and regulate their own performance. Indeed, as it is important to provide individuals with ways of doing so; otherwise, overdependency on supervisors or other colleagues may result. One man, for example, working as an accountant, was found to be taking an increasing number of short breaks during the day, and so he was asked to keep a record of these. This he did but no change in his behavior was observed. However, when his job coach suggested he should summarize the information in the form of a Power Point graph and display this graph clearly above his desk, he began to track his behavior much more carefully, and improvements were soon visible.

## Coping with Change

Unexpected changes in routine, staffing, work rotas, or even the office layout can cause considerable distress to employees with autism. Although forthcoming changes may have been discussed among other staff for weeks, the person with autism may remain totally unaware until the change actually takes place. Again, written information is usually much more effective than verbal, and if appropriate details of the proposed changes (e.g., new computer system specifications, architects' plans, or staff lists, etc.) are provided well in advance, the person with autism will feel fully informed and thus more in control.

The supported employment scheme run by the National Autistic Society places particular emphasis on the need for routine, consistency, and predictability in the workplace. Thus, difficulties in the early stages of the job are usually minimal. However, on occasion, clients have done so well, over time, that their problems in these areas are forgotten. If, subsequently, there is a move toward upgrading the job or giving the person with autism greater responsibility, the need for careful planning may be overlooked, which may trigger an upsurge in problems once more.

### Dealing with Anxiety

Beginning work for the first time or starting a new job, especially after a long period of unemployment, is highly stressful for most people. For anyone with autism, the anxiety generated by such a major life event can be particularly marked, and many clients lose their jobs within the earliest weeks. However, with appropriate support, a carefully designed work program, and a clear and consistent line management structure, so that any problems can be addressed immediately, stress can be kept to a minimum. Having sympathetic colleagues who understand the needs and difficulties of someone with autism is also a major advantage. Disseminating information about a member of staff with autism clearly requires sensitivity, and methods of doing so will vary from individual to individual. In some cases only immediate colleagues may need to be told, but where there is wider interaction with people from other departments, more staff will need to be involved. One man, who had started work as an accountant in a large banking company where he would have to deal with many clients, decided that the simplest thing to do was to send an e-mail to everyone, explaining that he had AS and giving them details of his own and other Web sites where more information would be available.

Although the need to minimize stress may be fully accepted when someone first begins work, it is important to recognize that promotion, too, can be very stressful. Promotions often involve increased *social* demands, and it is necessary to ensure that these will be within the individual's capabilities. If not, then it will be necessary to work out how the job role could be enhanced without requiring increases in managerial or administrative responsibility.

## CONCLUSION

Higher-functioning individuals with autism and AS experience considerable difficulties in their attempts to make progress at school, college, or in the workplace. However, this group also possesses many substantial and often unique assets. Follow-up studies, such as that by Lord and Venter (1992), suggest that the extent to which they are able to utilize their skills can depend crucially on the degree and appropriateness of support that is provided beyond the school years and into adulthood. Thus, although the focus of much recent research has been on the importance of early intervention programs (National Research Council, 2001), true social inclusion will only be possible if the long-term needs of this group of individuals are also fully recognized and adequately supported.

## REFERENCES

Ballaban-Gil, K., Rapin, I., Tuchman, R., & Shinnar, S. (1996). Longitudinal examination of the behavioral, language, and social changes in a population of adolescents and young adults with autistic disorder. *Pediatric Neurology, 15,* 217–223.

Bass, M., & Drewett, R. (1998). *Supported employment for people with learning difficulties.* Report from the Merseyside Project in Liverpool, Department of Psychology, University of Durham.

Beveridge, S. (1996). Experiences of an integration link scheme: The perspectives of pupils with severe learning difficulties and their mainstream peers. *European Journal of Learning Disabilities, 26,* 87–101.

Beyer, S., Goodere, L., & Kilsby, M. (1996). *The costs and benefits of supported employment agencies.* London: Her Majesty's Stationery Office.

Beyer, S., & Kilsby, M. (1997). Supported employment in Britain. *Tizard Learning Disability Review, 2,* 6–14.

Burack, J. A., Root, R., & Zigler, E. (1997). Inclusive education for children with autism: Reviewing ideological, empirical, and community considerations. In D. Cohen & F. Volkmar (Eds.), *Handbook of autism and pervasive developmental disorder* (2nd ed., pp. 796–807). New York: Wiley.

Carlberg, C., & Kavale, K. (1980). The efficacy of special versus regular class placement for exceptional children: A meta-analysis. *Journal of Special Education, 14,* 295–309.

Chung, S. Y., Luk, F. L., & Lee, E. W. H. (1990). A follow-up study of infantile autism in Hong Kong. *Journal of Autism and Developmental Disorders, 20,* 221–232.

Cumine, V., Leach, J., & Stevenson, G. (1998). *Asperger syndrome: A practical guide for teachers.* London: Fulton.

DeMyer, M. K., Barton, S., DeMyer, W. E., Norton, J. A., Allan, J., & Steele, R. (1973). Prognosis in autism: A follow-up study. *Journal of Autism and Childhood Schizophrenia, 3,* 199–246.

Deno, S., Maruyama, G., Espin, C., & Cohen, C. (1990) Educating students with mild disabilities in general education classrooms: Minnesota alternatives. *Exceptional Children, 57,* 150–160.

Farrell, P. (1997). The integration of children with severe learning difficulties: A review of the recent literature. *Journal of Applied Research in Intellectual Disabilities, 10,* 1–14.

*Further and Higher Education Act.* (1992). London: Her Majesty's Stationery Office.

Gilchrist, A., Green, J., Cox, A., Rutter, M., & Le Couteur, A. (2001). Development and current functioning in adolescents with Asperger syndrome: A comparative study. *Journal of Child Psychology and Psychiatry, 42,* 227–240.

Gottlieb, J. (1990). Mainstreaming and quality education. *American Journal on Mental Retardation, 95,* 16–17.

Graham, J. (1999). *The INTERACT Centre.* London: Hanwell Community Centre.

Grandin, T. (1991). Autistic perceptions of the world. In *Proceedings of the Autism Society of America Conference* (pp. 85–94). Indianapolis, IN: Autism Society of America.

Harris, S. L., Handleman, J. S., Gordon, R., Kristoff, B., Bass, L., & Fuentes, F. (1991). Changes in cognitive and language functioning of preschool children with autism. *Journal of Autism and Developmental Disorders, 21,* 281–290.

Harris, S. L., Handleman, J. S., Kristoff, B., Bass, L., & Gordon, R. (1990). Changes in language development among autistic and peer children in segregated and integrated preschool settings. *Journal of Autism and Developmental Disorders, 20,* 23–32.

Harrison, J. (1996). Accessing further education: Views and experiences of FE students with learning difficulties and/or disabilities. *British Journal of Special Education, 23,* 187–196.

Hill, M. L., Banks, P. D., Handrick, R. R. Wehman, P. H., Hill, J. W., Shafer, M. S. (1987). Benefit–cost analysis of supported competitive employment for persons with mental retardation. *Research in Developmental Disability, 8,* 71–89.

Howlin, P. (1997). *Autism: Preparing for adulthood.* London: Routledge.

Howlin, P. (2002a). Language ability and other behaviours in high functioning individuals with autism spectrum disorders: A comparison of adults with autism and Asperger syndrome matched for non-verbal IQ. *Journal of Autism and Developmental Disorders, 33,* 3–13.

Howlin, P. (2002b). Special educational provision. In M. Rutter & E. Taylor (Eds.), *Child and adolescent psychiatry* (4th ed., pp. 1128–1147). London: Blackwell.

Howlin, P., & Goode, S. (1998). Outcome in adult life for people with autism and Asperger syndrome. In F. Volkmar (Ed.), *Autism and pervasive developmental disorders* (pp. 209–241). New York: Cambridge University Press.

Howlin, P. Goode, S., Hutton, J., & Rutter, M. (in press). Adult outcome for children with autism. *Journal of Child Psychology and Psychiatry.*

Howlin, P., Mawhood, L. M., & Rutter, M. (2000). Autism and developmental receptive language disorder: A follow-up comparison in early adult life. II: Social, behavioural, and psychiatric outcomes. *Journal of Child Psychology and Psychiatry, 41,* 561–578.

Hoyson, M., Jamieson, B., & Strain, P. S. (1984). Individualized group instruction of normally developing and autistic-like children. *Journal of the Division for Early Childhood, 8,* 157–172.

Jolliffe, T., Landsdown, R., & Robinson, T. (1992). *Autism: A personal account.* London: National Autistic Society.

Jordan, R., & Jones, G. (1999). *Meeting the needs of children with autistic spectrum disorders.* London: Fulton.

Kanner, L. (1973). *Childhood psychosis: Initial studies and new insights.* New York: Winston/Wiley.

Keel, J. H., Mesibov, G., & Woods, A. V. (1997). TEACCH: Supported employment program. *Journal of Autism and Developmental Disorders, 27,* 3–10.

Kilsby, M., & Beyer, S. (1996). Engagement and interactions: A comparison between supported employment and day service provision. *Journal of Intellectual Disability Research, 40,* 348–358.

Kobayashi, R., Murata, T., & Yashinaga, K. (1992). A follow-up study of 201 children with autism in Kyushu and Yamaguchi, Japan. *Journal of Autism and Developmental Disorders, 22,* 395–411.

Kunce, L. J., & Mesibov, G. B. (1998). Educational approaches to high-functioning autism and Asperger syndrome. In E. Schopler, G. B. Mesibov, & L. J. Kunce (Eds.), *Asperger syndrome or high-functioning autism?* (pp. 227–262). New York: Plenum Press.

Larsen, F. W., & Mouridsen, S. E. (1997). The outcome in children with childhood autism and Asperger syndrome originally diagnosed as psychotic. A 30-year follow-up study of subjects hospitalized as children. *European Child and Adolescent Psychiatry, 6,* 181–190.

Lockyer, L., & Rutter, M. (1969). A five- to fifteen-year follow-up study of infantile psychosis. III. Psychological aspects. *British Journal of Psychiatry, 115,* 865–882.

Lockyer, L., & Rutter, M. (1970). A five- to fifteen-year follow-up study of infantile psychosis. IV. Patterns of cognitive ability. *British Journal of Social and Clinical Psychology, 9,* 152–163.

Lord, C. (1995). Facilitating social inclusion: Examples from peer intervention programs. In E. Schopler., & G. Mesibov (Eds.), *Learning and cognition in autism* (pp. 221–239). New York: Plenum Press.

Lord, C., & Venter, A. (1992). Outcome and follow-up studies of high functioning autistic individuals. In E. Schopler & G. B. Mesibov (Eds.), *High functioning individuals with autism* (pp. 187–200). New York: Plenum Press.

Lotter, V. (1974a). Factors related to outcome in autistic children. *Journal of Autism and Childhood Schizophrenia, 4,* 263–277.

Lotter, V. (1974b). Social adjustment and placement of autistic children in Middlesex: A follow-up study. *Journal of Autism and Childhood Schizophrenia, 4,* 11–32.

Lotter, V. (1978). Follow-up studies. In M. Rutter & E. Schopler (Eds.), *Autism: A reappraisal of concepts and treatment* (pp. 475–495). New York: Plenum Press.

Mawhood, L. M., & Howlin, P. (1999). The outcome of a supported employment scheme for high functioning adults with autism or Asperger syndrome. *Autism: International Journal of Research and Practice, 3,* 229–253.

Mawhood, L. M., Howlin, P., & Rutter, M. (2000). Autism and developmental receptive language disorder—a follow-up comparison in early adult life. I: Cognitive and language outcomes. *Journal of Child Psychology and Psychiatry, 41*, 547–559.

McCaughrin, W., Ellis, W., Rusch, F., & Heal, L. (1993). Cost-effectiveness of supported employment. *Mental Retardation, 31*, 41–48.

Mesibov, G. B. (1990). Normalization and its relevance today. *Journal of Autism and Developmental Disorders, 20*, 379–390.

Mesibov, G. B., Schopler, E., Schaffer, B., & Michal, N. (1990). Use of the Childhood Autism Rating Scale with autistic adolescents and adults. *Journal of the American Academy of Child and Adolescent Psychiatry, 28*, 538–541.

Meyer, R. N. (2001). *Asperger syndrome employment workbook: An employment workbook for adults with Asperger syndrome.* London: Kingsley.

Mittler P., Gillies S., & Jukes E. (1966). Prognosis in psychotic children: Report of a follow-up study. *Journal of Mental Deficiency Research, 10*, 73–83.

Morgan, H. (1996). *Adults with autism.* Cambridge, UK: Cambridge University Press.

National Research Council. (2001). *Educating children with autism.* Washington, DC: National Academy Press.

Noble, J., Conley, R. W., Banerjee, S., & Goodman, S. (1991). Supported employment in New York State: A comparison of benefits and costs. *Journal of Disability Policy Studies, 2*, 39–73.

Piven, J., Harper, J., Palmer, P., & Arndt, S. (1996). Course of behavioral change in autism: A retrospective study of high-IQ adolescents and adults. *Journal of the American Academy of Child and Adolescent Psychiatry, 35*, 523–529.

Pozner, A., & Hammond, J. (1993). *An evaluation of supported employment initiatives for disabled people* (Research Series No. 17). London: Department of Employment.

Rich, H. L., & Ross, S. M. (1989). Students' time on learning tasks in special education. *Exceptional Children, 55*, 508–515.

Rouse, M., & Florian, L. (1996). Effective inclusive schools: A study in two countries. *Cambridge Journal of Education, 26*, 71–85.

Rumsey, J. M., Rapoport, J. L., & Sceery, W. R. (1985). Autistic children as adults: Psychiatric, social, and behavioral outcomes. *Journal of the American Academy of Child Psychiatry, 24*, 465–473.

Rusch, F. R., Conley, R. W., & McCaughrin, W. B. (1993). Benefit–cost analysis of supported employment in Illinois. *Journal of Rehabilitation, 59*, 31–36.

Rutter, M., & Lockyer, L. (1967). A five- to fifteen-year follow-up study of infantile psychosis. I. Description of sample. *British Journal of Psychiatry, 113*, 1169–1182.

Rutter, M., Greenfield, D., & Lockyer, L. (1967). A five- to fifteen-year follow-up study of infantile psychosis: II. Social and behavioural outcome. *British Journal of Psychiatry, 113*, 1183–1199.

Sainsbury, C. (2000). *Martian in the playground: Understanding the school child with Asperger's syndrome.* Bristol, UK: Lucky Duck.

Saintano, D., Goldstein, H., & Strain, P. (1992). Effects of self-evaluation on preschool children's use of social interaction strategies with their classmates with autism. *Journal of Applied Behavioral Analysis, 25*, 127–141.

Sigafoos, J., Roberts, D., Kerr, M., Couzens, D., & Baglioni, A. J. (1994). Opportunities for communication in classrooms serving children with developmental disabilities. *Journal of Autism and Developmental Disorders, 24*, 259–280.

Simpson, R. L., & Myles, B. S. (1993). Successful integration of children and youth with autism in mainstreamed settings. *Focus on Autistic Behavior, 7*, 1–13.

Smith, M., Belcher, R., & Juhrs, P. (1995). *A guide to successful employment for individuals with autism.* Baltimore: Brookes.

Stein, D., Ring, A., Shulman, C., Meir, D., Holan, A., Weizman, A., & Barak, Y. (2001). Brief report: Children with autism as they grow up—description of adult inpatients with severe autism. *Journal of Autism and Developmental Disorders, 31*, 355–360.

Szatmari, P., Bartolucci, G., Bremner, R. S., Bond, S., & Rich, S. (1989). A follow-up study of high functioning autistic children. *Journal of Autism and Developmental Disorders, 19*, 213–226.

Szivos, S. E. (1990). Attitudes to work and their relationship to self-esteem and aspirations among young adults with a mild mental handicap. *British Journal of Mental Subnormality, 36*, 108–117.

Tuffreau, R., Richard, P., Chardeau, P., Fortineau, J., Morisseau, L., Labastire, P., Ross, N., & Fombonne, E. (1995, September). *The outcome of severe developmental disorders in late adolescence.* Paper presented at the 10th International Congress of the European Society for Child and Adolescent Psychiatry, Utrecht, Netherlands.

Venter, A., Lord, C., & Schopler, E. (1992). A follow-up study of high-functioning autistic children. *Journal of Child Psychology and Psychiatry, 33*, 489–507.

von Knorring, A.-L., & Hägglöf, B. (1993). Autism in northern Sweden: A population based follow-up study: psychopathology. *European Child and Adolescent Psychiatry, 2*, 91–97.

Wehman, P., Moon, M., Everson, J., Wood, W., & Barcus, J. (1988). *Transition from school to work.* Baltimore: Brookes.

Williams, J. (1995). In support of supported employment. *The Psychologist, 8*, 405–406.

Wolfberg, P. J., & Schuler, A. L. (1993). Integrated playgroups: A model for promoting the social and cognitive dimensions of play. *Journal of Autism and Developmental Disorders, 23*, 1–23.

Zetlin, A., & Murtaugh, M. (1990). Whatever happened to those with borderline IQs? *American Journal on Mental Retardation, 94*, 463–469.

# 13

# What Do We Know and Where Should We Go?

MARGOT PRIOR

The increasing professional and public awareness of Asperger syndrome (AS) as a not uncommon childhood disorder brings with it a number of benefits and many challenges. On the one hand, in the 21st century there appears to be a better chance that (1) families with children with AS will recognize early that development is not proceeding along the pathway they had expected, and (2) they will be able to find an expert professional who will help them to understand how and why their child is different. Although diagnosis of a disorder such as AS is a sad event for families, there can be positive outcomes, such as relief from the anxiety and puzzlement that comes from *not understanding* what has gone awry in the child's development; access to information to help explain the condition; opportunities to plan for their child's life in ways which best suit his or her needs; and access to specialist help which can make life easier for the whole family. On the other hand, it cannot be denied that life is not easy for young people with AS and their families; great efforts will be needed to equip them to cope independently and in a satisfying way with a sometimes unfriendly, and frequently opaque, world; and finding an educational milieu that meets their needs can be a challenging task.

In this book contributors have focused on the core aspects of AS (i.e., the understanding and managing of behavioral and learning difficulties) that must underpin efforts to provide children with AS with the best possible experience of education for an independent life. In the latter part of the book, contributors have applied the best of our current knowledge of the characteristics of the syndrome and the needs of the children to develop blueprints for structures, strategies, curricula, and teaching approaches. The final chapter provides a synthesis of this knowledge, highlighting signposts for future development in clinical, educational practice, and research domains.

## DIAGNOSTIC DEBATES
## AND THEIR IMPLICATIONS

Although there is no unanimity of opinion regarding the status of AS as a disorder that is, or is not, part of the autism spectrum, the consensus of the contributions to this volume is that a predominance of evidence indicates that AS is best considered as a variant of autism. Reviewing symptoms and behavior, language and communication difficulties, cognitive strengths and weaknesses, response to education, and school experiences and outcomes, as we have done here, provides substantial support for this perspective. The case for the overlap, if not equivalence, of AS and high-functioning autism (HFA) is made convincingly in the first chapter, with a summary of the most up-to-date evidence from extant research on this question. This case is reinforced in other chapters that consider the differential diagnostic issues in particular domains of functioning. Tager-Flusberg addresses this question directly in her chapter, and her thorough review indicates that children with AS or HFA do not differ in language or social domains, or in terms of their educational needs or their outcome. The label so often depends on the mental lens through which the labeler looks.

Questions about diagnosis and classification have abounded in the autism field for more than 50 years. New papers addressing these questions appear regularly in scientific journals. It is likely that the individual differences and behavioral diversity among children with a putative diagnosis of autism spectrum disorder (ASD), AS, classic autism, or any other such label, will always give rise to uncertainty, unless or until biological markers can be identified to provide a new level of "hard" evidence on such questions. In terms of developing the most successful ways of helping children with AS, we are fortunately not stalled by fallibility of diagnoses; we continue to understand more about the condition and to find increasingly better ways of meeting educational needs and managing the condition.

## SPECIFIC LEARNING DIFFICULTIES
## IN ASPERGER SYNDROME

It is reasonable to ask whether specific learning difficulties (SLDs) are a common feature of AS. Clinical experience and published clinical evidence suggest that they are, in that a significant proportion of children presenting at clinics for assessment of AS are found to have uneven and often idiosyncratic patterns of abilities and learning aptitudes, which are evident as they grapple with school curricula. As a group, young people with AS are extremely variable, with some doing poorly at school and others doing very well and progressing to university degrees. Nevertheless, most of these young people are vulnerable to SLDs of one kind or another, which usually become evident in the classroom after the early years of school. This is the time when more challenging demands involving abstract thinking and reasoning, cognitive flexibility, and lateral thinking characterize the curricula, which is also based on the expectation that sound basic literacy and numeracy skills have been established.

The definition of an SLD is still debated, with differing parameters and labels applied in different countries, and even within countries. In this book we have taken it to mean the presence of specific areas where learning is not progressing as we would expect, given the child's overall intellectual capacities and a context of a reasonable standard of school attendance and educational provision (Prior, 1996). An SLD is different from the delay or slow progress in learning evidenced by a child with a developmental delay, wherein the delay is consistent with that child's level of intellectual disability. This latter problem is often described as "learning disabilities" and does not carry with it the unexpected or inconsistent aspect that is central to an SLD.

Teachers are frequently very puzzled as they try to understand why these children can do so well in some academic areas and so atrociously in others (see Manjiviona, Chapter 2, this volume). By definition, children with AS have normal or near-normal IQ; indeed, sometimes they are very bright. Level of IQ is a powerful factor in the child's capacity to cope with learning of any kind, but academic progress is often influenced by a variety of particular neuropsychological deficits that may be identified through careful assessment. Although it is sometimes claimed that an ability pattern specific to an AS diagnosis exists, in fact, the evidence for a regularly appearing cognitive neuropsychological profile does not support this claim. For example, a myth that has developed in this field is that children with AS show a distinctive pattern of cognitive assets and weaknesses when tested on the Verbal and Performance scales of the Wechsler Intelligence Scale for Children (WISC). It has even become fashionable to try to use the presumed pattern (we are not sure what this pattern is, because it keeps changing) as an aid to differential diagnosis between AS and autism. Authors in this book who take up this issue (Reitzal & Szatmari, Manjiviona, and Kunce) are in agreement that reliably distinguishing profiles have not been identified, and all confirm the need for comprehensive assessment for every child. These children do have very different thinking and learning styles by comparison with their peers in school, but these different styles do not translate into diagnosis-specific cognitive patterns, as extracted by standard cognitive tests.

Moreover, the fact that patterns and profiles change with development, as noted by several authors, should caution us against considering intellectual capacities and variabilities as fixed. Mayes and Calhoun's study, reported in Chapter 1 of this book, demonstrated a reduction in the discrepancy between Verbal and Performance IQ over time in children with low and high IQs, as well as the effect of overall IQ on the kinds of ability patterns evident in their sample. The Canadian data reported in Chapter 4 and Manjiviona's (Chapter 3) case study of Dylan illustrate just how much children with AS may change with development and in relation to their initial level of abilities. In fact, diversity appears to be the norm in this group of children.

Although there is marked variation in reported patterns of cognitive strengths and weaknesses in children with AS (see Klin, Volkmar, Sparrow, Cicchetti, & Rourke, 1995; Manjiviona & Prior, 1999; Ozonoff & Griffith, 2000; Szatmari, Archer, Fisman, Streiner, & Wilson, 1995, for examples), it is unclear whether, or how, particular profiles directly relate to vulnerability to SLDs. Myles, Barnhill, Hagiwara, Griswold, and Simpson (2001) have provided a synthesis of the characteristics of young people with AS, including those associated with intellectual and academic domains. They note problems with abstractions, including metaphors and figures of speech, discriminating between relevant and irrelevant detail, language-based problem solving, and literalness. On the other hand, rote learning is a strength; they are usually very good with factual material. Although there is considerable variability in literacy domains, children with AS often become skilled readers, even though their comprehension may lag behind their word recognition abilities. Composition and the capacity to complete essays and assignments are extremely poor, often in contrast to their oral presentation abilities. Mayes and Calhoun (in press) reported that 63% of the children in their sample had a specific difficulty with written expression (see also Manjiviona case examples, Chapter 3, this volume; and Myles et al., 2001).

Other characteristics of AS can hinder a smooth passage through both primary and secondary level curricula. These include lack of cognitive flexibility, difficulties in generalizing, preoccupations with idiosyncratic interests (which may include overfocusing on only some parts of a school curriculum), social and emotional unease, subtle language impairments, noncompliant behavior, and poor teacher–child understanding and relationships.

Although it is frequently noted that some strengths are common in the profiles (e.g., rote memory and some visual skills), Manjiviona's case studies highlight the variability in cognitive functioning in children with shared symptoms, behaviors, and diagnosis. At 13 years Jack showed higher Verbal than Performance IQ, notable weaknesses in the Coding subtest of the WISC (with its attentional and writing demands), and had a disorder of written expression, while functioning well in other domains. Matthew had clear problems in Vocabulary and Similarities tests as well as in the Picture Arrangement test, wherein verbal reasoning is important, but his Coding score was well above average. His reading comprehension ability was below his word-recognition level, but at this age, at least, he was coping well with the three R's. In contrast, Dylan showed a specific difficulty with spelling, along with low-average word-recognition and math skills, and overall weak verbal comprehension. The Swedish group (Ehlers et al., 1997) attempted a comparison of abilities in HFA, AS, and their DAMP (disorder of motor control, attention, and perception) groups, using the Wechsler scales. Their findings lent no encouragement to those who claim that profiles have differential diagnostic import, although they claimed that the AS subjects were better on tasks measuring crystallized intelligence (and, by implication, have better capacities with acquired or learned material). However, circularity is an issue here: The higher the IQ of the AS subjects in most research studies means that their learning abilities will almost inevitably be higher than those of groups with lower Verbal IQs.

Reitzal and Szatmari's analyses of the existing studies comparing AS and HFA (Chapter 2, this volume) confirmed the conclusion that no specific ability or learning difficulty pattern is characteristic. Nor is there any evidence suggesting the presence of subtypes of LDs in children with ASD. The longitudinal follow-up of the groups diagnosed with AS or HFA, however, offered some evidence for differentiation between them. As the children grew older, those with AS improved in reading skills, including comprehension, and specific rather than general LDs were more common. The group with HFA appeared more static in their academic progress. The differences at follow-up, however, seemed to reflect the criteria for selection into the study: The children with AS were more advanced in language development initially, and this placed them on a more advantaged learning pathway across time.

This mirroring of selection criteria in reports of comparative studies of cognitive and academic outcomes in AS and HFA appears to be a common, and perhaps unsurprising, finding. Reitzal and Szatmari noted that it is inordinately difficult to find children with AS who do not also meet criteria for a diagnosis of autism (see also Leekam, Libby, Wing, Gould, & Gillberg, 2000), at least using current conventions for diagnosis. They offered a thought-provoking interpretation of their findings by suggesting that autism is actually AS with a superimposed specific language impairment (SLI). This argument can accommodate the shared social and information-processing impairments common in AS and HFA and take account of the greater deficiencies in language in the latter group. Certainly the work of the Canadian researchers confirms the need for further detailed follow-up studies of children with an ASD from the earliest developmental period, particularly those at the high-functioning end of the spectrum. It is also important to emphasize "spared abilities," which can influence the nature and implementation of effective learning and teaching strategies if their significance is recognized. Within the AS category are many and varied spared abilities, as seen in the heterogeneous profiles. In most (but not all) cases of ASDs, visual–spatial analysis and synthesis capacities, as elicited in the WISC Block Design subtest, are spared abilities. This test is said to represent "fluid intelligence" or innate ability, rather then learned capacity; hence the results of this test represent, at least in theory, a persistent and generalizable ability across a range of problems and tasks. For young people with AS, however, the "fluid" aspect of this intelligence is not always in evidence, as they struggle to find or adapt strategies to solve new problems (Prior & Ozonoff, 1998).

How best to assess these children is a key question, and there is also considerable diversity of opinion here, including national differences in preferred assessment methods. In their separate chapters, Kunce (Chapter 11), Manjiviona, and Reitzal and Szatmari comment upon the assessment process and note some useful and informative tests. Choice has increased steadily, with many new breeds of tests appearing in the 1980s and 1990s, and our assessment methods have become increasingly sophisticated (see Kaufman & Kaufman, 2001, for an up-to-date review, and in particular, their Table 13.1, which lists categories of cognitive functions and their apposite tests).

## NONVERBAL LEARNING DIFFICULTIES

Rourke and his colleagues have delineated a pattern of learning difficulties they call "nonverbal learning disabilities" (NVLD) and have likened children with this syndrome to those with AS (Rourke & Tsatsanis, 2000) in their impairments in social behavior. NVLD is characterized by notable deficits in nonverbal problem-solving skills and problems with visual–spatial, and tactile-perceptual tasks, with concomitant strengths in psycholinguistic skills, rote verbal learning, and phoneme–grapheme translation skills. According to these authors, children with this syndrome read and spell very well but have difficulties with mathematics. In addition, Rourke and colleagues have described a pattern of psychosocial difficulties that includes deficits in nonverbal aspects of communication, repetitive verbosity, poor capacity to deal with novel situations and "patterns of exchange," with reliance on rote learning of social rules and sometimes inappropriate behaviors; deficits in social perception, social judgment, and interaction skills; and risk for development of "internalizing" disorders in adolescence. They see this pattern of social and behavioral impairments (with its obvious flavor of AS) as associated particularly with NVLD. Comparing their findings with those of others in the field, especially the study of Klin and colleagues (1995), they claim to find an overwhelming concordance between children with AS and those with NVLD, using the defining criteria of the latter (see also Ehlers et al., 1997). But the close replications of this research that are needed to support such claims have not been forthcoming. Moreover, the longitudinal data on cognitive and academic outcome reported by Reitzal and Szatmari in Chapter 2 of this volume, do not confirm a NVLD pattern in their samples.

Although the parallels in cognitive and behavioral impairments between these two childhood syndromes have been described as striking, it is difficult to know how to interpret their meaning. There have been very few independent studies confirming Rourke's claims of a distinctive and empirically reliable NVLD category among children with an SLD. In clinical practice as well as in the countless studies of subgroups of children with an SLD, boundaries between subgroups are actually hard to find—if present at all, they are blurred—and the patterns of cognitive and academic difficulties are very diverse. A large proportion of children has multiple rather then specific difficulties across learning domains. Moreover, children with LDs are vulnerable to emotional and behavioral problems, especially if they are boys (Prior, Smart, Sanson, & Oberklaid, 1999). The question of whether the behavioral difficulties precede or follow the onset of learning difficulties remains controversial (see McGee, Prior, Williams, Smart, & Sanson, 2002; McGee, Share, Moffitt, Williams, & Silva, 1988; Smart, Sanson, & Prior, 1996), and difficult to establish, except via prospective longitudinal studies. Both internalizing and externalizing behavioral problems are common (Hinshaw, 1992). Indeed, there is frequently a complex mix of adjustment difficulties with ill-understood relationships to each other. Furthermore, the cognitive difficulties characteristic of various samples of children with AS are diverse rather than prototypical.

Nevertheless, the notion that AS could be related to, or characterized as, an SLD subtype (with accompanying social/communicative problems) is an interesting one but needs further large sample studies across a range of settings, laboratories, and clinical research groups. Rourke and Tsatsanis themselves note that their NVLD syndrome is associated with a range of neurological disorders that involve damage to various parts of the brain, sometimes including right-hemispheric dysfunction. Hooper and Bundy (1998) suggest that the NVLD model offers an opportunity to examine more closely the interaction between neurological and neuropsychological influences that may be associated with the distinctive behavioral features of AS, either directly or indirectly. Hooper and Bundy also took up the question of whether it is possible to distinguish between AS and HFA in terms of learning characteristics. Their review indicated few differences of a very subtle nature. Moreover, they concluded that most educational interventions available were not diagnosis-specific; they applied equally well to individuals on the spectrum (or with NVLD), taking into account the level of abilities. Bringing these speculations up to date in this volume, Reitzal and Szatmari conclude that their follow-up study of children with AS does not support the notion that children with AS have the NVLD profile of specific problems with visual–spatial processing, visual–motor skills, or motor incoordination.

In sum, the answer to the question of whether children with AS are prone to show SLDs is probably yes, but no specific subtypes or patterns of either cognitive capacities or difficulties in particular academic domains are reliably or distinctively characteristic of the disorder. Hence it is adaptive, as argued many times in this book, to treat each child as an individual and provide a comprehensive assessment that can be translated into an individualized educational program suited to that child's specific needs.

## CLUMSINESS

Clumsiness, or motor incoordination, which is associated with many developmental disorders, has been claimed to have particular diagnostic significance in AS (Gillberg, 1989). Asperger described his original four patients as clumsy, with poor coordination and balance and unusual gait and posture. In a recent review of the evidence for specific associations between motor clumsiness and AS, Ozonoff and Griffith (2000) attempted to distinguish between AS and HFA in this domain of development (see also Smith, 2000). The most common findings in the relatively small literature on this topic are that children with AS as well as HFA show a greater degree of clumsiness when compared to nonautistic psychiatric controls and normal children. However, they probably do not differ as subgroups (Eisenmajer et al., 1996; Gillberg, 1989; Manjiviona & Prior, 1995; Szatmari et al., 1995). Gillberg (1989) and Klin and colleagues (1995), though, reported more clumsiness in children diagnosed with AS than in those with HFA; and

Tantam (1991) has reported clumsiness as characteristic of most of the AS subjects he has studied. It is difficult to draw conclusions because of the variation in diagnostic criteria used in the various studies, as well as differing methods of assessing clumsiness, some of which have not employed standardized and currently validated neurodevelopmental or motor function tests (Ghaziuddin, Tsai, & Ghaziuddin, 1992; Smith, 2000). Some research does not take IQ into account when making between-group comparisons, despite the fact that motor and mental development are interrelated. Children with intellectual or learning disabilities are also prone to show motor clumsiness; hence it is important to look at associated features of the child's overall development.

An additional interesting question is whether SLDs are reliably associated with clumsiness. In this case it would be important to separate out the connections between the AS-related symptoms and the SLD-related influences. Thus far, this comparison does not seem to have been made. It is common for children with AS to have handwriting difficulties, in part, because of their motor difficulties. Hence, the handwriting difficulties are significant factors in regard to learning difficulties and often need expert attention from an occupational therapist. In general, the significance of clumsiness remains unclear, and given the absence of evidence for its import in diagnosing, understanding, and treating/teaching children with AS, it has not been specifically reviewed in this volume. Any putative role of motor incoordination in the etiology of AS remains to be fully examined.

## SENSORY SENSITIVITIES

Another area of particular interest which has been noted in some chapters concerns the common proclivity for some children with an ASD to have unusual sensory sensitivities. In her chapter, Wendy Lawson (Chapter 8) writes poetically and with deep feeling about how sounds, light, visual patterns, colors, tactile sensations, and other sensory experiences can make strong impressions on her, and affect her adaptation to many situations. Her vividly recalled memories of her early school experiences, such as her reaction to the clothes worn by her first teacher, highlight just how powerful these sensations can be for the child with an ASD. Crowded noisy places can be extremely disturbing for some individuals, meaning that standard classrooms can be continuously stressful, and situations such as milling around in the locker room can provoke extreme outbursts of anger and distress. Hence it is critical that people having any level of care and responsibility for a child with AS should know and understand how significant these sensitivities may be to the child. Furthermore, such features should be considered in assessment and educational planning for the child. Good communication between family and school can save a great deal of trouble, as the nature of the problem and some strategies to deal with it can become shared knowledge between home and school.

## SOCIAL AND BEHAVIORAL ISSUES

The challenges of understanding and managing social and behavioral problems in children with AS was a central theme of this book. The social impairments of AS are universal, primary, serious, and resistant to treatment. Although there are a number of very valuable systematic programs and strategies for addressing the difficulties, almost all researchers and professionals point to the intransigent problems of achieving generalization of taught social skills. The ever-changing context of social interactions, along with the subtleties inherent in human interpersonal communication, are extremely challenging. Although children with AS can learn "the rules," their pedantic and rote style of operating means that learned rules are not always useful as lubricants for social interaction. They get it wrong despite their best efforts. They complain of being friendless and alone.

Shaked and Yirmiya (Chapter 5) provide a comprehensive summary of the nature of social difficulties, which have been more extensively researched, perhaps, than any other features of AS. They remind us of the fact that older children with AS are often considerably aware of, and frustrated by, their differences and difficulties; they want to overcome them and be accepted by their peers, but they feel helpless about doing so. In the school setting, the need for guidance and supervision is always present in an array of complex social learning situations. Their chapter provides a review of the range and variety of intervention methods that have been developed to assist children with ASD to develop social skills. These methods need to be matched to the age and the cognitive functioning of the particular children involved.

Because a key goal of these interventions is fostering satisfying relationships with peers, and because skills must be practiced *in vivo* to be learned successfully, peer interaction is a critical ingredient of any intervention. Peers can fulfill many roles: as teachers alongside children with AS, as mentors or buddies, as members of designated Circles of Friends, as one-to-one or group companions, and as partners in interactions in which the child or adolescent with AS can have the role of the tutor. Two-way reciprocal interactions are the desired outcomes, not long-term dependence for the child with AS. There is no need to repeat the comments of Shaked and Yirmiya on this significant topic. But, as they concede, there is little evaluation of the outcome of any of the social skills training programs.

An increasing number of interventions for young children with autism has been evaluated (Attwood, 2000; see also October 2002 issue of the *Journal of Autism and Developmental Disorders*, which contains a cluster of evaluation papers; and the [U.S.] National Academy of Sciences booklet *Educating Children with Autism* [2001]). The fact that attending to the needs of children and adolescents with AS is a recent phenomenon, and the fact that these children are intelligent and articulate and therefore require rather different approaches from those developed for more impaired children, means that we can conclude little about long-term effectiveness of social interventions at this stage. However, parents and children find many of these programs to be positive, pleasurable, and valuable experiences that can be extremely worthwhile, even if the longer-term gains are limited. Evaluation of interventions (educational and social skills programs) for individuals with AS, especially over the long term, is much needed.

It has become apparent over the past decade that circumscribed interests, which are often obsessively pursued by young people with AS, are a marked feature of the disorder. The nature, function, and extent of these intense interests have received relatively little investigation and analysis in the literature. Attwood (Chapter 6, this volume) and others (e.g., Bashe & Kirby, 2000; Tantam, 2000) have suggested that the preoccupations serve a number of functions for the child. They can give a sense of order in a confusing world; they can reduce the uncertainties inherent in their social world, which are persistently troubling for these children; they can reduce anxiety and stress by allowing some escape from difficult situations and demands; they can evoke a feeling of happiness in the child from the great pleasure in focusing on the much loved topic/activity; and they allow a young person to achieve something noteworthy by developing an unusual degree of knowledge and skill in a particular domain. On the other hand, parents and teachers worry that the preoccupations may result in the child's withdrawal from other important learning experiences and thus may limit the potential for a more expansive life.

Attwood describes a raft of strategies (e.g., controlled access) that can maximize the positive aspects of these special interests. He outlines the many constructive applications that might be possible for a special expertise, such as motivating more learning, serving as a bridge to making friends, and facilitating employment. Gill too gives examples, within her school experience, of how preoccupations and special interests can be used to motivate and manage attention to learning. Howlin (Chapter 12, this volume) shows us how, in adulthood, special interests, with the accompanying expert knowledge, can sometimes enhance employment outcomes, if they can be fitted in to an appropriate and well-managed role for the adolescent or adult with AS.

As Tantam notes in his chapter (Chapter 7, this volume), children with AS are people first and children with AS second. They present with a variety of adjustment difficulties that overlap those seen in the non-AS population. Among the most salient of these are attention deficits, and sometimes overactivity and overarousal. These are commonly part of the picture in younger children with AS and require the same level of care and management as they do in other children with attention-deficit/hyperactivity disorder–type problems. Psychiatric disorders, including anxiety and depression, may arise in adolescence and adulthood particularly, although an elevated level of anxiety is also often observed in younger children with AS and may contribute to their agitation, hypersensitivity, attention problems, and social withdrawal.

Some children present with what Tantam calls "catastrophic reactions," whereby they become aggressive and violent toward themselves and others in response to some external (or internal) stimulus. These reactions are a major challenge to professionals trying to help families and teachers with management strategies, as they can be so extremely disruptive and ungovernable and may sometimes become habitual reactions to the slightest frustration. Tantam recommends avoiding situations and triggers for these reactions, where possible, and reducing stimulation and maintaining calmness when eruptions do occur. Attention to these rages is likely to make the situation worse. It is well known that children with AS can react very badly to changes in their routines, including major transitions such as change of school and unforeseen crises. Wise carers and teachers have learned to spend time and effort preparing their charges for changes and new experiences; this preparation is usually very helpful in reducing trauma. Tantam discusses a range of treatments for the psychological difficulties characteristic of AS, from judicious use of medication to strategic management designed to protect the child from him- or herself, as well as to enhance the capacity for learning to self-manage.

The normal array of developmental challenges faced during adolescence is also present in people with AS. The additional stresses related to their social deficits, however, may tax and even overwhelm their already stretched self-management resources. In this context, Tantam discusses problems relating to developing sexuality, which can become major dramas for some adolescents, young adults, and their families. He provides an illuminating case example illustrating a confident, rational, and successful way of dealing with a sexual obsession in a young man with AS. This illustrative case of a direct but calm and reasonable approach to inappropriate behavior reinforces Howlin's (Chapter 12, this volume) recommendation for clear, calm, and straightforward communication about the interpersonal or job-related problems that may arise in the workplace.

Recently it has become apparent that cognitive-behavioral therapy (CBT) is a treatment that holds some promise for young people with AS. CBT is a well-known and effective psychological treatment, particularly for mood and anxiety disorders, in older children, adolescents, and adults in mental health settings. Attwood has developed some modifications to CBT (see his Web site, "Modifications to CBT to accommodate the unusual cognitive profiles of people with Asperger Syndrome," at *http://trainland.tripod.com/ tony.a.htm*) to make it more suitable and flexible for people with AS. In his chapter in this volume (Chapter 6), he briefly reports on this approach in the context of dealing with preoccupations and special interests.

The key components of CBT—namely, problem assessment; affective education; perceiving the connections between thoughts, feelings, and behaviors; and discovering how the individual constructs and appraises a situation, and how this appraisal affects behavior—can be taught to people with AS. Exercises and activities incorporating stress management, cognitive restructuring, self-appraisal, and a graded schedule of opportunities to learn and practice new skills then can be applied. Hare (1997, case study) and Hare, Jones, and Paine (1999) have reported on the use of CBT to treat adjustment problems in patients with AS. This approach has the potential for further development and is likely to find a place in both individual and group-based treatments for people with AS who present with adjustment difficulties. As with all psychological and psychiatric treatments, we need treatment evaluation studies to provide sound evidence for the effectiveness of CBT with the kinds of problems that typically distress people with AS.

CBT is not the only useful intervention, of course; many young people benefit from counseling and interpersonal, interactive-type therapies, which give them the opportunity to air their problems and discuss ways of coping with challenges and stress. Stoddart (1999) has reported case studies in which he utilized both family systems therapy and individual therapy to treat family adjustment difficulties for three boys with AS. These approaches proved very helpful in addressing problem-solving issues at home, family conflict, parenting strategies, as well as a range of adolescent problems associated with self-esteem, self-concept, peer problems, social ineptness, school system barriers, and the expression and regulation of feelings. Since family conflict is almost inevitably associated with the challenges of raising a child with AS, the theories and methods from various family therapy orientations can be called upon to help child and family manage common stresses in more adaptive ways. The incorporation of medication in the treatment of two of Stoddart's cases was a helpful adjunct. Tantam's chapter in this volume (Chapter 7) also provides information on the kinds of medication that can be helpful for symptoms that are severely troubling and that may require pharmacological treatment.

## EDUCATIONAL SYSTEMS

A very common theme throughout the literature is the notable lack of education system support for children with AS. Although there have been considerable improvements in the provision of services, including early intervention and specialized teaching for children with autism, high-functioning children with an ASD (i.e., good learning and adaptive capacities) have not been considered eligible for special support, despite the clear evidence of their considerable deficits in social, emotional, and learning domains across all developmental stages. While acknowledging that service provision varies from country to country and even across regions within countries, the general tendency for services to be either unavailable or insufficient for children and young people with a diagnosis of AS contributes to the fact that they often are very unhappy at school, suffer from teasing and bullying, come into conflict with peers and teachers, and may not reach their intellectual and academic potential.

The term *stress* comes into almost every chapter in this book, leaving the reader in no doubt that this is an almost universal experience for children and adolescents with AS, as they progress through primary, secondary, and, in some cases, tertiary education. The risk of suffering at school is vividly described by first-person accounts of people with AS, such as Lawson (Chapter 8, this volume), Jolliffe (Jolliffe, Landsdown, & Robinson, 1992) and Grandin (1992), to name but a few. Other contributors in this book refer to the problems with self-esteem, which are almost universal in school-age young people with AS, as they find themselves not fitting in with their peers whose interests and interactive modes are so very different from their own.

The fact that young people with an ASD usually look normal and can behave quite normally for some of the time, coupled with their apparent language facilities, can work to their disadvantage, because educators find it hard to reconcile these apparent normalities with the unexpected and often incomprehensible social, communicative, and learning deficits that undermine these students' seeming suitability for mainstream classrooms. To some extent, theirs is a "hidden disability" that is not as likely to elicit the sympathetic and empathic understanding of teachers and peers as do children with clearly observable (and comprehensible) disabilities. As Attwood (Chapter 6, this volume) notes, these children sometimes project a "little professor" image, with their stores of detailed information on favored themes; this ability also can mislead others, at least until perspicacious teachers recognize and adapt to the limitations of this "expertise." Few teachers in the regular educational system have knowledge of AS, and the level of autism-specific training may be low even for specialist teachers. Kunce (Chapter 11, this volume) documents the striking mismatch between the characteristics of AS and the characteristics of regular classroom settings into which children with AS must fit. It is worth pointing out here that children with AS often fit more comfortably into small rural schools, where their particular needs can be met in a more benign fashion and where there is greater flexibility in curriculum, with children of mixed ability and different academic levels within the one room. That is, diversity is normal for this setting, and accommodating to individual differences is inherent in the school program. In urban areas, small private schools may be able to provide more flexibility and individual attention than larger state schools with many hundreds of pupils.

Kunce's integrated model captures the need for (1) accepting and knowledgeable people who are able to collaborate in the interests of the child; (2) assessment to be followed by individualized education plans; (3) sources of support across all domains; and (4) the planned curriculum to reflect both short- and long-term goals of the child's education. It is important to include explicit goals regarding adaptive outcomes (e.g., independence in all or some aspects of living) as part of that educational plan, including goals for self-management and preparation for work.

## INCLUSION/MAINSTREAMING CONTROVERSIES

The field is characterized by a paucity of studies documenting and evaluating the effectiveness of mainstreaming education for children with AS. This lacuna is in contrast to the rapidly accumulating literature regarding interventions for children with autism at the lower-functioning end of the spectrum. Studies of young people in secondary education settings (Howlin, Chapter 12, this volume) are particularly scarce. The huge variation in educational and employment outcomes for older adolescents and adults is graphically illustrated in Howlin's review. In general, the results do not encourage us to claim that mainstreaming is the "right" approach to adopt, although there is little doubt that inclusion is an admirable principle and should be an ideal goal for all children with disabilities. To be an achievable goal, however, would require a massive injection of system-wide support and adequate protection of these students' social, physical, and educational needs. All children are entitled to access to mainstream curricula and the full range of educational experiences, both academic and social, but given the special problems in AS, alternatives are clearly needed. Specific kinds of alternatives or adjunct programs have been mentioned, albeit in the context of children with normal-range abilities who are expected to attend regular schools.

One example of an alternative pathway is Gill's school (Chapter 9, this volume), which provides a "special" environment for young children with

AS, in which, for a period of time (defined according to the social and educational needs of the individual child) in small classes staffed by autism experts, they may be prepared for later mainstreaming. In this facilitative environment that combines high levels of teacher understanding, parent
liaison, and a flexible curriculum, children learn important skills they can
employ when they move on to regular schools. The transition is carefully
planned and gradually implemented, with increasing periods of time spent
in the mainstream setting. Ongoing support is provided by teachers from
the special school, who visit the new schools and coach the mainstream
teachers as well as the child with AS for as long as needed (albeit, diminish-
ing over time). In addition, this school provides a broad outreach service to
many schools attended by children and adolescents with AS, and manages a
special education unit within a secondary school that provides part-time integration of adolescents with AS or an ASD. The school also provides what
are called "respite days," when mainstreamed children may come on a regular basis to receive expert attention in a more relaxing and sympathetic
environment than the one they find in regular schools.

Consultation with expert staff can help solve many puzzles for mainstream teachers, who may be more receptive to being "coached" about autism by teaching colleagues than they would be to outside professionals
who do not always share the language, culture, and mores of school systems. Teachers struggling to understand the special needs of young people
with AS often worry that treating them with special consideration or
marked flexibility would not be fair to the remaining children and would
be perceived as favoritism, "spoiling" a particular child, or relaxing discipline too much. This kind of situation requires negotiation between the
teacher and the class, which many teachers find exceedingly difficult to accomplish without support and mentoring from expert colleagues.

The problems for teachers in mainstream schools who do not have expertise in autism, who are constantly puzzled and challenged by these unusual children, and who must manage a class of perhaps 25 or more other
individuals are noteworthy. Communication is a challenge highlighted in
many chapters in this book. It is hard for mainstream teachers to remember
that children with AS are not just being "smart alecks" or cruel in their objectionable comments, but are employing, as Gill puts it, "language files"
of ruled-based data that do not include the kind of flexibility, subtlety, and
creativity in responding to classroom situations and the behavior of others
that is normally exhibited. Since students with AS lack a well-developed capacity to "read" other subtle personal signs, such as body language and facial expression, this further deprives them of communication finesse (see
Tager-Flusberg, Chapter 4, and Shaked & Yirmiya, Chapter 5, this volume). Wendy Lawson's (Chapter 8, this volume) account of the difficulties
she experienced attempting to comprehend the communications of her

teachers and peers, along with the extreme literalness that so greatly affected her school experiences, helps us imagine the pain this disability can cause a misunderstood child.

There is universal agreement that the policy of integration or inclusion should be supported, that the requisite resources for doing so must be available, and that these services are needed across the continuum of education at various levels, and on into the employment arena (see Howlin, Chapter 12, this volume). Kunce's comprehensive model (Chapter 11, this volume) of the ideal educational situation encompasses strategies for all of the behavioral and educational challenges raised by the authors in this book. Although she writes in the context of the inclusion principle, since this is the most likely context for the majority of children with AS, she recommends a continuum of settings and is clear about the resources that would be needed to provide for the needs of this group of children in a satisfactory manner. Without adequate support, these children risk receiving what Jordan (Chapter 10, this volume) termed "travesties of inclusion." It also must be conceded that mainstreaming is not for everyone; it may be too hard for some children, given their high levels of sensitivity and reactivity and poor self-regulation skills. No matter how laudable the principle of inclusive education might be, it is damaging to expose children with an ASD to the experience of failing in a mainstream setting.

Existing barriers to inclusion include inflexible organizations, inadequately trained staff, rigid curricular demands, insufficient or inexpert support, communication and teaching styles that may be a mystery to children with AS, as well as the rough-and-tumble and, sometimes cruel, ways of children on the average playground. These factors all conspire to give children with an ASD a tough time at school.

It is acknowledged that parents know more about their children than any of the "experts," and a collaborative relationship between teachers and parents can be a valuable and effective resource throughout the school years. Parents can even act as coaches for their children. Even at tertiary levels, where lecturers and tutors may be completely unaware of the difficulties faced by students with AS, advocacy, coaching, and consultation from parents is likely to be needed.

There is some diversion of opinion regarding the need to modify educational curricula for children and adolescents with AS. Manjiviona notes (Chapter 3, this volume) that such modification can be important and that there may be a need for parents to advocate for their children on this issue when they are clearly struggling. Jordan (Chapter 10, this volume) prefers that opportunities to cover all curriculum offerings should be available, and is less positive about excluding some subjects. The underlying factor, of course, is individual difference. Some young people will be less stressed and more successful at school if they are able to use an adapted curriculum that excludes areas and subjects where they have very negative experiences. The policy of modification may extend to curriculum areas in which these students are unable to get along with a particular teacher. Others thrive on being able to deal with all or most subject areas and take pride in remaining, at least on the surface, fully mainstreamed in academic areas. The ability level and profile of the individual, his or her specific interests, and the developmental stage of the child or adolescent will influence decision making on this issue.

## OTHER ARENAS OF CONCERN

Gill (Chapter 9, this volume) describes homework as "horror territory" for some children and families. The difficulties with organization, time management, concentration, and motivation that are part of the challenges in this territory can be especially severe and may create considerable stress and emotional outbursts. Gill offers a number of practical suggestions for minimizing and dealing with this conflict arena, although it has to be conceded that, in practice, it is parents who will have to sustain a great deal of the stress when their children arrive home after a hard day at school (as, indeed, they often do with their nonimpaired children). Consultation and understanding between home and school is critical to negotiate a work program that is feasible and tolerable for the child and family at home.

The school playground presents severe challenges for children with AS, and strategies to assist with this problem have been suggested by several authors. Lawson's memories of bullying provide a first-person account of just how appalling a time some children experience. Bullying is an endemic problem in schools and is not confined to children with AS. Fortunately we have developed heightened awareness of the problem and greater willingness to deal with it, rather than dismiss it as part of the hurly-burly and "toughening process" of normal school experience. For anyone on the playground, being different is often tantamount to an instigation to bullying. There is no clear set of solutions to this situation, but intervention is mandatory. Some degree of protection can be afforded through (1) greater staff presence on the playground, (2) the reliable availability of a support peer or teacher, and (3) by teaching children how to respond to, and cope with, bullies in a self-protective way. In addition, alternatives to the playground area, which can provide a refuge for children with AS, must be available. These alternatives typically include the library, computer room, a separate part of the playground, a part of staff offices, or any other area that affords some degree of shelter and protection.

A further difficulty encountered by some students and their families is the students' vulnerability to being "led astray." Naiveté coupled with a keen desire to be accepted in the social group can mean that the young person is at risk of being led into bizarre behavior or antisocial or delinquent acts, drawn along by children with a propensity for such behaviors. They are easy targets, with their typically immature grasp of social mores and moral reasoning, and their desire for acceptance that makes them easy to influence. Lawson describes what she calls her gullibility, the victimization she suffered at school because of it, and how it got her into trouble (see also Tantam's work, Chapter 7, this volume). These kinds of problems have been documented in the recent literature; in the saddest cases, young people with AS have become involved with legal systems as pawns of such influences. Part of their educational provision thus needs to ensure that they are protected from the risk of such destructive experiences.

## EMPLOYMENT

Howlin's review (Chapter 11, this volume) indicates relatively poor prospects for continuing employment for people with AS. Nevertheless, it is instructive and encouraging to read of the supportive employment systems that have been developed, including the one currently managed by the National Autistic Society in the United Kingdom, which has produced much better results than schemes tried in earlier years. The principles in this scheme include matching jobs to clients; providing alternatives to standard job interviews via such methods as coaching, short-term job trials, or written presentations; and job coaching for employers as well as employee. Such approaches can be taken up more widely to deal with this ever-increasing problem as more and more young people with AS emerge from their educational institutions, seeking work, identity, and independence.

An important issue raised by Howlin concerns the need to give direct feedback on job-related performance problems, both social and work-related, since the person with AS is not able to "take hints" or to perceive the subtle signs of people's dissatisfaction. He or she does not grasp the unwritten rules of behavior that are normally followed in the world of work. Use of clear written information about expectations and performance also can enhance understanding and responsiveness for the employee with AS.

## A DIAGNOSIS OF ASPERGER SYNDROME: WHOM SHOULD WE TELL?

The question of to whom it is advisable to reveal a diagnosis of AS was raised in the introduction to this volume. There is no research from which to draw knowledge about whether such a revelation has positive or negative effects. On the basis of her extensive experience, Gill notes (in Chapter 9, this volume) that there are no rules. Some autism experts maintain that it is essential for the school staff to have a clear understanding of the problems encountered by children with AS, in order to be able to help them achieve their learning potential. It is hard to argue with this assertion. However, decisions depend on the views of parents, teachers, and children and are best made on a joint basis. Some parents are relieved by the opportunity to explain to people why their child behaves in an odd or unexpected way, perhaps at last able to deflect criticism by their relatives about their management difficulties. Others are determined to pursue as normal a pathway as they possibly can, and will make every effort to teach their child to behave as normally as possible at all times, to "expect" the child to behave normally, and to minimize the risk of adverse comment. An opinion poll on this topic would almost certainly lead to the opinion that "it depends" on the nature of the child and of the family and the features of their social and community environments.

In many cases the need to label conditions and disorders is driven by health and educational systems and hence may diminish personal choice. Writing in reference to resources for children with SLDs, Kaufman and Kaufman (2001, p. 449) describe "the blatant unfairness of a legal system that requires categorisation and labelling before funds are available to provide help that is obviously needed." Unfortunately, in the case of AS, funds are often not available even with the diagnosis and the label; hence this statement has particular poignancy for this group. Tantam takes up this issue (Chapter 7, this volume), noting that the commonest reaction to diagnosis is acceptance and relief by the parents, and rejection by the young person with AS. Giving full information and explanation is critical as long as the child is old enough to comprehend what is being said and is able to discuss the implications. Giving the child a written explanation which he or she can digest alone and over an extended period of time is often helpful. The National Autistic Society in Britain has developed a helpful information brief, which parents and young people find very valuable. However, the issue of diagnosis and labeling is a contentious one, and some professionals and families may prefer to manage the situation by focusing on and finding ways to deal with the specific problems that are evident in the child's life, rather than focusing on the "disorder" per se.

## FOR THE FUTURE?

What major implications from the reviews and recommendations in this book could inform further clinical, educational, and research endeavors relating to AS?

## Diagnostic Dilemmas: Spectrum or Subgroup?

Debates around diagnosis and classification of ASDs (HFA and AS) continue, and the recurring themes were discussed, in detail, in the first sections of this book. There is the minimally researched issue of whether the original conceptualization of AS as a personality disorder by Asperger himself (1944/1991) should be revisited. Definition and diagnosis of personality disorders are themselves problematic exercises, which have always challenged psychiatric practice. However, there is scope for at least an examination of whether this question could usefully be considered further, in light of current knowledge about AS. The pragmatists among us find it more satisfactory to focus on the symptoms and behaviors of AS that create social adaptation problems and on ways to ameliorate these difficulties. With regard to the question of whether AS is a variant of autism, the research literature suggests perhaps an uneasy truce among researchers at the moment, with this conceptualization probably best fitting the current picture we have of the disorder.

The circularity of research that seeks to identify and/or compare subgroups of children with an ASD but which preselects the groups in ways that almost ensures how they will differ has been evident in some of the material reviewed in the book. What is also evident is that current strictures to reserve an AS diagnosis for children with "normal" language development does not work. A consensus is emerging that AS is a variant of autism, and that it represents the upper end of a spectrum of similar disabilities. Reitzal and Szatmari (Chapter 2, this volume) proposed that AS is the key disorder and that severe language impairments (which are present in the majority of cases) can be added to the existing autism disorder. Demonstrating that the prevalence of AS greatly exceeded that of AS plus specific language impairment (i.e., autism) might warrant further investigation in the future. The most parsimonious way of conceptualizing the situation currently seems to be to consider cases of AS as representing a lesser degree of impairment in the disorder we call autism. Chapters in this book add weight to calls for a rethinking of current diagnostic and classificatory recommendations, so that the status of AS as a disorder can be clarified, and so that the current risk of woolly and confusing diagnostic practice can be reduced.

## Educational Provision

It seems undeniable that the vast majority of children with AS has learning difficulties of one kind or another. Few would disagree that education within the mainstream system is the ideal if the special needs of this population can be met. There is insufficient data, however, to back up claims that inclusive education is preferable, and that it leads to greater success and happiness in the long term. There is a fair body of data to confirm that most children need specialized help in social, psychological, and learning domains, in whatever setting they are educated. A clear solution based on traditional quantitatively based evaluation methods is unlikely, because finding the right "horses" for the right "courses" is so important in a group as diverse as the group of children with AS. The principles and strategies outlined by Kunce (Chapter 11, this volume) provide the signposts for this quest. It is essential that educational systems understand and accommodate the needs of these children and adolescents, which translates into enhanced teacher support and the allocation of financial resources. In addition, providing special training and continuing education for those teachers working with students with AS is a priority, if these young people are to more successfully navigate their way through our educational systems.

## Outcome for People with Asperger Syndrome

Long-term follow-up of people with AS is an area of research that should take priority. Not only is better documentation of social and educational outcomes needed, but information about employment opportunities and barriers, and lifestyle outcomes, including achievement of well-being, is also critically important. Many people with AS form relationships and may marry, producing families of their own. How do they and their partners and children cope with intimate relationships and the normal gamut of family stresses and triumphs? What developmental factors are conducive to good outcomes, and which are associated with poor outcomes? Long-term follow-up studies could resolve some of the diagnostic dilemmas, if a substantial body of outcome data on carefully diagnosed and well characterized samples were available to contribute to the debate.

## Therapeutic Approaches

Much has been learned about the particular adjustment problems common in AS, and some promising treatments for young persons with AS have been developed. Perhaps the most substantial progress is evident in training and educating younger children with this disorder. But adolescents and adults, in particular, are greatly in need of help to deal with their aspirations and needs in relation to the demands and expectations of adjusting to an independent and satisfying life. Achieving a sense of competence and well-being is as critical for them as for any other members of society. Recent examples of the use of approaches such as CBT, social skills training, and family therapy have been noted. These and other promising strategies deserve further investigation and evaluation in order to finds ways of maximizing the strengths that people with AS undoubtedly possess.

## REFERENCES

Asperger, H. (1991). Autistic psychopathy in childhood. In U. Frith (Ed.), *Autism and Asperger syndrome* (pp. 37–92). Cambridge, UK: Cambridge University Press. (Original work published in German 1944)

Attwood, A. (1998). *Asperger's syndrome: A guide for parents and professionals.* Philadelphia: Jessica Kingsley.

Attwood, A. (2000). Strategies for improving the social integration of children with Asperger syndrome. *Autism, 4*(1), 85–100.

Attwood, A. (2002). *Modifications to cognitive behaviour therapy to accommodate the unusual cognitive profile of people with Asperger syndrome* [Online]. Available: *http://trainland.tripod.com/tony.a.htm*

Bashe, P., & Kirby, B. (2000). *The oasis guide to Asperger syndrome.* New York: Crown.

Ehlers, S., Nyden, A., Gillberg, C., Dahlgren-Sandberg, A., Dahlgren, S.-O., Jelmquist, E., & Oden, A. (1997). Asperger syndrome, autism, and attention disorders: A comparative study of the cognitive profiles of 120 children. *Journal of Child Psychology and Psychiatry, 38,* 207–217.

Eisenmajer, R., Prior, M., Leekam, S., Wing, L., Gould, J., Welham, M., & Ong, B. (1996). Comparison of clinical symptoms in autism and Asperger's disorder. *Journal of the American Academy of Child and Adolescent Psychiatry, 35,* 1523–1531.

Ghaziuddin, M., Tsai, L., & Ghaziuddin, N. (1992). A reappraisal of clumsiness as a diagnostic feature of Asperger syndrome. *Journal of Autism and Developmental Disorders, 22,* 651–656.

Gillberg, C. (1989). Clinical and neurobiological aspects of Asperger syndrome in six family studies. In U. Frith (Ed.), *Autism and Asperger syndrome* (pp. 122–146). New York: Cambridge University Press.

Grandin T. (1992). An inside view of autism. In E. Schopler & G. Mesibov (Eds.), *High functioning individuals with autism* (pp. 105–126). New York: Plenum Press.

Hare, D. J. (1997). The use of cognitive-behavioural therapy with people with Asperger syndrome: A case study. *Autism, 1*(2), 215–225.

Hare, D. J., Jones, J. P. R., & Paine, C. (1999). Approaching reality: The use of personal construct assessment in working with people with Asperger syndrome. *Autism, 3*(2), 165–176.

Hinshaw, S. P. (1992). Externalizing behavior problems and academic underachievement in childhood and adolescence: Causal relationships and underlying mechanisms. *Psychological Bulletin, 111,* 127–155.

Hooper, S., & Bundy, M. (1998) Learning characteristics of individuals with Asperger syndrome. In E. Schopler, G. B. Mesibov, & L. G. Kunce (Eds.), *Asperger syndrome or high-functioning autism?* (pp. 317–342). New York: Plenum Press.

Jolliffe, T., Landsdown, R., & Robinson, T. (1992) *Autism: A personal account.* London: National Autistic Society.

Kaufman, A., & Kaufman, N. (2001). Assessment of specific learning difficulties in the new millennium: Issues, conflicts, and controversies. In A. Kaufman & N.

Kaufman (Eds.), *Specific learning disabilities and difficulties in children and adolescents: Psychological assessment and evaluation* (pp. 433–461). New York: Cambridge University Press.

Klin, A., Volkmar, F. R., Sparrow, S. S., Cicchetti, D. V., & Rourke, B. P. (1995). Validity and neuropsychological characterization of Asperger syndrome: Convergence with nonverbal learning disabilities syndrome. *Journal of Child Psychology and Psychiatry, 36,* 1127–1140.

Leekam, S., Libby, S., Wing, L., Gould, J., & Gillberg, C. (2000). Comparison of ICD-10 and Gillberg's criteria for Asperger syndrome. *Autism, 4*(1), 11–28.

Manjiviona, J., & Prior, M. (1995). Comparison of Asperger Syndrome and high functioning autistic children on a test of motor impairment. *Journal of Autism and Developmental Disorders, 25,* 23–39.

Manjiviona, J., & Prior, M. (1999). Neuropsychological profiles of children with Asperger syndrome and autism. *Autism: International Journal of Research and Practice, 3*(4), 327–356.

Mayes, S. D., & Calhoun, S. L. (in press). Ability profiles in children with autism: Influence of age and IQ. *Autism.*

McGee, R., Share, D., Moffitt T., Williams, S., & Silva, P. (1988). Reading disability, behaviour problems and delinquency. In D. H. Saklofske & S. B. G. Eysenck (Eds.), *Individual differences in children and adolescents: An international perspective* (pp. 158–172). London: Hodder & Stoughton.

McGee, R., Prior, M., William, S., Smart, D., & Sanson, A. (2002). The long-term significance of teacher-rated hyperactivity and reading ability in childhood: Findings from two longitudinal studies. *Journal of Child Psychology and Psychiatry, 43*(8), 1004–1017.

Myles, B., Barnhill, G., Hagiwara, T., Griswold, D., & Simpson, R. (2001). A synthesis of studies on the intellectual, academic, social/emotional, and sensory characteristics of children and youth with Asperger syndrome. *Education and Training in Mental Retardation and Developmental Disabilities, 36,* 304–311.

National Academy of Sciences. (2001). *Educating children with autism.* Washington, DC: Author.

Ozonoff, S., & Griffith, E. M. (2000). Neuropsychological function and the external validity of Asperger syndrome. In A. Klin, F. R. Volkmar, & S. S. Sparrow (Eds.), *Asperger syndrome* (pp. 72–96). New York: Guilford Press.

Prior, M. (1996). *Understanding specific learning difficulties.* Sussex, UK: Psychology Press.

Prior, M., & Ozonoff, S. (1998). Psychological factors in autism. In F. R. Volkmar (Ed.), *Autism and pervasive developmental disorders* (pp. 64–108). Cambridge, UK: Cambridge University Press.

Prior, M., Smart, D., Sanson, A., & Oberklaid, F. (1999). Relationships between learning difficulties and psychological problems in preadolescent children from a longitudinal sample. *American Academy of Child and Adolescent Psychiatry, 38*(4), 429–436.

Rourke, B. P., & Tsatsanis, K. D. (2000). Nonverbal learning disabilities and Asperger syndrome. In A. Klin, F. R. Volkmar, & S. S. Sparrow (Eds.), *Asperger syndrome* (pp. 231–253). New York: Guilford Press.

Smart, D., Sanson, A., & Prior, M. (1996). Connections between reading disability and behavior problems: Testing temporal and causal hypotheses. *Journal of Abnormal Child Psychology, 24*(3), 363–383.

Smith, I. M. (2000). Motor functioning in Asperger syndrome. In A. Klin, F. R. Volkmar, & S. S. Sparrow (Eds.), *Asperger syndrome* (pp. 97–124). New York: Guilford Press.

Ssucharewa, G. E., & Wolff, S. (1996). The first account of the syndrome Asperger described? [Die schizoiden Psychpathien im Kindesalter]. *European Child and Adolescent Psychiatry, 5*(3), 119–132.

Stoddart, K. (1999). Adolescents with Asperger syndrome: Three case studies of individual and family therapy. *Autism, 3*, 255–271.

Szatmari, P., Archer, L., Fisman, A., Streiner, D. L., & Wilson, F. (1995). Asperger's syndrome and autism: Differences in behavior, cognition, and adaptive functioning. *Journal of the American Academy of Child and Adolescent Psychiatry, 34* 1662–1671.

Tantam, D. (1991). Asperger syndrome in adulthood. In U. Frith (Ed.), *Autism and Asperger syndrome* (pp. 147–183). Cambridge, UK: Cambridge University Press.

Tantam, D. (2000). Adolescent and adulthood of individuals with Asperger syndrome. In A. Klin, F. R. Volkmar, & S. S. Sparrow (Eds.), *Asperger syndrome* (pp. 367–399). New York: Guilford Press.

# Index